HYPNOTHERAPEUTIC TECHNIQUES

John G. Watkins, Ph.D.

The Practice of Clinical Hypnosis
Volume I

 IRVINGTON PUBLISHERS, Inc., New York

Irvington Publishers, Inc.,
Executive offices: 522 E. 82nd Street, Suite 1, New York, NY 10028
Customer service and warehouse in care of: Integrated Distribution Services,
195 McGregor St, Manchester, NH 03102, (603) 669-5933

Library of Congress Cataloging-in-Publication Data
Watkins, John G. (John Goodrich), 1913-
   The practice of clinical hypnosis.

   Contents: v. 1. Hypnotherapeutic techniques.
   Bibliography: p.
   1. Hypnotism—Therapeutic use. I. Title.
[DNLM: 1. Hypnosis—methods. WM 415 W335p]
RC495.W35 1987   615.8'512   87-2597
ISBN 0-8290-1462-4 (v. 1)

Printed in the United States of America

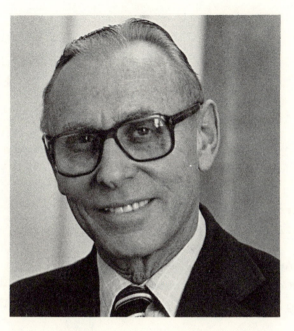

About the Author

John G. Watkins received his Ph.D. from Columbia University. He is a clinical psychologist and is also accredited as a psychoanalyst by the National Accreditation Association for Psychoanalysis. Dr. Watkins has served as President of the American Board of Psychological Hypnosis, Division 30 (Hypnosis) of the American Psychological Association and the Society for Clinical and Experimental Hypnosis, which he co-founded. Dr. Watkins is also Professor Emeritus and former Director of Clinical Training at the University of Montana, and has held faculty appointments at Washington State University, University of California Los Angeles, Northwestern University and The University of Oregon Medical School. For sixteen years he was the Chief Clinical Psychologist of various Veterans Administration facilities. He and his wife Helen, also a psychologist, live in Missoula, Montana.

OTHER BOOKS BY *John G. Watkins*

Objective Measurement Of Instrumental Performance
Hypnotherapy of War Neuroses
General Psychotherapy
The Therapeutic Self
We, the Divided Self (Irvington Publishers)

Audio Tapes
Hypnotic Induction Techniques   John G. Watkins
Raising Self Esteem   Helen H. Watkins

TABLE OF CONTENTS

Preface

With many good books on hypnosis available today, what is the justification for still another? A brief overview of the market may help to explain.

Some of the available books are designed to picture the current state of the field to the reader who is relatively naive in this area (Marcuse, 1964; Wolberg, 1972) or show the nature of the hypnotic modality (Shor & Orne, 1965). Others outline for the general medical practitioner techniques and approaches valuable in the treatment of a wide variety of problems (Crasilneck and Hall, 1975; Crasilneck and Hall, 1985; Kroger, 1977; Schneck, 1963; Wolberg, 1948; Cheek and LeCron, 1968). Some are aimed at the psychotherapist, often from a psychodynamic orientation (Edelstien, 1981; Gill and Brenman, 1959; Schneck, 1965; Watkins, 1949; Wolberg, 1945). Scientific works reporting controlled research studies (Fromm and Shor, 1979; Hilgard and Hilgard, 1975; Kline, 1963) have appeared at various intervals. A few books have aimed to portray the comparative development of hypnosis in various parts of the world (Marcuse, 1964). A number are devoted to the theoretical controversies which raged between exponents of different viewpoints (Barber, 1969; Sheehan and Perry, 1976; Sarbin and Coe, 1972). Several are primarily general and aim at the entire range of hypnotic theory, research and practice (Ambrose and Newbold, 1958; Frankel and Zammansky, 1978; Gordon, 1967), while others emphasize treatment techniques (Erickson, Hershman and Secter, 1961; Haley, 1973; Weitzenhoffer, 1957). Some texts are behavioral in their orientation (Gibbons, 1979; Dengrove, 1976; Kroger and Fezler, 1976). In some works the treatment procedures are focused about the needs of a specific class of patients (Gardner and Olness, 1981; Duke, 1984; Moss, A., 1952; Shaw, 1958). Applications in legal practice are now receiving attention (Hibbard and Worring, 1981; Reiser, 1980; Udolf, 1983). With all this variety just why is another work needed?

Unlike many other treatment modalities it is difficult to get training in hypnotherapy today. Only a small minority of medical schools and graduate schools of psychology offer courses in hypnosis. The two major scientific societies in the field, The Society for Clinical and Experimental Hypnosis and The American Society of Clinical Hypnosis do offer workshops, normally about three days in length, at their annual meetings and during the year at various centers about the country. These are usually "cram" courses where the beginner is immersed within a very short time in a strange and baffling field which is foreign to his previous experience, often fascinating, but with demands upon his[1] own personality and its defenses that may provoke anxiety. The skilled surgeon, calm and collected in the face of observable physical pathology, may practice his skills with high concentration and equanimity. Yet this same person confronted with apparently "magical" happenings for which he has no tangible, objective rationale, quails and avoids as if he were asked to stay in a haunted house. On the other hand, the objective scientific researcher who has dealt with concrete, observable behavior as variables, and who can trace intricacies of stimulus-response with the aid of complex designs and mathematical analysis often finds himself wishing to avoid a modality which lends itself to objective formulations only with the greatest of difficulty. Behavioral theories today are inadequate to account for the esoteric phenomena induced in the hypnotic situation.

There are not many competent instructors in this field. Most medical schools, as well as most university graduate schools, do not have a faculty member who is prepared to offer regular courses in this discipline. Furthermore, there is tremendous ignorance on the part of many physicians and psychologists concerning hypnotic phenomena, which is manifested by suspicion and distrust of workers in the field. Psychoanalysts continue parroting objections to hypnotherapy based on unverified theoretical positions voiced by Freud and his associates over half a century ago. Accordingly, it is no wonder that so few professionals are skilled in the use of hypnosis as a treatment modality. The bottleneck seems to be that skill in hypnotherapy is limited to a few psychotherapists as compared to the many practitioners who have mastered other approaches for dealing with mental illness.

Now that hypnosis has been officially recognized as a legit-

[1]Throughout this work the words "he" and "him" are often used in the broad sense of "person." They are used solely for convenience; no brief is held for concepts of masculine superiority, and the strivings of women for full economic and political equality have our utmost support.

imate scientific and treatment modality by the American Medical Association, the American Psychological Association, as well as the American Association for the Advancement of Science and the World Federation for Mental Health[2], it should be taught in medical schools along with other accepted methods of treatment. Likewise, the phenomena of hypnosis should be studied in psychology departments the same as other aspects of personality functioning, such as learning, motivation and perception. In the field of clinical psychology hypnotherapy should be as much a part of the curriculum as the cognitive or behavior therapies.

The professor of psychiatry or psychology who undertakes to teach a solid course in clinical hypnosis or hypnotherapy will find many articles and reference works available. However, not one of these today seems to have been specifically designed as a *teaching textbook*. The topics, although often well discussed, are not arranged in the same systematic way as one would expect in a general textbook in physiology—or in zoology. Units of instruction should be outlined with consideration of the typical 3–5 hour course for an academic quarter or semester. Lecture and discussion need to be interspersed with practicum exercises which gradually initiate the new student into the various hypnotic phenomena and the techniques for eliciting them. Presentations must range from the simple to the more complex. Theories of hypnosis, often thrown at the reader in great profusion, should be simplified and directly related to hypnotic experiences. The history of hypnosis needs to be presented in a way which allows the newcomer to identify with the struggles and difficulties pioneers had when investigating these phenomena, developing their treatment techniques, and dealing with hostile opposition from colleagues. For indeed the history of hypnosis is one of repetition. One worker after another has gone through the same sequence of skepticism, observation, conviction, over-zealousness, fight to maintain scientific respectability, and problems of "selling" his approaches to associates and the public. The history of any field, and especially of hypnosis, ought to be presented in such a way

[2]The American Medical Association officially approved the clinical use of hypnosis in 1958, the American Psychological Association in 1960, and the two major hypnosis societies, SCEH and ASCH hold membership in both the American Association for the Advancement of Science and the World Federation for Mental Health.

that the newcomer can identify with the stream of its development, its heroes and innovators. In such training he can experience within himself the same changes of perception and understanding which characterized the professional careers of his predecessors.

The student will pass through the initial amazement the same as did his teacher. Whether this "turns him on" to the field or scares him off will depend on whether his initiation is systematic and step-wise, permitting him to cognitively master new experiences, integrate them into his previous professional background, and develop assurance in the skills of hypnotic induction and therapy.

During the past 40 years I have taught hypnotherapy to many hundreds of physicians, dentists, psychiatrists, psychologists and other psychotherapists. A number of them have become quite proficient in the modality. A few are now distinguished clinical and experimental contributors to the field. But unfortunately, many left the courses, the workshops, or the institutes in which the instruction was given, interested, fascinated, promising themselves that they would really learn to utilize these techniques, but finding themselves many years later using only non-hypnotic procedures. Somehow, their early anxieties and personal blocks were never overcome.

Many of us who have served as teachers in this area have met former students who report that they enjoyed the course, gained a great deal in understanding personality dynamics, improved their doctor-patient relationships and developed a greater comprehension of the role of psychogenic factors in causing mental and physical disfunction. But they then state that, "I always intended to practice hypnosis, but I never felt at ease with it." If a student has not started using hypnosis within a month or two after completing a course he usually never employs it. There is thus a great waste in the teaching of this modality since only a minority of those who take workshops become active hypnotherapists or hypnotic researchers.

Here at the University of Montana a course in hypnotherapy has been a regular part of doctoral training for clinical psychologists for twenty years. Starting as a two-hour seminar it has grown into an instructional unit which combines two hours a week of supervised practicum with three hours of formal classroom presentations. Films, audio, and video tapes are widely used. Demonstrations before the class are continuously integrated with the lectures. In spite of all this, we found that only about a third of our students were actively using hypnosis in their treatment two or three years later. Students begged for additional supervised training with actual patients, and accordingly an advanced "hypnotherapy team" was established in the Clinical Psychology Center for those who had completed the course. Our results show that initial courses, however well organized, can whet the professional appetite of practitioners and can inculcate a great deal of theoretical knowledge, but that if these students are to profit from advanced seminars they need much more actual experience in utilizing the hypnotic modality.

In our training students serve both as subjects and as hypnotists. They work with screened volunteer subjects of known hypnotizability; they participate in both group and individual inductions. They study the literature and relate it first to their experiences in hypnotizing subjects and later to their understanding of clinical cases. Only in this way do they seem to acquire the assurance which permits them to employ hypnosis regularly as a continuous technique in their therapeutic armamentarium.

It is from this background that it seemed to us that a "teaching text" in hypnotherapy was needed which would address itself specifically to the problems of teaching and learning, and to the personal needs of students wrestling with this new modality. This book is, accordingly, designed with a focus on the clinical professor and his students. It aims to include that which can be learned, and no more, within a typical academic year. Broader background, familiarization with a wider variety of techniques, acquaintance with the many nuances of theoretical controversy, and polished finesse in the practice of hypnotic skills will come later.

After having acquired certain basic procedures, having thoroughly convinced himself of the potential effectiveness which hypnosis can demonstrate in the treatment situation, knowing at least a number of clinical problems within his practice which are amenable to hypnotic approaches, and having mastered his initial awe to the point where he feels some confidence in his hypnotic abilities, the clinician can then develop further through individual reading of the literature plus attendance at legitimate workshops and scientific meetings. This work, therefore, is dedicated to getting the student over the initial hurdle and furnishing the starting impetus necessary to make him into a functioning practitioner in the field of hypnotherapy. He, himself, must subsequently develop his skills further if he is to be an artist, a master of the discipline, and more than a journeyman practitioner.

Most books are written objectively. The writer knows certain facts and skills. He writes in an effort to pour his experience, his wisdom into the student—the big jug and the little mugs theory of education. I also have written a number of earlier books, book chapters and articles in this field which were presented specifically from that point of view—that of the instructor.

In this book the effort will be made to do a bit differently. A theory of therapeutic relationship presented in an earlier work (Watkins, J., 1978) posited two viewpoints from which we may view another person: the objective and the resonant. When we are objective we observe the actions of a patient from a vantage point outside of him, much as we might look at a specimen under a microscope. The other is an "it", not ourselves, and our responsibility for "its" actions are minimal. But if we temporarily identify with the other, perceive the world as if through his eyes—even view our own self as he might—then we are resonating.

Resonance is that process by which an individual (therapist) attempts to replicate within his own self a close facsimile of another's experiential world. It is approaching a problem from the inner perspective of the other rather than from that of our own. The practice of resonance can be as valuable in the field of education as in therapy. The teacher whose presentations are developed from the viewpoint of the student struggling to master the material should be more effective than the professor who simply "doles it out" and places on the student the burden of mastery. Insofar as it is possible we shall try to incorporate the resonant point of view in writing this book. This means that when designing each unit we shall try to think, not "What is it we wish to tell the students? What should they learn?" Rather we will endeavor to ask ourselves continuously the question, "if I were a new student what would I want to know, what help would I need to master both my own insecurities in this new modality and the techniques necessary to use it skillfully?" Whenever possible the student's frame of reference will be assumed, and the material written accordingly.

The writer's theories (Watkins, J., 1963, 1967, 1978a; Watkins & Watkins, 1981) of psychotherapy emphasize a balance between objectivity and resonance. Therapy is only a kind of education or re-education, often at unconscious levels. But a good therapist is a good teacher. Here we are not trying to "treat" problems of a student, but to inculcate techniques, manners, and approaches effective in the treatment situation.

If this approach can be effectively used in teaching hypnotherapy, then perhaps a beneficial "spill-off" will also occur. We learn by modeling. Those of us who are psychotherapists often copied our manner and skills from the master, the professor or the analyst with whom we studied. As the clinical instructor is to his students, so will his students be in relation to their students—their patients. Manners are contagious, so perhaps the manner of presenting our material may prove of benefit first, objectively, as the student learns, practices, and masters the necessary skills, and secondarily, through resonance, as he incorporates some of the indirect manners of suggestion, persuasion, and interpretation which might be transmitted by the written as well as the spoken word. Hypnotherapy may be learned as a science, but it is practiced as an art.

Every specialized discipline has its "lingo." Psychoanalysts talk in "psychoanalese." Behavior modifiers write in "behaviorese" terms, etc. Without wishing to offend the psychologist, the psychiatrist, or other professionals, the terminology in this book will be kept as clear and simple as possible. Where technical or professional terms are used it will not be assumed that the student understands them. Since the physician, the psychiatrist, the psychologist, psychoanalyst, and the dentist each have their own unique vocabulary we will try to couch the language here in terms that would be easily understandable to the intelligent layman. Specialized terms will be explained and illustrated. Repetition will not harm the sophisticated reader; failure to explain may leave the professional from another discipline confused.

Explanations should be concrete, illustrations and case examples frequent, and specific wordings presented. How often have you read a good psychoanalytic case presentation where the statement was made that, "At this point I interpreted his negative transference?" And how often have you wondered, "Yes, you did. But just what did you say? Exactly what were the words you used, and why did you choose those specifically? Why did you decide to interpret the negative transference at this time? What specific reactions did your patient show to your interpretation—in his next remark, his behavior during the rest of the session, in the hours and days which followed?" The statement that, "At this point I interpreted his negative transference," may have satisfied the writer. It was objective, but it was not resonant since it did not meet the needs of the student to understand. It did not answer the questions which were on the reader's mind, and it did not develop his learning much so that he, too, would know just how to interpret the negative transference of his patient when required. That is why we will try to make this book as concrete and specific as possible. Pictures and diagrams will be used. Reference to films, audio, and video tapes which have been published will be made when these could aid the learning process. Study questions and practicum exercises are designed to develop the stages of learning and to maximize both retention of factual knowledge and acquisition of technical skill. As much as possible, induction techniques and case material will be presented verbatim, together with explanatory notes.

Hypnotherapy must be learned and practiced as a meaningful discipline, not as a collection of scientific facts nor as a cookbook of recipes for handling various clinical problems. Elements must not be learned in isolation from one another, but an integrated whole of understanding should emerge within the student as it is increasingly put together. As in other professional treatment disciplines, the hypnotherapist should become a clinician, not a technician.

The study of hypnosis usually makes a clinician a better psychologist, physician, or other more understanding student of human nature. Perhaps nowhere in the behavioral sciences does the interplay of psychological cause and effect show more clearly than in the psychodynamic movements revealed by hypnosis. Whatever has been one's skepticism about the reality of unconscious processes, no other experience, unless it be that of intensive psychoanalysis, is so convincing as to the reality of covert interactions within the human psyche.

The orientation will be psychodynamic-eclectic in this treatise. That is, it will be psychoanalytic to the extent that it accepts the existence of unconscious behavior, considers that it is mediated within psychodynamic mechanisms (such as projection, identification, displacement, rationalization, etc.)

and believes that these interactions play significant roles in the etiology of pathological symptoms and maladaptive behavior. However, since many contributions to the treatment of clinical problems have stemmed from the recent investigations of behaviorists and have been incorporated in the technology of behavior modification and behavior therapy, this work will also be eclectic. It is the opinion of this writer that some clinical problems are best approached from a psychoanalytic viewpoint, others from the perspective of behavioral therapy, etc. Furthermore, the significant, broad and long-range goals targeted by the humanistic-existential therapists, such as the development of meaningfulness, authenticity, and spontaneity in the self, often are required if other than temporary relief is to be granted to many of our patients.

Accordingly, this book will not be "purist." Rather it will try to draw from a number of psychological approaches those conceptions and skills which, practiced within the hypnotic modality, promise maximal therapeutic leverage.

Some information will be given concerning the major scientific hypnosis societies and how to affiliate with them. They can furnish a continuing education for the initiate (as well as the expert) in the field. There are legitimate national and international societies concerned with research and practice in hypnosis, and ethical codes governing its use. Unfortunately, certain other organizations with lowered professional and ethical standards attract those whose power and exhibitionistic needs exceed their professional sense of responsibility for the amelioration of mankind's ills.

Clinical Hypnosis is divided into two parts, *Volume I Hypnotherapeutic Techniques,* and *Volume II Hypnoanalytic Techniques.* Volume I is designed to serve as a basic text for an introductory course. The material included should be sufficient for a single quarter or semester course in graduate school or medical school or for an intensive introductory workshop. It is accompanied by an *Instructor's Manual* which can assist the teacher in organizing a systematic course, selecting practice subjects and providing practicum exercises. The manual also includes sources for audio-visual instructional materials, such as films, plus audio and video tapes.

Volume I provides a background in the history of hypnosis, theories, suggestibility tests, induction, and deepening techniques. These are followed by chapters on suggestive methods of treatment within the various branches of medicine, dentistry, and psychology. In these will be presented a number of therapeutic techniques practiced by the author and his wife and colleague, Helen H. Watkins, plus approaches which have been utilized by many other well-known hypnotherapists. We have tried as much as possible to link theory, research, and practice and to provide meaningful rationales for the procedures described.

Volume I concludes with a chapter on "Precautions, Dangers and Contra-Indications." The practice of hypnotherapy represents a significant psychological intervention into physical and mental processes. To the extent that it has validity and potency it also requires ethical responsibility to insure maximum benefit and minimum harm to one's patients. This chapter presents some of the issues involved.

The number of clinical and experimental studies being currently published is enormous. Accordingly, the bibliography of references included can in no way be exhaustive. Many excellent books and articles must of necessity be over-looked. However, we have tried to refer to many of the most significant works, and the serious student will wish to read further in this vast literature.

Volume II Hypnoanalytic Techniques, picks up where Volume I leaves off. It considers those more complex and "analytic" treatment approaches which seek basic changes in personality structure—more than the suggestive alleviation of symptoms. In a more general work in psychotherapy this author (Watkins, 1960) tried to outline all the treatment approaches current twenty-five years ago. These were organized under the two major headings of "Supportive Techniques" and "Reconstructive Techniques." The "Supportive" therapies included "those methods which aim at relieving symptoms by the use of motivation, supression, ego-strengthening and re-education without the altering of basic personality structure." Some 26 different approaches, ranging from reassurance, suggestion, and advice through behavior therapy, music therapy, art therapy, bibliotherapy, etc. were included under this heading. Under "Reconstructive" therapies were placed "those methods which aim at the indirect relief of symptoms through a reorganization of the patient's basic attitudes toward self and his customary modes of personality interaction with others." "Insight" was considered to be a distinguishing component. Psychoanalysis, some 13 variations and modifications, plus 22 other "analytic" systems comprised this category. Although this distinction is no longer considered to be as significant or clear-cut as it was when psychoanalysis and its variations were contrasted with therapies which did not "reconstruct" the ego, nevertheless, the difference between "hypnotherapy" and "hypnoanalysis" as divided between these two volumes, retains something of the above meanings.

Forensic hypnosis, although not concerned with the treatment of patients, does involve the evaluation of witnesses and victims. It is best practiced by psychological and psychiatric clinicians, who have had much experience in treatment, and have acquired additional expertise in the needs of the courts and the legal profession. As a sub-specialty within clinical hypnosis it has been receiving both great interest and controversial criticism. Accordingly, we have included a chapter on this discipline, outlining its possibilities, weaknesses, and its current legal status. There should be increased opportunities, both in practice and in research in this area—and much research is greatly needed.

In Volume II we will be much more concerned with "depth," with "insight," and with efforts to achieve profound changes in the personality, even though there are many references to patients' "insights" and understandings in Volume I and many "supportive-suggestive" aspects of hypnoanalytic procedures. The difference between the two volumes is one of degree along a continuum of technique complexity and theoretical formulation.

Volume II may well serve as a textbook in an advanced course which those students who have completed an introductory course or workshop may wish to take, after they have acquired skills in suggestive approaches to treatment, and feel sufficiently comfortable working in hypnosis to commit more of themselves to its practice.

For those readers who are just starting their acquaintance with clinical hypnosis, welcome aboard and bon voyage. It will be an exciting and challenging experience. And for those of you who are already working in the field, you know what I mean by the fascination of probing deeper into the mysteries of human existence.

As a little boy I always was thrilled by the tales of exploration of Columbus, Balboa, Magellan, etc. As an adolescent my imagination was stirred by the possibilities for exploring outer space. Alas, only a few of us will probably be privileged to walk upon the surface of the moon, or gaze through a porthole window as the terrain of an unknown planet unfolds beneath. But as you work with hypnosis perhaps you, too, like many of us who began its study earlier, will experience the same intriguing sense of wonder as you see the amazing phenomena which it continuously reveals within "inner space," the universe of behavior and experience which constitute the "self" of every person.

Chapter 1

The History of Hypnosis and its Relevance to Present Day Psychotherapy

Imagine that you have discovered a great new healing principle. As a doctor who has devoted his life to the study of human illness, you have happened by good luck on a new approach that seems to have miraculous results in relieving pain and curing many conditions which have defied the best efforts of your country's most distinguished practitioners. You have watched hundreds of sufferers lose their pains, throw away their crutches, see when blinded, and resume normal living after being invalids for years. As to the effects of your new technique there can be no doubt.

Furthermore, to account for this therapeutic power, you have developed a theory which is related to what is known scientifically about the operations of natural law. Your waiting room is besieged by patients from near and far. Your reputation as a great healer is established throughout the land. Only one cloud shadows your present; your colleagues are jealous of your success. They refuse to listen to you, learn your procedures, and verify them on their own patients. How would you feel? What would you do?

Perhaps in your eagerness to share this great discovery with the rest of the world and to be scientifically recognized for your contribution, you would welcome an official hearing. Let some highly respected members of the medical and scientific societies investigate your practice and see your therapeutic achievements first hand. Their skepticism will be erased. They can announce to your colleagues and to the rest of the world the truth about your great discovery.

1

Suppose that finally the government appoints such a commission, consisting of several of the most respected names in science, and that furthermore this group actually visits your treatment office, studies your charts, observes your therapeutic procedures, and interviews your patients. Now you surely will be vindicated. Their long awaited report is finally published and—you are devastated. They have ignored the concrete examples of your healing. They have paid little attention to the reports of your many patients who attest to their cures. They only criticized the theory by which you attempted to explain your therapeutic achievements, then said that any reported results must be due to "imagination." How would you feel now? Could you carry on being scorned by colleagues and patients alike? Or would you, like Franz Anton Mesmer, leave the country in disgrace, filled with shame and bitterness?

The Discoveries of Mesmer (1781)

Mesmer, born in 1734, secured a degree in medicine in 1766. His doctoral thesis, *De Planetarum Influsu*, attempted to relate changes in human functioning to gravitational and other forces in the surrounding universe. After all, if the position of the moon could so move the oceans of the world would not such powerful forces also have significant impact on the operations of living organisms, especially humans?

Mesmer was a brilliant man of great imagination. His interests were indeed broad. A musician himself, he was a friend of Mozart, of Gluck, and of Haydn. Vienna of that day was a city in which the arts blossomed as much as the sciences. But Mesmer was equally a scientist and physician, and as such had been made a member of the Bavarian Academy of Science.

The mid-eighteenth century was a time of great ferment. The impetus for new advances, which two centuries before in the Renaissance had broken the frozen grip of medievalism and stimulated a new flowering in all the arts, especially in Italy, now swept on into the realms of natural science. Newton, Galileo, Copernicus, Kepler, and others had made significant breakthroughs in understanding the universe and its laws. Gravity, chemical reactions, electricity and magnetism were being discovered as great natural forces, energies which were soon to be harnessed and enormously increase man's standard of living. The Western world was on the verge of an industrial revolution.

And speaking of revolutions, explosive social forces were at work which would soon sweep through America and Europe. Monarchies tottered before the increasing clamor of the many common people demanding their rights for liberty, equality, and fraternity.

It was in such a world that Mesmer learned from the Royal Astronomer in Vienna, a priest named Maxmilian Hell, the principle of the magnet. If one would hold a bit of magnetized metal before the eyes of a subject he would become transfixed. Moving and acting as if in another realm, he was especially susceptible to healing suggestions which could be administered to him at that time. His pains could be made to leave. Many other complaints could also be banished under the spell of the magnet.

However, Mesmer soon made a most puzzling discovery. A priest named Gassner had been practicing a form of healing much like "magnetism" which involved passes of the hands without the use of metal magnets. Mesmer observed Father Gassner's work and found that he, himself, could also accomplish the same results merely by placing his hand near his patients even without holding a piece of magnetized metal.

How could this be? It had been established that a magnet has about it a field which influences other pieces of metal, and when held close to a patient it obviously influenced him too, since he would then relinquish pain and other symptoms. There must be something of the same energy inhering in the hand of the doctor. Therefore this great healing power apparently was not limited to metals; it could also be found in bodily tissues. So Mesmer coined the term "animal magnetism" to represent a universal force which might account for the healing achieved by "the laying on of hands."

How normal, how natural it was that a brilliant thinker with the seeking, searching mind of Mesmer could arrive at such an explanation. Yet here we see an example of what has occurred often in science where through faulty reasoning an invalid theory is formulated even though based on sound observational data. Accordingly, Mesmer established his clinical practice on a concept which several years later would be invalidated by scientists who were more careful and rigorous in their experimental controls.

Mesmer was not the last to advocate the theory of a fluid, magnetic energy to account for healing effects. A century and a half later a brilliant, creative psychoanalyst, Wilhelm Reich (1945), formulated theories about the concept of the "orgone," a life energy which could be concentrated in a box and focused back upon the human body with healing results. He also treated patients according to his theory and was jailed for refusing to obey a desist ruling of the Federal Food and Drug Administration in America. He died in jail, but perhaps that idea even now has not been put finally to rest. Recent "Kirlian" photographs (Krippner & Rubin, 1973) have shown that there is an "aura" of radiation about plant and animal tissue and that alterations in it are correlated with healing effects. Maybe, just maybe, Mesmer and Reich were not entirely wrong.

Mesmer's Controversial Case of "Restored" Sight

Maria Theresa Paradis, a young singer and pianist, had been blind since the age of three. The best physicians had not been able to restore her sight. She was brought to Mesmer, who developed a strong interest in her case. With her parents' consent, he took her into his home and treated her. Although a number of prominent physicians had diagnosed her condition as due to destruction of the optic nerve, there was considerable evidence that the blindness may have been hysterical.

Maria had played before Empress Maria Theresa who, being favorably impressed with the girl, had provided for her education and granted her parents a pension. At first, the treatment seemed to be successful, and the girl apparently was able to see again. However, the case created consternation within the conservative medical profession of Vienna. If Mesmer really had such powers the other doctors might lose their patients to him.

Several influential physicians were able to convince her parents that her "cure" was not genuine, and they suggested that if she was no longer thought to be blind the parents might lose the pension. As a result she was removed by her parents from Mesmer's care and returned to her home—after which her "blindness" returned.

Here we see an experience from history which is so frequently repeated today, one which society prefers to ignore, but which complicates enormously the task of the healing arts practitioner, namely, attempting to treat a patient who has more to gain by remaining ill. Huge malpractice suits are won; workman's compensation, disability payments, and the pensions of neurotically ill veterans are awarded to those who can successfully establish and retain symptoms in the face of treatment, psychological or physiological. To his great chagrin, Mesmer learned about secondary gains and reinforcements in the maintenance of illness long before the investigations of such factors by psychoanalysts and behaviorists. This case example also serves to warn us that the first therapeutic question is not *how* we should treat the patient, but whether the patient should be treated at all.

Mesmer's Theory of Disease

Mesmer held that since the human body was composed of the same elements as those which made up the universe it should be subject to the same laws that govern other bits of matter, including the planets. It, too, should be influenced by light, heat, electricity, and changes in gravitation and even by influence from celestial space. He believed that the two halves of the human body acted in relation to each other like two poles of a magnet, and that phsyiological processes were disrupted when there was a lack of harmony because of the improper distribution of magnetism.

Animal magnetism was viewed as a kind of fluid which could penetrate all matter, which could be concentrated and reflected, and which could be invested by the human will into various parts of the body. Mesmer believed that he could direct this magnetic fluid through his presence, the passes of his hands, the waving of a metallic rod, and contact with the baquet.

The baquet was a large wooden tub about a foot high which he had constructed within his clinic. It was filled with bits of metal, bottles systematically arranged in concentric rings, broken pieces of glass, and water. It was large enough so that a number of patients could sit around it. From its upper lid there projected several iron rods. This baquet was supposed to concentrate the magnetism (like a kind of eighteenth century cyclotron) which could then be transferred by patients to their afflicted members through rubbing against the rods. Being a musician (and undoubtedly somewhat of a showman) Mesmer felt that the experience would be enhanced if the clinic room was darkened and music was playing while he, in a long flowing purple robe, passed among his patients rubbing their bodies from time to time with his metal rod.

Since patients were expected to go into crises (hysterical seizures) when the concentration of "magnetism" became sufficiently great, it is not surprising that every so often one would writhe and fall into a "fit," thus further impressing the others as to the potency of the treatment. When the number of patients seeking Mesmer's help exceeded the capacity of his clinic he would magnetize a tree in a nearby park by stroking it. People could then stand around it basking in its "magnetism" and occasionally going into crises.

Mesmer's Reception by Colleagues

The same suspicion and criticism by medical colleagues which had plagued him in Vienna continued in Paris, and the greater his successes, the greater became the hostility of the other doctors. In 1784, because of the conflicting claims, King Louis XVI appointed a distinguished commission, whose members were suggested by the French Academy of Science, to investigate Mesmer's practice. It is most interesting to note who was included among its members. There was doughty old Benjamin Franklin, he who had discovered with his kite the relation of lightning to electricity. At that time he was American ambassador to France. There was Lavoisier, the first to isolate the element of oxygen. There was Jussieu, an eminent botanist, and finally (not without symbolic significance for the future of Mesmer's practice) the inventor of that device for amputating the head—Dr. Antoine Guillotine.

Mesmer's therapeutic zeal was exceeded only by his tendency for exaggeration, his lack of caution in theoretical generalization, and his arrogance, a trait not uncommon in good hypnotists. The commission was soon able, through simple but well-controlled experiments, to conclude that the changes in the symptoms of Mesmer's patients could not have occurred through the action of an hypothesized magnetic field. Their report stated flatly that there was no such thing as "animal magnetism" and that, since it did not exist, reported cures could only be the result of fraud or "imagination." Rejected by colleagues and patients alike, Mesmer left Paris, and, after some wandering, settled in Switzerland near Lake Constance, on whose shores he had been born fifty years before. There he spent the rest of his days, unnoticed and unheralded.

How often does an individual who is beaten by the forces of life return to the scenes of his childhood? How often does he simplify his existence, relinquish his challenges to competitors, and cease his efforts to make further advance? We see it every day in many of our patients. We call it regression. Mesmer's star burst forth like a brilliant nova in the development of psychological treatment, but within a few short years it had returned almost to oblivion. Although personally discredited, broken and embittered, he left a legacy of findings and questions which have ever since fruitfully stimulated man's quest for more knowledge about himself. Mesmer reached to become God; he ended up very much human. Such strivings for power have often been the nemesis of practitioners of hypnosis, who, dazzled by the apparently unbelievable effects they achieve through the hypnotic modality, reactivate their own infantile yearnings for omnipotence. They sometimes lose their *raison d'etre* as practitioners of the healing arts, as servants to men, and seek to use their new found skills to become masters of men. The history of hypnosis has many lessons to teach the would be therapist—and history tends to repeat itself.

The development of modern hypnosis is considered to have started with Mesmer. However, the use of hypnosis in treating human ills is probably as old as the history of medicine. There is evidence that most of the hypnotic phenomena were known to ancient man. Eighteen hundred years before Christ, hypnosis was apparently practiced in China. The Old Testament Hebrews employed the trance state in the making of prophecies. And the Druids would put suspects into a "sleep" to induce them to tell the truth. In the fourth century B.C., temple cults developed in Greece during which an induced "sleep" was combined with other forms of suggestion for the treatment of illness. Through the dances of whirling dervishes, the ancient Egyptians induced states of trance and ecstasy, during which hypnotic analgesia could be achieved.

Mass hypnosis accounts for the rage of tarantella dancing which swept through Europe during the late Middle Ages. Hundreds of people were seized by the fury and gyrated in wild abandon until they collapsed in a state of exhaustion. In India the Hindus practiced more passive forms of hypnotic meditation which have continued today in the exercises of the Yogis. Many Indian tribes in America utilized the trance for purposes of both prophecy and medical treatment. For those wishing to delve further in this area, Williams (1968) presents a more detailed and documented account of the various hypnotic practices among primitive peoples. It is sufficient here to note that hypnosis (although called many different names) has been known for many centuries by both primitive and civilized men, and was employed to treat human ills in every part of the world long before it became a serious object of scientific inquiry.

The Development of Hypnosis after Mesmer

Let us return to trace the history of this interesting phenomenon during more recent years. One of Mesmer's students, the Count Maxime de Puysegur, is credited with having been the first to discover the phenomenon of somnambulism, wherein the hypnotized subject can walk, talk, and engage in many activities, yet still remain in a trance state. After Mesmer, a number of people continued to practice in the field, calling themselves magnetists or mesmerists. Some of these, such as de Puysegur, while employing Mesmer's therapeutic techniques, were not convinced that the phenomena were due to an invisible magnetic fluid. They approached close to the more psychological etiologies now held. In 1821 Recamier in France reported a painless surgery accomplished on a "magnetized" patient.

Although the practice of animal magnetism became almost extinct in France following the discrediting of Mesmer, workers in Germany, especially during the 1840's, continued to employ it. Their efforts were apparently aimed at gaining respectable medical and scientific acceptance, and in fact in 1818 the Berlin Academy of Science offered a prize for the best thesis on the phenomena. However, little more was done to bring new discoveries to the field, and none of these men left enduring marks on its development. Sporadic attempts were also made by disciples of Mesmer in France to re-activate interest. They were able to induce the French Academy of Medicine on several occasions during the early 1800's to appoint a commission to examine the therapeutic claims of magnetism. The results were usually inconclusive or negative, and it was not until many years after Mesmer's death in 1815 that renewed study of the phenomena awakened attention.

Perhaps this illustrates the repetitive nature of the history of hypnosis which has occurred again and again up until the present. Each episode started as a reputable physician or scientist observed hypnotic demonstrations by another worker, often a lay person. The physician's incredulity changed to belief and enthusiasm. He adopted these techniques in his practice and tried valiantly to convince his professional colleagues. Students and disciples flocked around him, and his center became a beehive of practice and investigation. He frequently became overly arrogant and pretentious in his therapeutic claims, thus antagonizing more conservative scientific colleagues who then tried to discredit him. His over-enthusiastic followers attempted to treat all conditions, both organic and functional, by hypnotic techniques. They made of their leader a god, and tried to emulate him. Inevitably they became disillusioned, and interest in the field died down, only to be revived again similarly by a new "messiah."

A critical psychiatrist once remarked, "Hypnosis has been tried and abandoned by the human race many times. Why should we study it now?" To which the only appropriate reply is, "No matter how many times hypnosis has been abandoned, people keep coming back to it."

The cycle of skepticism, discovery, application, and over-enthusiasm leading to abandonment, has not only characterized different times and the physicians of different countries; it is a typical experience today by the newcomer who is taking his first course or workshop in the field. In fact, you who are now reading this may go through these same stages. You undertake a course in hypnosis because of curiosity or the recommendation of a colleague. Initially you have many doubts and reservations about its reality or potency. You observe the induction of a number of subjects into a trance state and learn how to do it yourself. You watch demonstrations of deep trance phenomena, such as hypermnesia, regression, perceptual distortions, and hallucinations. You are astounded. Why had you not been taught these marvelous powers before? Here you have the "magic bullet" that medicine has always sought to cure human ills. You enthusiastically apply the procedures to your own practice with more or less success. If you now seek perfection and omnipotence sooner or later you will be disappointed. Many of you, will forsake the field as did most of Mesmer's followers. First stage, skepticism. Second, over-enthusiasm. But if you can persevere through to the third stage you may reach the point where you recognize that hypnosis is not the magic wand, that it cannot cure all conditions, that it has limits and that it does not always work. You will then perceive it as simply another useful technique in your therapeutic armamentarium which can often help in the successful treatment of many sufferers. You will find that with this tool you can at times do some things you could not otherwise accomplish, or at least not without a much greater expenditure of time and effort. You are then no longer merely "a hypnotist." You are a mature member of the healing arts professions who knows how to use this modality along with many others for the benefit of his patients. These are a few of the lessons which the study of scientific hypnosis teaches us.

It is 1837 in England, and history is about to be repeated. John Elliotson (1843), a very attractive and brilliant physician, has just observed demonstrations by Monsieur Depotet, a visiting French mesmerist. Elliotson was known for his tremendous energy, his willingness to experiment with new concepts, his unorthodoxy. He had been the first physician in England to use a stethoscope. He had translated Blumenbach's *Physiology*, a major text of the day. He had many other original contributions to his credit. He had discovered the value of such drugs as potassium iodide and prussic acid in the treatment of various conditions. Moreover, he was First Professor of the Practice of Medicine in London University and President of the Royal Medical and Chirurigical Society.

Obviously, such an inventive and innovative man would be fascinated with the phenomena of hypnosis. He began practicing and writing about it. He and his students published a journal, *The Zoist*, devoted to the reporting of cases treated by mesmerism. He immediately incurred the anger and scorn of his medical colleagues and was singled out especially for attack by the editor of *Lancet*, the medical journal. Elliotson believed in the magnetic theories of Mesmer and was inveigled into an experiment where he intended to demonstrate that a silver coin (since it contained magnetism) would induce the trance state, while a lead coin would fail. Unfortunately, one of his opponents switched coins. The subject was hypnotized by the lead coin, hence responding to Elliotson's words and not to the "magnetized" coin.

Elliotson was bitterly attacked. He continued his work against all opposition, but he was denied the pages of the medical journals and forced to resign his post on the staff of the University Hospital. He was especially noted for his treatment of children, with whose sufferings he could so well identify. Ridiculed, despised, and abused he died in 1868, vainly attempting to interest his medical colleagues in the practice of mesmerism and to regain his scientific respectability.

Times are better now for clinicians and researchers interested in hypnosis. Courses in the modality are offered in many medical schools and in graduate departments of psychology. One can specialize in this area and retain professional acceptance. But even yet the shades of reactionary ignorance linger on. If you return to your hospital or clinic and practice what is taught in this book do not expect to be received by your more conservative colleagues with open arms. And if you are an academic professor of psychology your department may well indicate it would prefer that you study such respectable areas as learning theory, motivation, or perception. Appointments and promotions in prestigous universities are not likely to come your way if you are too closely identified with hypnosis.

The time is 1845 and the place Calcutta, India. A skilled surgeon by the name of James Esdaile (1957) has been conducting dozens of operations using mesmerism as his anesthesia. He induces profound trance states in his patients and during a period of seven years has performed over two thousand painless operations. Some three hundred of these would be classed as major surgery. They involved amputations, removal of scrotal tumors, cataracts, etc.

At first, Esdaile attracted favorable attention, especially from the Deputy Governor of the State of Bengal. Through his auspices Esdaile was given a hospital devoted to mesmeric practice. He even succeeded in convincing a number of prominent physicians of the validity of his work. However, when he returned to Scotland in 1852 he, too, was the recipient of the rejection which had been hurled at Elliotson. In Calcutta hypnoanesthesia was for the first time practiced on a grand scale. True, scattered operations had been reported earlier in America, England, France and Germany, but no one had before employed mesmerism for the wholesale relief of pain in hundreds of surgical cases—and no one has employed it so extensively since that time. Ether and chloroform were discovered. The more general applicability of chemo-anesthesias, coupled with the unreliability of the mesmeric trance and the greater skill required for its use, soon settled the matter. However, at least one finding of Esdaile's has not been challenged to this day and is deserving of much further research. While a high proportion of surgical cases died in surgery (or shortly afterward) of shock, almost none of those whose operations were conducted under mesmerism did so. This favorable ratio held even when compared to surgeries conducted under chemical anesthesias.

One other great contributor of the day came from the English-speaking world. James Braid (1843) was a Scottish ophthalmologist. In November of 1841 he visited the demonstration of a French magnetist, La Fontaine. Initially skeptical, he denounced the first "seance." But he stayed and changed his mind. Within a year he had presented a paper to the Medical Section of the British Association in Manchester, which was rejected.

Braid received attacks, not only from the medical profession, but also from the clergy with whom he got into a controversy as to whether the effects of mesmerism were due to the influence of "Satanic agency." Braid could not accept the magnetic theories of Mesmer. He was the first to insist that the phenomenon was psychological in nature and due to "suggestion." In an effort to place this on a neurological basis he coined the term "neuro-hypnotism" or nervous sleep. Soon he referred to it as simply "hypnotism" and the one who practiced it as a "hypnotist." Braid derived the word from the Greek term which means sleep. However, hypnosis is not a true sleep although sometimes it shows a superficial resemblance to that state. Braid initially thought it was a kind of ocular reflex until he found out that he could hypnotize blind patients. He was the first to untie the phenomenon completely from an untenable magnetism theory and place it clearly within the field of psychology. As such, he was a significant forerunner of Freud and perhaps should be credited with being the first true practitioner of psychosomatic medicine.

Braid did not suffer as much from the darts of jealous colleagues as did Mesmer and Elliotson. But then he was not a man who was driven to seek prestige as much as the others, nor was he as argumentative in his claims. His career leaves us with a constructive thought. He who returns from his first acquaintance with hypnosis to trumpet enthusiastic claims for its superiority as a therapeutic modality can expect the mobilized opposition of his colleagues. Resistance is not engendered nearly as much when assertions of its value are tempered.

It should be mentioned that magnetism had reached into the United States. During the 1830's and 40's a number of operations under trance were reported, and in 1845 there was an active society of mesmerists in New Orleans. Phineas Quimby practiced hypnosis in America, but he is not as well known as his most celebrated pupil, Mary Baker Eddy, who founded Christian Science. Although this method of healing greatly resembles hypnotic suggestion, its founder and followers insisted that it has nothing to do with hypnosis (see Janet, 1925).

Almost a half century after the death of Mesmer, the focus of hypnotic practice returned to France. In 1864, Antoine Liebeault, a poor man's doctor, settled in Nancy. He had finished his medical degree in 1850 at the University of Strasbourg. After reading a book on mesmerism during his medical studies, he had been successful in hypnotizing several subjects. However, it was not until 1860 that he began to practice the modality seriously.

Liebeault was a simple and modest man. In order to induce his French peasant patients to submit to hypnotic treatment (since they were accustomed to drugs and physical manipulations), he offered to treat them free with hypnosis while charging for the more traditional therapies. He acquired much respect among the poor people of the area and is pictured as a great humanitarian, interested in the welfare of others regardless of recompense to himself. Would that we had more practitioners of his type today. Bramwell (1956) describes a typical incident which he observed in Liebeault's clinic.

"Two little girls, about six or seven years of age, no doubt brought in the first instance by friends, walked in and sat down on a sofa behind the doctor. He, stopping for a moment in his work made a pass in the direction of one of them, and said; "Sleep, my little kitten," repeated the same for the other, and in an instant they were both asleep. He rapidly gave them their dose of suggestion and then evidently forgot all about them. In about twenty minutes one awoke and, wishing to go, essayed by shaking and pulling, to awaken her companion— her amused expression of face, when she failed to do so, being very comic. In about five minutes more the second one awoke, and, hand in hand, they trotted laughingly away."

Liebeault believed that the phenomena were psychological

in nature and completely discarded the magnetic theories. After two years of hard work he published a book entitled *Du sommeil et des états analogues, considérés surtout au point du veu de l'action de la morale sur le physique*. (On sleep and Related States, Considered Especially from the Point of View of the Action of the Mind on the Body). Only one copy of the book (Liebeault, 1866) was sold then. He continued treating as the poor man's doctor, unknown, for some twenty more years, when recognition belatedly came his way.

Liebeault practiced actually and figuratively on "the wrong side of the tracks." On the other side lay the great University of Nancy. And at its medical school resided an eminent doctor, Hippolyte Bernheim, Professor of Neurology. Liebeault was successful in treating a patient who for many years had resisted Bernheim's therapeutic efforts, and the eminent professor decided to pay a visit to Liebeault. Highly skeptical at first, Bernheim must undoubtedly have felt that he was carrying out this investigation for the purpose of exposing a quack.

However, if he came to jeer, he stayed to cheer. Liebeault's work interested him greatly, and he became one of the country doctor's best friends. In 1886 he published his own textbook, *Suggestive Therapeutics* (See Bernheim, 1964), describing the techniques and giving due credit to Liebeault. After that, visitors from far and near flocked to Nancy to observe and study with Liebeault and Bernheim. Even though now famous and even though many purchased his book, Liebeault preferred to treat the poor for little or no fees, and he apparently never profited financially from his new-found status. He and Bernheim developed what came to be known as "the Nancy School," a center for hypnotic practice and instruction which emphasized the concept of suggestion and taught that hypnosis was a psychological phenomenon, not a magnetic one.

Another "school" developed to the North in Paris under the leadership of the distingished neurologist, Jean Martin Charcot (1889). Charcot practiced at the Salpetriere Hospital and opposed the views of the Nancy group. He believed that hypnotic phenomena were pathological and found only in hysterical people. Although he was aware of the factor of suggestion and of psychological influence he still tried to revive interest in the old magnetic theories.

Liebeault and Bernheim were soon drawn into a controversy with Charcot, and a number of joint experiments were set up to test the relative claims of each. The views of the Nancy group prevailed, and magnetic theories of hypnotism

Fig. 1:1. A Demonstration of Hypnosis by Charcot

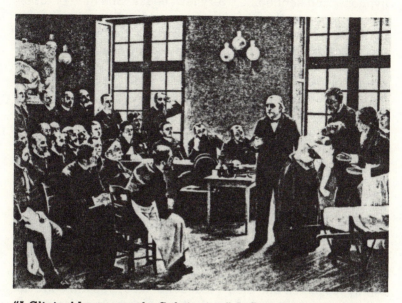

"A Clinical Lecture at the Salpêtrière." A. Brouillet's painting
shows Charcot at the height of his fame, demonstrating a case of
"grande hystérie" to an elite audience of physicians and writers;
behind him is his favorite disciple, Babinski. The painter has
involuntarily shown Charcot's fatal error: his verbal explanations
and the picture on the wall suggest to the patient the crisis which
she is beginning to enact; two nurses are ready to sustain her
when she falls on the stretcher, where she will display her full-
fledged crisis. *(From Le Salon de 1887, Paris, facing page 62.)*

were no longer seriously voiced after that time.

Pierre Janet (1925) studied with both Bernheim and Charcot
and was a prolific practitioner of the hypnotic art. He considered that it was a form of dissociation and likened hypnosis to
hysteria. He reported an interesting case of a young woman
who suffered from anorexia and a glove anesthesia over most
of her body. She would only eat while under a state of hypnosis. Once, while Janet was absent from the clinic, he left her
under hypnosis so she could be fed. In the hypnotic state she
appeared so normal that when her family came to visit that
day they concluded she was cured and took her home. After a
week or two the hypnosis wore off, and her symptoms returned. She was hypnotized by Janet again and sent home

once more. During the next eight years she was placed back in hypnosis and sent home every few weeks. She died of tuberculosis, apparently having spent eight years existing in a permanent hypnotic state. Janet was aware of unconscious processes and wrote about them. However, since it was Freud who described these processes in more detail, Janet was not given the credit as their discoverer.

Up to this time hypnosis had been used as a general therapeutic method for attacking all types of symptoms, whether they were organic or psychogenic in nature. Hypnoanesthesia and the relief of pain were its most common uses. Also, until this time psychiatric illness was considered by most practitioners, if not simply malingering, to be organically caused. Even Charcot subscribed largely to this point of view. But now the time was ripe for the discovery that many disorders were psychologically, not physiologically caused, and hypnosis was to play an important role in the vanguard of these advances.

Josef Breuer was a general practicing physician in Vienna, highly respected and also a teacher of medicine although not a "professor." He was conservative in nature and given to much equivocation and doubt in pursuing a remarkable discovery he had made. Hypnosis had been primarily used to suppress or suggest-away symptoms. Thus Bernheim and Liebeault would hypnotize their patients and instruct them to relinquish their illnesses. Often this was effective; often not. Breuer treated by suggestive hypnosis a young woman known as Anna O., who suffered from an hysterical disorder. He was not successful in relieving her symptoms at first. However, when he induced her to "abreact," or re-live early traumatic situations in her life in which she both remembered and expressed feelings, the symptoms left. Breuer and Freud were close friends. In fact, Breuer helped Freud financially during his early medical studies, which enabled Freud to get married. Both Breuer and Freud had studied with Dr. Ernst Brücke, a psychiatrist who espoused a strong physical-chemical approach to the understanding of mental disorders. Freud was most intrigued with Breuer's abreactive method, but he received no encouragement from Charcot when he described it to this teacher, and Brücke was most violently opposed to hypnosis, which he regarded as rank charlatanism. Accordingly, although Freud had observed Breuer's work as early as

1882, he, himself, did not take up the practice of hypnotism until 1887.

Freud's experience with hypnosis brought him to the discovery of unconscious processes and provided the great breakthrough in psychiatric thinking which was to dominate this discipline for the next half century (Breuer & Freud, 1957). However, for a number of reasons he relinquished his use of this technique. In the first place, he was not a very good hypnotist. He was unable to induce a deep state in many of his cases. This may have been due to the fact that Freud, a brilliant, impatient young genius, was not sensitive in interpersonal relationships, nor sufficiently patient to involve himself in the induction process long enough to secure a profound hypnotic state. Furthermore, Breuer, the modest old conservative, was quite embarrassed when Anna O. developed strong love feelings for him as a result of the treatment. This caused him to break off his therapeutic relationship with her. Freud, himself, was embarrassed when a female patient threw her arms about him. He had not at that time discovered the meaning of transference and did not know how to deal with such manifestations. Also, many patients who relinquished their symptoms under hypnotic suggestion or abreaction would reinstate them again, and Freud despaired of achieving permanent results by this modality.

At any rate, he developed a slower and less spectacular method of cathartic release by pressing his hand on the patient's forehead and asking him to freely associate, that is tell everything which came to his mind. As we will see later, this may have actually constituted the induction of a light hypnotic state, but the material which emerged was less emotionally laden. Freud was better able to handle it and understand it. Perhaps this was best for the development of psychoanalysis since it brought to therapy a slower and more rational approach. This enabled him to study the process more logically and with less emotional distraction.

Unfortunately, Freud masked his own inadequacies at working within the hypnotic relationship by maintaining that psychoanalysis only began with his discarding the hypnotic method and introducing that of free association. The daughter (psychoanalysis) rejected its mother (hypnosis), and it was the parent which was regarded as illegitimate during the next few decades. Most of the objections which Freud raised about hypnosis, such as that its results were temporary and that it "by-passed the ego," have since been disproved by investigators in the field.

It should be noted also (See Kline, 1958) that when Freud practiced psychoanalysis he was content to listen passively to the associations of his patients, but that when he used hypnosis his own manner of treatment changed. He became the authoritarian and commanded the symptoms to disappear. In fact, he himself said that he became bored with the monotonous arbitrary prohibitions used in treatment by suggestion. Whether Freud's different therapeutic manner when he used hypnosis compared to when he was psychoanalyzing was due to his having been taught that hypnosis was an authoritative approach involving command and entreaty, or whether something within his own counter-transference needs was stimulated by the hypnotic relationship, we will probably never know. Hypnosis gives the hypnotist the illusion of great power, and many a modest man has been seduced by power into becoming a tyrant. At least it does teach us that therapeutic hypnosis is much more than an altered state of consciousness achieved by manipulations of the operator. In the treatment situation it is a sensitive mode of communication, and its effective use is subject to the quality of the interpersonal relationship between hypnotherapist and patient. Freud's failure with hypnosis was largely due to his personality rather than to an inherent weakness in the modality. Would that this point was known by more analytic psychotherapists. But the aura of Freud, the great master of psychoanalysis, remains and still keeps many of his disciples from learning to recognize that his prejudices withheld from the psychoanalytic field a most fruitful technique, which can uncover repressed material, assist in its ego integration, and frequently produce permanent results in a much shorter time than can free association.

In spite of his rejection of hypnosis Freud could never quite abandon it completely. Time and again he would toy with the idea, although he personally could not bring himself to re-examine his postion and use it again on his patients. In 1919 he wrote that in applying psychoanalysis to numbers "hypnotic influence might find a place in it again." He also stated (Freud, 1953, Vol. II, p. 402) that the practical psychoanalysis might constitute an alloy of "the pure gold of analysis" with the "copper of direct suggestion"—meaning hypnosis.

The days of the 1890's were a time of boom for hypnotic practitioners. Everybody hypnotized everybody for every known disorder. Carcinomas, brain tumors, viral diseases, etc. were subjected to hypnotic suggestion—of course, with a high number of failures. Doctors who wished for omnipotence and thought that they had arrived there became disillusioned. With the rising interest in psychoanalysis among physicians hypnosis fell once more into disuse. Only a few isolated practitioners and lay entertainers continued to employ the modality.

A Harvard psychiatrist, Morton Prince (1906), investigated multiple or dissociated personalities by hypnosis, and in World War I, Simmel in Germany and Hadfield (1940) in England employed it to treat war neuroses. Simmel (1944) developed a modified abreactive technique in which his German soldier-patients were induced to release their angers by tearing to pieces under hypnosis a dummy wearing a French uniform. Hadfield integrated hypnosis with psychoanalytic techniques and was probably the first to coin the term, "hypnoanalysis."

Modern Hypnosis*

In 1933 Clark Hull, a distinguished experimental psychologist, published the first book which presented controlled, research investigations on hypnotic phenomena. He and his associates looked into such matters as the relation of postural sway to hypnotizability, age differences in hypnotizability, the relation of hypnotizability to general intelligence, the ability of subjects under hypnosis to transcend normal motor and sensory abilities, etc. These were the first carefully controlled investigations. Up to that time nearly all data about hypnosis had been secured from clinical observations on patients. Such reports had inherent in them the subjectivity and biases which are characteristic of case studies. Hull was the first to map out hypnosis as a legitimate field of study by modern experimental science.

*For a detailed account of the development of modern hypnosis in this country, see "Hypnosis in the United States", pp. 265–290 by Watkins in *Hypnosis Throughout the World*, edited by F.L. Marcuse (1964). The remainder of this chapter is a brief condensation of that report but brought up-to-date.

The world of academia proved to be just as conservative as the province of medicine, and Hull was the recipient of much criticism by other psychologists, who regarded hypnosis as within the field of magic and not science. Hull's pioneering studies did much to break down academic prejudice against investigators in this area, since his own scientific credentials were impeccable. He was widely renowned as a researcher and theorist in the field of learning, and in 1936 served as President of the American Psychological Association. Hull and his students were a powerful influence in making hypnosis respectable among experimental scientists just as Bernheim and Charcot had been in relation to the medical profession.

During the 1930's another boost to physicians and psychotherapists came as a flood of innovative papers emerged from the pen of Milton H. Erickson (See Haley, 1967). This psychiatrist experimented with a wide variety of ingenious techniques for inducing hypnosis and eliminating symptoms. He became a master in the art of using language to communicate with his patients at unconscious levels. Erickson did not subscribe to the psychoanalytic goals of achieving insight into the causes of neurotic disorders. Rather, he would by-pass resistances and make his patient's defenses untenable, thereby forcing a relinquishment of symptoms. As first president of the American Society for Clinical Hypnosis, and as the first editor of the *American Journal of Clinical Hypnosis*, he achieved worldwide recognition. He was also a controversial figure during the societal quarrels which broke out among hypnotic specialists during the late 1950s and early 1960s. That is another story which we will describe later.

During World War II this writer (Watkins, J., 1949), while at the Welch Convalescent Hospital in Daytona Beach, Florida, was given the unusual opportunity of developing a hypnotherapy program for returning soldiers. The abreacting of war experiences had been found valuable by Grinker and Spiegel (1945), but in their work they, as well as most other military psychiatrists, relied on the use of such drugs as sodium amytal and sodium pentothal to induce the altered state of consciousness which would permit emotional release. At that time only a few military practitioners were employing hypnotic techniques in the treatment of war neuroses (called "shell shock" in World War I). The Welch Hospital in 1945 included some 2500 soldiers who were psychiatric casualties, and an entire "company" of patients was allocated to treatment either by hypnotherapy or "narcosynthesis," the term Grinker and Spiegel (1945) applied to their approach. Much latitude was given in this "Special Treatment Company" to develop and experiment with a wide variety of hypnoanalytic procedures.

During the years immediately after the war there was a great upsurge of interest in the applications of hypnosis to dental practice. The anxieties and dental phobias shown by many patients have always been a source of difficulty to these practitioners. Hypnosis offered an approach for dealing with them. In addition, hypnotic anesthesia might prove of value either in replacing or supplementing chemo-anesthesias for the relief of dental pain. Burgess (1952) and Heron (1953), two psychologists in Minnesota, taught hypnotic techniques to many dental practitioners. "Hypnodontia" societies were organized, and there were over 300 dentists within that state using hypnotic procedures almost before dentists in other parts of the country had heard of such procedures.

A pioneering group of some twenty-five psychologists and psychiatrists organized the Society for Clinical and Experimental Hypnosis in 1949. The leaders in this group were Jerome M. Schneck, a psychiatrist and psychoanalyst, who served as its first President, and Milton H. Kline, who became the editor of the *Journal for Clinical and Experimental Hypnosis* published by the Society. In order to counter the criticism focused on hypnosis by psychoanalysts, conservative physicians, and academic psychologists, membership in this organization was purposely restricted by insisting on extremely high requirements. To become a member one was required to have had many years of experience and have published significant contributions. Accordingly, the organization grew very slowly, and during the following eight years it did not number more than one hundred.

In 1955, a report by a lay hypnotist was published which described a subject who, under hypnotic regression, purported to be the re-incarnation of a young Irish woman called Bridey Murphy. Bridey gave many details of her "life" of a hundred and fifty years earlier. Although reputable scientific study (Kline, 1956) could find no realistic basis for this claim, the case attracted much public attention. *Time, Life, Look* and many other magazines devoted space to it. Both lay people and many professionals were intrigued. The publicity given to

Bridey Murphy tended to emphasize the unscientific and spectacular claims which had so often in the past brought repudiation of hypnosis by reputable physicians and scientists. It smacked of Mesmer's showmanship. Interest in hypnotic "re-incarnation" died down, but a number of scientists and mental health practitioners were induced to commence serious study of the therapeutic potentialities in hypnosis.

Milton Erickson organized a teaching team which gave three-day seminars throughout the United States to physicians, psychologists and dentists. Many new recruits to the field received their initial training at these courses. However, these newcomers found that they did not have the extremely high requirements for membership in SCEH (The Society for Clinical and Experimental Hypnosis). They were considerably dissatisfied at their inability to affiliate with the only hypnosis society existing at that time.

After a battle over efforts to lower the entrance requirements for SCEH Erickson and his associates organized, overnight, a new society called ASCH (The American Society for Clinical Hypnosis). Filled from the ranks of the students in seminars, this organization grew rapidly and became much larger in size than SCEH. A bitter conflict ensued between the parent group, centered in New York, which insisted on the high standards of membership, and the new vigorous young ASCH, centered in Chicago, which argued that hypnosis was too valuable a modality to be so restricted. This split occurred in 1957 and was followed by over five years of bitterness, name-calling, and raiding of each other's membership. Competition for new members, especially of those who had achieved status in the field, was keen. SCEH prided itself on its "quality" and had at that time the better established journal. ASCH, with its large and increasing membership, was much stronger financially, had a built-in recruitment system for new members in the seminars and held out its shingle as "the most representative" organization in the field.

SCEH, threatened by the large membership and financial solvency enjoyed by ASCH, countered in 1958 by developing two new organizations which were to make significant impact. Specialty boards existed in the field of medicine, dentistry, and psychology, which certified practitioners who could demonstrate certain high-level qualifications. Thus medicine had the American Board of Obstetrics and Gynecology, the American Board of Psychiatry and Neurology, the American

Board of Surgery, etc. Specialty certification existed in such dental fields as periodontia and orthodontia, and in psychology the American Board of Examiners in Professional Psychology certified highly qualified practitioners in the fields of clinical, industrial, and counseling psychology. These usually involved five years of specialized experience plus examinations.

Accordingly, SCEH undertook to organize and launch "The American Board of Clinical Hypnosis" with three sub-boards: The American Board of Medical Hypnosis, the American Board of Hypnosis in Dentistry, and the American Board of Examiners in Psychological Hypnosis; this latter issued separate certificates in clinical and in experimental hypnosis.

Reception of these boards was mixed. The Psychology Board was approved by the American Psychological Association, and its "diplomates" were officially listed in the APA Directory. The Medical Board did not receive official recognition by the American Medical Association although the AMA had approved hypnosis as a legitimate medical discipline. The Dental Board did not receive the approval of the American Dental Association, nor would the ADA even recognize hypnosis as legitimate study for dentists.

To complicate the picture of conflict further the American Medical Association, stimulated by its psychiatric members, tried to restrict the use of hypnosis only to medical practitioners and to exclude psychologists from the field, especially clinical psychologists who were employing it psychotherapeutically. In general, this effort was not successful except for a few states where medical practice laws were ammended to limit the use of hypnosis to physicians. Within the two societies, SCEH and ASCH, physicians, psychiatrists, psychologists, and dentists enjoyed a close, congenial relationship and quarrels between disciplines were largely avoided.

The second move by SCEH at that time was in organizing ISCEH (The International Society for Clinical and Experimental Hypnosis). ASCH had been more successful in developing the field within the United States, but its very name limited its member-getting ability in other countries. Accordingly, the ISCEH, with SCEH as its U.S. Division, soon initiated "divisions" in some thirty different countries. Bernard B. Raginsky, a Canadian psychiatrist who was President of SCEH at the time, requested this writer to form and chair the International

Organizing Committee. The Committee contacted leading workers all over the world to become the international directors of the new society and to organize the various national divisions. Raginsky, who was also a president of the Academy for Psychosomatic Medicine, was a distinguished contributor to the field and had published numerous papers, especially on the applications of clinical hypnosis to the treatment of psychosomatic disorders (1963a). Widely known and respected, his leadership as the first president of the International Society was strongly instrumental in getting it accepted on a worldwide basis. This writer served as its Executive Secretary during the first four years and later also as its President.

ASCH initially perceived the Boards and the International Society as inimical to its interests and boycotted both organizations. However, as time passed, and as the bitterness of competition between SCEH and ASCH declined, it became rather inevitable that these two groups were complementary to each other and that each had something constructive to offer the field. ASCH had many more members, a solid treasury, and a continuous educational program. SCEH had the Boards, the ISCEH, and a widely accepted journal, whose name was now changed to "The International Journal for Clinical and Experimental Hypnosis." Many people who were members of both societies pressed for unification. As of this time, 1986, such a uniting has not taken place, but the old quarrels, the bitterness, and the competition have largely disappeared. The two societies now cooperate in many matters and occasionally arrange contiguous meetings where participants can go from one to the other. Reports of each other's conventions and papers are published in both the *American Journal of Clinical Hypnosis* and the *International Journal of Clinical and Experimental Hypnosis.*

The International Society held meetings about every two to three years (Chicago, 1958; Sao Paulo, Brazil, 1960; Portland, Oregon, 1962; Kyoto, Japan, 1967; Mainz, West Germany, 1970; Uppsala, Sweden, 1973; Philadelphia, 1976; Melbourne, Australia, 1980; Glasgow, Scotland, 1982; Toronto, Canada, 1985). In 1973 it was reorganized and its name changed to the International Society of Hypnosis. Both ASCH and SCEH are now affiliated with it.

The Institute for Research in Hypnosis was also originally organized by SCEH as a training and research unit. It was chartered by the Board of Regents of the State University of

New York as a non-profit educational foundation and served as the medium through which a number of courses, workshops and international congresses were presented. The Institute developed a treatment facility in New York City called the Morton Prince Center for Hypnotherapy. In the American Psychological Association, Division 30 was organized to promote research and practice in the field of hypnosis. Both SCEH and ASCH sponsor workshops in hypnosis, as do various local hypnosis societies. A number of medical schools and graduate departments of psychology now offer training in hypnosis.

Today, hypnosis has largely overcome the prejudices in the medical profession and academia and is accepted (albeit with some suspicion) as a legitimate scientific and treament modality. A great deal of research in the field is currently going on, especially in certain psychology departments. Laboratories, such as those headed by Ernest Hilgard at Stanford, Martin Orne at the University of Pennsylvania, and Theodore X. Barber at the Medfield Foundation have received much grant support from the National Institute of Mental Health and other organizations. The national conventions of SCEH and ASCH are attended by hundreds of members where the latest research papers, clinical studies, symposia, and training workshops on hypnosis are presented. Awards are annually made to outstanding contributors. It seems as if hypnosis may have outgrown its boom or bust cycles and is here to stay, intriguing legitimate scientists into investigating its strange phenomena and converting reputable clinical practitioners within the medical, psychological, and dental professions into using it to help their patients.

As a final note we should remember that this current stage of growth and acceptance was only achieved at the cost of much conflict. The pioneers in this field fought hard to secure its recognition and to maintain their own professional status. Mesmer, Elliotson, Braid, and Esdaile battled constantly with the establishment of traditional medicine. Liebeault treated for twenty years in obscurity. Charcot engaged in bitter controversy with the Nancy practitioners. Freud drew from hypnosis his first understanding of unconscious processes and then abandoned it. His followers rejected it. Professional quarrels raged over the question of training. Hypnosis societies battled over standards of membership and fought for respective status. The practitioner or investigator in this field survived and flourished only if he could demonstrate outstanding abilities and could maintain his professional integrity in the face of attacks and pressures from many directions. Perhaps this resulted in a selecting process which was all to the good, because the field today is peopled by many able clinicians and scientists. Both the major societies, plus the international organization, now number among their members many outstanding contributors who are continuously adding to our knowledge of this fascinating modality and developing an effective therapeutic technology. If humanity is to survive, the understanding of man's inner space may be of greater importance than his conquest of outer space, and in this realm, hypnosis can play a significant role.

Outline of Chapter 1.   A Chronological Outline of the History of Hypnosis

Pre-historic period	Hypnosis probably used by primitive man as almost his only "medical" treatment.
Ancient historical period	"Hypnosis" used in India by Yogis and in Greek temples as "sleep therapy."
Medieval Period	Trance states involve dancing frenzies and cures by the "laying on of hands."
1775-1784	Mesmer develops and practices his theories of animal magnetism.
1784	The French Commission evaluates and rejects Mesmer's theories.
1784	de Puysegur discovers the state of somnambulism.
1821	A painless surgery reported in France by Recamier on a "magnetized" patient.
1837-1868	Elliotson fights for scientific and medical acceptance.
1841	Braid develops the term "hypnotism" as a *psychological* phenomenon.
1845-1853	In Calcutta, India, Esdaile performs over 2000 operations under hypno-anesthesia.

1864	Liebeault begins his practice of clinical hypnosis in Nancy.
1864	Phineas Quimby practices hypnosis and teaches it to Mary Baker Eddy, founder of Christian Science.
1882	Bernheim visits Liebeault and is converted to the value of hypnosis.
1882	Freud observes Breuer's abreactive method.
1885	Bernheim publishes his book *de la Suggestion*.
1886	The "Nancy" school of Liebeault and Bernheim prevails over the "Paris" school of Charcot, and hypnosis is established as a psychological, not "magnetic" phenomenon.
1887	Freud takes up the practice of hypnotism.
1894	Freud abandons hypnosis and begins the development of psychoanalysis.
1906	Morton Prince treats a case of dissociated personality with hypnosis.
1933	Hull publishes the first book on experimental hypnosis, *Hypnosis and Suggestibility*.
1933	Milton Erickson begins publication of a series of papers reporting unique and innovative approaches in hypnotherapy.
1945-1946	Watkins develops hypnoanalytic techniques in the treatment of war neuroses.
1947	Dental hypnosis begins in the State of Minnesota.
1949	The Society for Clinical and Experimental Hypnosis is founded.
1953	The Journal for Clinical and Experimental Hypnosis begins publication.

1956	The Case of Bridey Murphy excites much public attention.
1957	The American Society of Clinical Hypnosis is formed.
1957	The American Board of Clinical Hypnosis with three sub-boards, The American Board of Medical Hypnosis, The American Board of Hypnosis in Dentistry, and The American Board of Examiners in Psychological Hypnosis is formed.
1957	The International Society for Clinical and Experimental Hypnosis is founded.
1957-1962	Much strife between the two hypnosis societies, SCEH and ASCH.
1958	The therapeutic use of hypnosis by physicians is approved by the American Medical Association.
1960	The American Board of Examiners in Psychological Hypnosis receives the official approval of the American Psychological Association.
1973	The International Society of Clinical and Experimental Hypnosis is re-organized, broadened in membership and re-named "The International Society of Hypnosis."

Chapter 2

Theories of Hypnosis

My first intimate acquaintance with hypnosis took place in August 1941, about two months after the beginning of the war, in Lemberg where I was a prisoner of the Germans. I was taken into a prisoners' camp, where several thousand people, live, dead and wounded, were together on an area of two square kilometers, under the open sky, not receiving food or even water during weeks, where all the grass had been eaten and there had been some cases of cannibalism. There, people died every day from emaciation or wounds in geometric progression and new prisoners were brought in their place.

On my first night, I casually lay on the ground beside somebody whose hand was wrapped in a rag with clotted blood, who at certain moments had crises of intense pain, pressing the hand and writhing on the ground—then he calmed down. In one of his calm moments, this person turned to me and said, 'countryman, take from my pocket a package of tobacco. I don't smoke. But if you can, ease my pain. This should be very simple, do as you believe my mother would have done if she were here; reveal compassion, calm me, suggest to me that I will not suffer.'

This was my first rapidly successful induction of a hypnotic trance, though I only came to know it, to my considerable surprise half a year later. Then I began to apply the same procedure more decidedly to cases of amputation and war neuroses among the war prisoners, with greater or lesser success.[1]

[1]Excerpt of a letter from Dr. Anatole Milechnin, noted Uruguayan hypnotherapist.

It is in the nature of man to seek explanations for natural phenomena, especially when they seem to be foreign to common-sense experience—as is hypnosis. Accordingly, it is not surprising that there are many theories which have been proposed to explain it. Most of these are merely descriptive; some only deal with one aspect of the modality. A few attempt to account for hypnotic phenomena by relating them to other psychological concepts which are already in use. In fact, each, like the blind men and the elephant, appears to have a bit of truth about hypnosis but is not sufficiently comprehensive to include all manifestations which are ordinarily meant by the term. We must conclude that as yet there is no completely adequate definition or explanation of hypnosis which is satisfactory to all serious workers in the field. But then we still lack an adequate definition of the term "personality" even after all the years that psychologists have wrestled with this concept. So we should not be surprised that, although there is much agreement as to the phenomena which can be evoked, we have not as yet been able to pin it down so that we can define in all that should be included, and rule out that which is not hypnosis. Perhaps this is because hypnosis may not be a single, unitary entity. Hence, hypnosis between operator A and subject B may not be the same psychological process as between operator C and subject B or even between A and B from one time to the next. We may have been trying to give a single definition to a whole range of complex psychological interactions within subjects and between hypnotist and subject.

Let us now survey the more common theoretical views which have been proposed. We will omit the "animal magnetism" concept of Mesmer which has been described in the previous chapter, since it has been discredited.

Hypnosis as a "trance" or Sleep-Like State

The word "sleep" has often been used during the hypnotic induction. Liebeault moved through his clinic from patient to patient, often uttering only this word to induce in them a deep trance state. Furthermore, when one views the typical hypnotic subject immediately after the state has been initiated he looks as if he were asleep. Relaxation and passivity, combined with the closing of eyes, are common behaviors related to hypnosis. Many hypnotists, especially those engaged in clinical work, seek to get their subjects into a profound state of relaxation. it should be noted that the term "hypnosis" was coined by Braid from the Greek word "hypnos" meaning sleep. The level of deep hypnosis is also called "somnambulism," hence, walking in one's sleep, and subjects who act-out behaviors suggested to them while in this state often appear as if they were performing while asleep.

Pavlov (1923) held that sleep, hypnosis and simple inhibition were different degrees of the same qualitative process and that hypnosis represented a partial sleep. He believed that these phenomena occurred because of an inhibition of the higher brain processes. Therefore, hypnosis was defined as a state of partial cortical inhibition.

A number of the earlier workers, such as de Puysegur, Abbe Faria, and Bernheim considered sleep and hypnosis identical. Bernheim reported that he had established hypnotic "rapport" with a sleeping patient and could elicit the same response to suggestions as he could from a hypnotized subject.

Hull (1933) examined this concept at considerable length and quoted a number of studies such as that by Bass (1931) and others which showed rather conclusively that hypnosis and sleep were not identical. Bass measured the height of the kick in the patellar reflex on a number of subjects in the waking, the hypnotic, and the sleep state. Invariably, the response in the hypnotic state approximated that in the waking condition.

The apparent conflict between Bass's studies and the reports of Bernheim have been resolved by the discovery that it is possible to change sleep to hypnosis and vice-versa. By speaking to a sleeping subject we may "awaken" him in the sense that, although he does not open his eyes, he enters an hypnosis state and becomes suggestible. On the other hand, hypnotized subjects may simply go to sleep in the absence of stimulation.

Many of the early workers noted that some apparently hypnotized subjects appeared to be alert and active, hence, "somnambulists." Others entered a "lethargic state." They considered these two different kinds of hypnosis. Hull believed that the lethargic state was simply sleep and not hypnosis. Later theories attempt to account for these differences by a multi-factor explanation of hypnosis. Hull, on the basis of his studies (which were conducted during the 1920's and 1930's) concluded that "hypnosis is not sleep," and that "it has no special relationship to sleep."

The relationship between these two states, however, has continued to intrigue researchers, since they appear to have so much in common behaviorally. The most recent and complete studies in this area have been reported by Evans (1979). We shall not attempt in this introductory text to pursue the many interesting findings that have so far emerged, but a few of the significant ones should be mentioned.

With the invention of the electro-encephalograph much more sensitive measures of sleep are now possible. We know that the EEG patterns under hypnosis do not resemble those under a true sleep, thus confirming Hull's earlier studies. However, the incidence of both sleep-walking and sleep-talking correlates significantly with hypnotizability. Considerable interest has centered about the alpha, or slow wave activity, which characterizes the onset of sleep or the awakening from it. In spite of isolated reports to the contrary, the consensus of findings is to the effect that hypnosis and alpha activity are unrelated.

One very interesting finding, which has had verification both experimentally and clinically, is the extent to which post-hypnotic suggestions can influence the content of dreams (Moss, C.S. 1967; Sacerdote, 1967). Hypnoanalysts have used this phenomenon to initiate and analyze "unconscious" answers in dream form to therapeutic questions which were posed to their patients.

Behavior which can be suggested under sleep is similar to that which can be induced under hypnosis—even as Bernheim had reported. However, this is believed to result from the subject's "awakening" into hypnosis when spoken to and then returning to sleep. In true sleep the subject becomes lethargic, does not attend, or respond to spoken words. In hypnosis there is considerable evidence of active underlying mental processes. However, subjects who did respond to questions while apparently asleep proved to be more hypnotizable than those who did not.

The investigations on the relation between sleep and hypnosis are continuing, but perhaps we can best summarize our present state of understanding in the words of Evans (1979), "there is no interchangeability of sleep and hypnosis. The EEG during hypnosis and sleep are basically different. For this reason, it is perhaps not surprising that hypnosis cannot be used as an effective substitute for sleep." One interesting finding has been noted, however, by Sherman (1971). Under very deep trance all EEG activity came to an almost complete stop, almost like that approaching death. Naruse (1962) related hypnotic tance to "meditative concentration."

Physiological Theories of Hypnosis

Pavlov's Theories

Pavlov, of course, is best known for his work on conditioned reflexes (1957). It is not surprising, accordingly, to find that the partial cortical inhibition, which he believed to be hypnosis, was described by him as a conditioned reflex. The word or gesture used in the induction process was seen by him as constituting the stimulating cue which elicited the reflex of hypnosis. He believed that there was a process of radiation of inhibitions throughout the cerebrum as a consequence of monotonous stimulation. His theory, although not validated or commonly accepted in the West, does provide some rationale for such phenomena as "highway hypnosis," that trance-like state whcih is often induced in the bored auto driver who is going along a very straight highway at night, focusing on the center line, or responding to the monotonous swishing of a windshield wiper. Certainly, the conditioned reflex theory of hypnosis does not explain such phenomena as regression, hypermnesia, post-hypnotic hallucinations, and many other manifestations of somnambulistic trance.

Schneck's Theory of Hypnosis as a Primitive Psychophysiological State

Schneck (1963) held that most theories of hypnosis simply describe the phenomena which can be induced under hypnosis or during the induction process itself; they do not get at the basic underlying condition which constitutes hypnosis. To him, hypnosis is a primitive form of psychophysiological awareness in which consciousness is eliminated, and the ability of the self to differentiate itself from the environment is at an absolute minimum. Under this condition awareness of time, person, and place would be absent. Such a state would approach the most primitive biological state of organic functioning.

Neurological Theories of Hypnosis

Although no complete neurological theory of hypnosis seems to have yet been broached, Crasilneck and others (1956) cite evidence to support the view that the hippocampus is involved in whatever neural circuits underlie hypnosis. West (1960) has suggested that hypnosis is a state of "altered awareness maintained through parassociative mechanisms mediated by the ascending reticular system."

Hypnosis as an
Altered State of Consciousness

There seems to be much broader agreement that in hypnosis a state of altered awareness is manifested, whether this is physiologically or psychologically caused. It would be easy at this point to get immersed in the old philosophical controversies regarding mind and matter, but nothing would be gained. Accordingly, "psychological" theories of hypnosis as contrasted to "physiological" ones simply mean that no observable physiological processes associated with the phenomenon have yet been spotted and that the "state" is apparently caused by verbal, educational, or interpersonal relationship impact.

The essential propositions of the "state" theory of hypnosis have been stated succinctly by Barber, the theory's most ardent critic. As a prelude to the presentation of his own, and competing theory (which we will discuss later), he lists these as follows (1969):

a. There exists a state of consciousness—The hypnotic state or trance—which differs from both the waking and the sleeping state.

b. The hypnotic state can be elicited by many procedures, especially by those commonly termed hypnotic induction.

c. The hypnotic state is a casual factor in producing suggested analgesia, hallucination, age regression, amnesia, and other hypnotic phenomena.

d. The greater the degree or depth of the hypnotic state, the more readily are hypnotic phenomena elicited.

This "state" theory hypothesizes that consciousness or awareness can be changed by the suggestions administered during the induction process, and that the "hypnotic state" which emerges as a consequence has certain unique characteristics which enable the hypnotist to elicit unusual behaviors and perceptions that cannot be activated during the normal, conscious mental state.

A number of writers have mentioned this altered awareness or altered consciousness aspect of hypnosis (Marmer, 1959; Spiegel & Spiegel, 1978; Tart, 1969). Hilgard (1977) notes that subjects who are hypnotized experience themselves differently than at other times. They may report that they have been "in a fog," "spaced-out," "not myself," being under the "influence" of outside forces, "feeling strange," etc.

Kline (1958) holds that the "state" of hypnosis is characterized by a lowered criticality. In some ways the "state" may at times resemble the "state" of drunkenness wherein a person loses some of his controls and engages in speech, agressive or sexual behavior which he would normally inhibit. Not that the uninhibited behavior is so often spontaneous when the subject is hypnotized, but rather that suggestions can be given him to display such behavior and he is more likely to execute them.

A controversy has raged between workers in the field who believe that hypnosis is such an altered state, and that this state must be "induced" before the "hypnotic" behaviors can be elicited, and those who feel that there is no need to posit an intermediate "state." These latter individuals, notably Barber (1979) and Sarbin & Coe (1972) hold that the hypnotic behaviors are elicited directly in the subject through adequate suggestions and motivation. A number of studies have been devised to test the hypothesis of a state or no-state (Barber, 1979; Orne, 1979a). Orne used "simulators," hence subjects who were told to "fool" the hypnotist by acting like hypnotic subjects. Although they successfully elicited most of the phenomena found in the hypnotic subjects, there were specific differences. The "reals," hence "hypnotized" subjects, were more impervious to pain stimuli, emerged from hypnosis more slowly at the termination of the experiments, and often continued to behave like hypnotized individuals after the hypnotist left the room. Not so, the simulators.

Hypnosis as a State of Hyper-Suggestibility

The most common definitions given in psychological and

psychiatric dictionaries stress the aspect of suggestibility in hypnosis. It will be recalled that this was also the explanation proposed by Braid, and espoused by Liebeault and Bernheim, although both de Puysegur and the Abbe Faria, early disciples of Mesmer, had come close to this formulation in their own views. This was an early effort to account for hypnotic phenomena as purely psychological in character. Such a view has been predominant since that time. The increase in suggestibility is perhaps the most noticeable trait of hypnosis. Hypnotized subjects will carry through bizarre suggestions and perform actions suggested to them which they would reject with indignation if presented under other circumstances. Often these suggestions can involve the transcending of normal physiological functioning, such as insensibility to pain, alteration of the time sense, hallucinations, restoration of previously lost memories, etc. Since only under hypnosis can these behaviors normally be elicited it is not surprising that hypnosis has so commonly been described as a state of heightened suggestion.

Since the days of Braid, Liebeault and Bernheim there has been no shortage of observations and studies linking suggestion and hypnosis. Probably, the potentiating of suggestions administered during hypnosis represents its single most marked characteristic. In fact, many writers seem to define hypnosis as equated with suggestibility but involving a more extreme degree of it.

Weitzenhoffer (1953) attempted to carry the term "suggestion" further by describing various forms of it. He felt that hypnosis could be explained by the operation of three different types of suggestion: *homoaction, heteroaction and dissociation.*

By homoaction he meant the process by which the suggestion facilitated the acceptance of another of similar nature. Hence, if the subject accepts the suggestion that his eyelids are becoming heavy, it is much easier for him to respond positively to a following one informing him that his eyes are closing.

In heteroaction the acceptance of one suggestion modifies the reactions of the subject to subsequent suggestions even though they are of a different type, hence, each suggestion which is followed increases his general suggestibility.

By dissociation Weitzenhoffer meant that suggestions tend to operate concretely so that one behavior could be split off from another, thus reducing the integration and coherence with which the entire human organism functioned.

Defining hypnosis as a state of heightened suggestibility, however, simply tells us what can be accomplished with it. This definition is more descriptive than explanatory. Many writers have been impressed with other aspects of the hypnotic process. Today, among the serious scholars in the field, attention does not focus so much on its component of suggestibility, which has been well substantiated, but on other features which may more significantly constitute its true "essence."

Behavioral Theories of Hypnosis

The Ideo-Motor Theory of Hypnosis

If an individual is asked to describe a spiral staircase he will very often respond by tracing one in the air with his finger. It has been noted that thoughts of an act often initiate a tendency to perform that act, and that these manifest themselves by tiny muscular contractions in the appropriate muscles. This theory has been used to account for such hypnotic phenomena as arm levitation or postural sway, two induction techniques which will be described in detail in later chapters. Unfortunately, this theory, like so many others, is related only to a small segment of hypnotic behavior. It provides no rationale for age regression, the lifting of repression, dreams, and fantasy under hypnosis, etc. This theory might be classified as "cognitive-behavioral" since it involves the initiating of overt behaviors (hypnotic) by ideational stimuli.

Barber's "Task Motivation" Theory of Hypnosis

Barber (1979) has pointed out that although the concept of a "hypnotic state" has been predominant for over 100 years its existence as a necessary and sufficient variable in eliciting the various hypnotic phenomena has little actual proof. Its existence has been largely taken for granted. When the bizarre and unusual behaviors characteristic of hypnosis are initiated they are assumed to stem from an "hypnotic state." The behaviors are considered as evidence for the reality of the state. However, on the other hand the "state" is considered necessary for the eliciting of the behaviors. He has sought a more parsimonious explanation of the "hypnotic" phenomena whose reality he fully accepts.

He began his studies from the position that a careful charting of the *antecedents* to "hypnotic" behavior are required and that the *consequences* associated with these antecedents must be specifically described. Such antecedents should be classified into the smallest number possible to account for the hypnotic phenomena.

Proceeding in this way he concluded that the concept of a "hypnotic state" was neither necessary nor sufficient to account for the elicited behaviors. In a number of his studies he was able to activate the unusual behaviors traditionally associated with hypnosis (such as analgesia, post-hypnotic suggestions, hypermnesia, regression, amnesia, hallucinations, etc.) without the formal hypnotic induction usually considered essential to induce "trance" or "hypnotic state." He called this alternative procedure "task motivation" and so defined it to his experimental subjects.

Barber has maintained that most of the *hypnotic* behaviors (italics his) can be explained as determined by five antecedent variables: "(a) subjects' attitudes toward the specific test situation, (b) subjects' expectations concerning their own performance on assigned tasks, (c) subjects' motivation to cooperate, not to resist, and to try to perform the suggested behaviors and to experience the suggested effects, (d) the tone and wording of the specific suggestions that are administered, and (e) the tone and wording of the questions that are designed to elicit reports of the subjective experience."

Role-playing Theories of Hypnosis

White (1941) described hypnosis as "meaningful, goal-directed striving, its most general goal being to behave like a hypnotized person as this is continually defined by the operator and understood by the subject." This does not explain unusual spontaneous phenomena which often arise during hypnoanalysis.

Sarbin (See Sarbin and Coe, 1972) developed White's position further by proposing that hypnotic behaviors are essentially role enactments, the subject manifesting those behaviors which are imposed by his expectations, skills and the social demands of the situation. This can account for many hypnotic reactions. However, it is difficult to explain hypnotic analgesia and anesthesia (during which major surgery is possible) simply on the basis of "role-playing." Perhaps role-taking should be considered as one significant aspect of hypnosis, rather than its essence.

Hypnosis as an Interpersonal Relationship Process

Although trance states can be self or mechanically induced the usual procedure involves suggestions between a hypnotist and subject or patient. Thus, it becomes an interpersonal relationship experience. As such, it manifests the various feelings, distortions, defenses, blocks in communication, and irrational understandings which are a part of all relationships between people.

This concept has been especially emphasized by those who do not subscribe to the theory that hypnosis is an altered state of consciousness. If hypnosis is a "state of consciousness," then it inheres within the subject. The role of the hypnotist is simply that of evoking within his subject a process in which the subject is capable of engaging to a greater or lesser degree. The emphasis falls on the subject. The relationship theorists point out that if hypnosis is viewed as a bi-polar situation, something which occurs in a social situation, then equal attention must be given to the hypnotist as to his subject. Subjects are not simply hypnotizable, non-hypnotizable, or partially hypnotizable. Rather, they are responding to a socially stimulating intervention by another person with whom they have at the time an intensive communication relationship, not necessarily by some altered "state," but simply by behaviors which are being demanded of them by the social aspects of the hypnotic situation. As noted before, Barber and his colleagues especially have attacked the concept of "state" and endeavored to conceptualize hypnosis as a relationship process in which the subject behaves in certain ways because of the demand characteristics placed upon him by the hypnotist.

The Early Psychoanalytic Theory of Hypnosis

Freud was intrigued with hypnosis by his observation of Breuer's use of hypnotic abreactions in the treatment of hysteria. Freud's period of using the modality occurred before he had developed his understanding of the dynamic processes involved in interpersonal relationships. He soon found himself involved in a medium which he did not understand, could not master, and which confronted him with such complications in dealing with his patients that he abandoned its use. His stated reasons for doing so have been frequently noted by psychoanalytic writers and have had the effect of discouraging psychoanalysts from employing hypnosis. However, his subjective reasons, which were based on problems with Freud's own personality, have been intensively analyzed by Kline (1958). They seem to have been unique to Freud himself, and to personal dynamic needs of other similar therapists. His objective reasons for abandoning the technique, namely, that hypnosis by-passes the ego, masks the resistance, and obscures the underlying psychodynamic inter-play, thus making the loss of symptoms only temporary, have been discredited by modern research and clinical practice.

However, Freud did make efforts to understand the phenomenon. His first efforts apparently were to link hypnosis with hysteria as had Charcot and Janet. Thus he states (*Collected Papers*, Vol. I, p. 33) "Under hypnosis we discover painful ideas of precisely this (repressed) character underlying the hysterical phenomena (e.g., in the hysterical deliria of saints and nuns, of abstinent women and well brought-up children)". In fact, the basic concept of psychoanalysis which holds that therapy consists of bringing into consciousness previously repressed ideas simply extended into the area of cognition that which Freud had learned from hypnosis in dealing with repressed emotion. Thus, he also wrote (*Collected Papers*, Vol. I, pp. 40-41) "By providing an opportunity for the pent-up affect to discharge itself in words the therapy deprives of its effective power the idea which was not originally abreacted; by conducting it into normal consciousness (in light hypnosis) it brings into associative readjustment or else dispels it by means of the physician's suggestion as happens in cases of somnambulism combined with amnesia." Freud here was describing hypnosis as a modality for gaining access to repressed material—which it indeed is but in more complex ways than he envisioned at that time.

A misconception about hypnosis first promulgated by Freud and emphasized by Anna Freud (1946) has been most instrumental in turning psychoanalysts away from using it. This was the view that hypnosis obliterated the ego and made impossible the integration of unconscious material uncovered during it. This conception has been shown to be in error (Gill & Brenman, 1959) and is no longer held by those analysts who are knowledgeable and experienced with hypnosis.

Freud was very close to the theories which view hypnosis as a special relationship or transference, and in fact later (Freud, 1922) he stated that, "From being in love to hypnosis is evidently only a short step."

"Father Hypnosis" and "Mother Hypnosis"

Ferenczi (1926) specifically depicted hypnosis as a form of transference, describing it as a parent-child relationship. He further delineated two different types which he called "father hypnosis" and "mother hypnosis." The first exemplified that kind of relationship exhibited during stage demonstrations where the hypnotist dominates his subject. This was related to the typical German family of that time wherein the father exercised a commanding power over his wife and children. Thus, this characterized hypnosis when induced by command and direction.

"Mother" hypnosis was typical of that used in clinical treatment where the practitioner maintains a more gentle and persuasive attitude, where the soft voice is used to lull the subject into a trance state, and the therapeutic suggestions are couched in a diplomatic manner—the way Victorian mothers were reputed to handle their children. Viewed from this standpoint hypnosis becomes a special type of relationship which facilitates the suggestive modification of behavior.

This writer (Watkins, J., 1954) at one time attempted to equate the hypnotic state with transference, but later (1963) modified this and maintained rather that hypnosis was not itself simply transference, but that transference needs in the hypnotic subject and counter-transference motivations in the hypnotist determined whether a hypnotic state could be induced easily, with difficulty, or not at all, and whether that state was light or deep.

Kline also has pointed out the interdependence of the hypnotic "state" on the quality and intensity of the interpersonal relationship between hypnotist and subject. Thus he states (1958) "There is no constancy of itself to the hypnotic relationship, although there may be a constancy to the hypnotic trance state. The trance state is a very basic and fundamental reorientation in perceptual and object relationship. The form that it takes is a reflection of the dynamic interaction between the two persons involved."

The point Kline was making was that hypnosis is not a unitary "something," an "either-or." It exists both quantitatively to different degrees and in different depths and qualitatively in different forms depending on the nature of the unique relationship inhering between the two parties before, during the induction, and afterward during the therapeutic interventions. We must conclude from this that the state of hypnosis induced in subject A by hypnotist B is not the same as that induced in the same person by hypnotist C; that it is not the same in subjects A and D when both are induced by hypnotist B; and that it is not the same in subject A when induced by hypnotist B at one time and at another time. The differences in each of these cases are both quantitative and qualitative in nature. Therefore, hypnosis cannot be regarded simply as a unitary state without considering the relationship setting in which it occurs, just as a figure cannot be evaluated independently of its ground.

The theory of hypnosis as a special kind of relationship accounts for the fact that many subjects may become more hypnotizable after they are better acquainted with the hypnotist, while at other times they may be responsive to strangers onto whom they can project unrealistic transference feelings. It also explains the observation made by many experienced hypnotists that a number of the research studies which show negative results with hypnosis are often conducted by unsensitive investigators who are more knowledgeable in the intricacies of experimental design than they are experienced in the subtle interpersonal relationships involved in working with hypnosis. Such experimenters crudely read off standardized inductions, secure some degree of relaxation, and then conclude that hypnotic phenomena are not "real." Perhaps they never succeeded in activating a genuine hypnotic state-relationship.

It has long been a belief of this writer that while there may be a pure entity which can be called a hypnotic "state," such a concept has little value in clinical hypnotherapy in which the human interpersonal factor is always a most essential part.

Hypnosis as Dissociation

While some writers have described hypnosis as being characterized by regression other workers have perceived its most notable feature as being *dissociation*. During dissociation certain behaviors and experiences seem to be split off from others. In psychoanalytic terms there is a division in the ego which separates it into two or more different states. If the dissociation is severe we have multiple personalities in which each of the entities is oblivious of the existence of the other. These two different personalities may take turns being "executive." Hence, during the period when personality A is functioning B is dormant, asleep, or unconscious. When B appears it is amnesic to the period during which A was active.

These alternating multiple personalities had been observed by Janet (1907) and classified as a form of hysteria. Charcot, who had been Janet's teacher, had always regarded hypnosis as being equated with hysteria. Since the phenomena of hypnosis was so similar to the symptoms of hysteria it was but natural that Charcot perceived hypnosis as being a psychopathological condition rather than a normal personality phenomenon.

Janet noted that in hypnosis the behavior and perceptions which were suggested seem to be dissociated, hence, split off from normal ego functioning. According to him, both hysteria and hypnosis represented dissociated behaviors. He also was one of the first to use hypnotic techniques in the treatment of multiple personalities. Since that time some form of hypnomanipulation or hypnoanalysis is the preferred approach in dealing therapeutically with these cases (Prince, 1906, Thigpen and Cleckley, 1957, Watkins and Johnson, 1982).

It is hard to quarrel with the view that hypnotic behavior is dissociated from normal responses in an individual, and that the induction of any hypnotic state permits dissociative reactions such as are otherwise seen only in the hysteric, the amnesic or the multiple personality. However, again we are confronted with a theory which emphasizes a single prominent feature but still does not tell us precisely what hypnosis is nor just how such phenomena are produced, even though it relates these to a psychiatrically distinguishable category of mental illness.

Hilgard's Neo-Dissociation Theory of Hypnosis

After the early work of Janet and Charcot the dissociation theory of hypnosis fell into disregard. However, it has had a recent revival of interest as a consequence of the experimental studies of the Hilgards at Stanford University. (Hilgard, E.R., 1977).

Hilgard's original purpose was to investigate the hypnotic relief of pain. These involved primarily the administration of hypnotic suggestions of analgesia in an arm which was placed in ice water. Apparent pain-free responses were elicited in which the subjects evinced no overt pain behaviors and reported that they did not feel pain. Such phenomena, of course, have been well documented since the time of Esdaile. However, when questioned under hypnosis as to whether there was "some part" of the person which experienced the pain most subjects responded affirmatively. Communication was established with this "part" by the automatic writing method—in which a hand is dissociated from the rest of the body and asked to write independently. Because of the slowness of this procedure the communication was shifted to "automatic talking" in which the voice is dissociated and speaks for this "part" independently and separate from the rest of the person.

The studies of the Hilgards showed that although there was often little evidence of *overt* pain when analgesic suggestions had been hypnotically inculcated, both the experience of pain and memories of it were being *covertly* recorded and could be reported by this "part" as a "hidden observer" (1975). Later, Hilgard became more explicit and proposed that the human personality was divided into "cognitive control systems," and that the covert pain was being recorded by a secondary cognitive control system which did not normally have communication either with the outside world or with the other primary system which had been hypnotized. He hypothesized that this secondary cognitive control system was separated by "barriers" from the primary one and from communication with the outside, but that under hypnosis these barriers could be broken through the techniques of automatic writing or automatic talking, thus making it possible to verify the existence of "covert" pain in the absence of normal overt indicators.

The Hilgards noted both physiological and psychoanalytic explanations for this phenomenon, ranging from consideration of the duality of right and left hemisphere action within the brain, to "temporary partial structures within the ego" similar to multiple personalities. They suggested that the hypnotic suggestions could apparently "shift controls from one system to another" and proposed that if these systems were more intensely investigated they would prove to represent "broader mechanisms than those applicable only to pain and suffering." Hypnotic procedures can then be employed to rearrange "the hierarchies of control over systems other than those involved in pain." These findings seem to carry significant implications for a reappraisal of what constitutes normal personality structure and functioning. Through these studies the Hilgards have revived the theory of hypnosis as a kind of dissociation.

Psychodynamic Theories of Hypnosis.

It was inevitable that many analytic-minded theorists should formulate conceptions of hypnosis which were related to the structure and function of the ego. Some of these have singled out a specific defense mechanism, a definite dynamic process, which they see as most characteristic of hypnotic phenomena.

Regression in the Service of the Ego

Gill and Brenman (1959), two analysts associated with the Menninger Clinic in Topeka, Kansas, developed the thesis that hypnosis is a temporary and non-malignant kind of regression. They characterized it as a "regression in the service of the ego." This is contrasted with "regression proper." Kris, a prominent psychoanalytic theorist (1951), described regression in the service of the ego as follows: "The ego enrolls the primary process in its service and makes use of it for its purposes." Primary processes, of course, are primitive, both cognitively and behaviorally, such as characterize the experience of the small child, and probably also that of the human race during its development from a lower species of animal. Ideas are accepted at face value and need not be integrated within a broader matrix of meaning. In psychoanalytic theory primary process characterizes the "id" wherein two totally opposing concepts can reside, yet not contact each other or struggle for resolution. Primary process thinking does not follow the principles of Aristotelian logic. The schizophrenic who groups a sink stopper and a cigarette together in an object assembly test, not because they both are round, but because a man he once knew "was smoking a cigarette while he was fixing a sink" is using primary-process logic. Primary process will not solve mathematical equations, but it may contribute to artistic creations—such as the paintings of Salvador Dali. According to Kris, the strong ego is able at times to relinquish its need for full integration and to "enjoy" the childhood play of a regression to primary processes, hence, a "regression in the service of the ego."

Gill and Brenman have summarized the characteristics of a regression in service of the ego as follows:

1. More likely to occur as the ego grows more adaptive and less likely to occur as the ego grows less adaptive.
2. Marked by a definite beginning and end.
3. Reversible, with a sudden and total reinstatement of the usual organization of the psyche.
4. Terminable under certain emergency conditions by the person unaided.
5. One which occurs only when the person judges the circumstances to be safe.
6. One which is voluntarily sought by the individual and is—relative to a regression proper—active rather than passive.

Both sleep and hypnosis fulfill the above conditions for a regression in the service of the ego. Psychosis would constitute a "regression proper" in that it may not have a definite end and is not normally terminable by the patient unaided.

Gill and Brenman held that hypnosis was a state of altered ego functioning which was brought about by transference, that is, the tendency for the hypnotized subject to regress into a more passive and childlike state in which the relationship with the hypnotist changes the nature of the subject's functioning so that it involves a greater degree of primary process thinking and behavior. This change, however, unlike that in the schizophrenic, is temporary and can be reversed at the will of the subject's ego, hence, voluntarily.

Gill and Brenman believed that in hypnosis a "sub-system"

of the ego is created, and that it is only this sub-system which regresses in transference with the hypnotist. The remaining part of the ego, the "central ego" simply becomes dormant but is available to terminate the regression and bring the individual back out of hypnosis if it feels that the situation is no longer "safe." They conclude that hypnosis is not a "kind" of psychotherapy nor a specific procedure. Rather it should be regarded as a special sort of interpersonal relationship which can be used in many ways to influence the course of treatment.

Hypnosis as an "Atavistic" Regression

Meares (1961) accepted the concept that hypnosis is a regression, but differed from the psychoanalytic point of view in that he focused not on regressed *behavior* but rather on regressed *mental functioning*. That is, the hypnotized subject, especially the deeply hypnotized one, thinks and functions at a primitive level much like that which is common to the most aboriginal peoples, or even like that which must have characterized humans during their phylogenetic development from animal to primitive man. He holds that in this early stage the process of suggestion must have determined the acceptance of ideas, hence intellectual functioning was at an archaic level. Logical thought in man developed later. Meares points out that it is precisely this logical thought which is set aside during the regression into a hypnotic state. This coincides with Kline's "lowering of criticality" as a characteristic of hypnosis.

Hypnosis as a Loss of Ego Boundaries

Kubie and Margolin (1944) have presented a theory of hypnosis from the psychoanalytic viewpoint which emphasizes the mechanism of identification. They distinguish specifically between hypnotic induction and the state of hypnosis which is the product of that induction.

Induction involves the gradual elimination of normal sensory-motor relationships. This initiates a sleep-like condition in which all channels of communication with the outer world are obliterated except one, that with the hypnotist. Through monotony and immobilization (eye-fixation, etc.) the subject is induced to withdraw all attention to exteroreceptive stimuli—except those presented by the hypnotist.

Finally, a fully developed hypnotic state is established in which the subject once more expands his ego to contact the outer world. This time, however, "his own ego" is changed by its incorporation of the hypnotist within it. The image (voice, behavior, etc.) of the hypnotist is now fused with the previously incorporated images of parents. It tends to replace or modify the super-ego. The voice of the hypnotist is like the voice of the parent within—and is obeyed as such. Hypnosis thus becomes an experimental reproduction of the natural developmental process which represented the early parent-child relationship. Kubie and Margolin suggested that hypnosis may be necessary in any psychotherapy which hopes to replace the authority of early critical super-ego figures with more benevolent re-parenting.

In this theory, as in that by Brenman and Gill, we see the concept of regression occupying a predominant position. However, while Brenman and Gill conceived of it as regression to an early state of thinking and behavior, Kubie and Margolin perceived it as regression to the earliest child-parent relationship. Furthermore, in their theory the incorporation of (identification with) the hypnotist by the subject accounts for the fact that the subject experiences and carries out the hypnotist's suggestions as if they were ego-syntonic, hence, originating within his own self.

Hypnosis as a Modality for Manipulating "Ego" or "Object Cathexes"

Paul Federn (1952) a close associate of Freud's, formulated a theory of personality structure which was never well understood by psychoanalysts or other psychologists, perhaps partly because of his difficulty in clearly expressing his views. Although Federn's theories were not aimed specifically at hypnosis but rather at the general structure and functioning of the ego, they appear to be especially relevant.

He held that the essence of "selfness" was an energy which he called "ego cathexis." Any physiological or mental process invested with this energy was experienced as belonging to "me." Hence, "my" hand is experienced as part of me because it contains ego cathexis. The same would be true of "my" thought. This ego energy is itself "the self" and is distinguished from "object" cathexis, a kind of non-self energy which can also activate various physiological and psychological processes. If my arm is invested only with object cathexis I experience it as not part of me, as if it were a board simply attached to my shoulder, or as it would be sensed if it had been hypnotically anesthetized and made immobile. It has no feeling and appears to be detached from the body ego. The arm is no longer "me" but has become "it." According to Federn's theory "me-ness" or "it-ness" depends upon whether an item (either physical or mental) is "cathected" with ego energy or object energy. Thus, an idea which breaks out of repression into the ego without being invested with ego energy is experienced as an object, as "not-me." In the schizophrenic such an idea (for example the thought of his dead mother) breaks into consciousness without being invested with ego cathexis. Accordingly, it is experienced as an hallucination, as if it had originated in an object outside the self. The schizophrenic experiences this as if he were "seeing" his dead mother, not "thinking" about her.

Federn, himself, did not write much about hypnosis per se. However, when through hypnosis we resolve an amnesia, initiate or remove a paralyzed limb, lift a repression, or inculcate within a subject suggestions which are acted upon as if they were his own ideas we are definitely manipulating object and ego energies as these have been defined by Federn. From his ego-psychology viewpoint hypnosis becomes a modality for the manipulation of cathexis, a way of reversing subject and object either in parts of the body or in ideas and perceptions.

Federn further delineated ego structure by hypothesizing that it is normally divided into states. Each "ego state" represents a body of self behaviors and experiences bound together by a common principle and separated by a boundary from other states which have been integrated about other factors. Thus, ego state A may represent those behaviors and experiences which are united by the common factor of having occurred when the subject was in the first grade. Ego state B may represent a similar set of items which are included within the concept of relationship to parent figures. Ego states may be large or small. They may overlap, just as the United States includes states, counties, cities, school districts and national forests, each organized around a central concept, including a set of items bound by a common jurisdiction, and separated by a boundary from other states.

Watkins, J. (1978) has modified and extended Federn's concepts to provide the rationale for a manner of psychotherapy which can be both hypnotic or non-hypnotic. He conceives of normal personality structure as being organized into ego states because of the economy of jurisdiction in the same way that the nation allocates to various local states, districts, and cities, the more specific responsibilities of government, leaving to the Federal authority the interaction of the entire nation with other countries.

Within the personality at any given time one state is usually "executive." It constitutes "the self" in "the now." It includes those behaviors and experiences currently being activated and which are being felt or acted-upon. At that time the executive state is the one most highly energized with ego cathexis. Other states, separated by a boundary from the executive state, are for the moment relatively immobilized. Their impact upon the entire individual is "unconscious." For example, when the individual is at a party one state is "executive" and one set of behaviors and experiences are operative. When he is at work the next day the "party state" has ceased to be executive and is replaced by another. He behaves and experiences differently.

From this position the hypnotized person is in a different state, so that a different set of behaviors and experiences are activated. Hypnosis, by its ability to manipulate cathexis, can de-activate a present state and make executive another, just as in regression to an early age the subject is induced to relive his earlier experiences and repress his present awareness.

The boundaries between ego states vary in permeability from person to person and probably within a single individual from time to time. At one end of the continuum there is almost complete communication between elements in different states. The boundaries are token, and the "federal" jurisdiction over all the person makes him highly integrated. At the other end are the true multiple personalities, wherein the boundaries between the respective states are so rigid and impermeable that "Mary" is completely unaware of the existence of "Joan," and when one is executive it is amnesic to the period during which the other was activated. Most people lie somewhere in between.

There is also partial dissociation, and there are many *latent* multiple personalities. Such an ego state or covert multiple personality might account for Hilgard's "hidden observer." Hilgard and Hilgard (1975) wrote that "It does not mean that there is some sort of secondary personality with a life of its own—a kind of homunculus lurking in the shadows of the conscious person. The 'hidden observer' is merely a convenient label for the information source tapped through experiments with automatic writing, and here through the equivalent, automatic talking." They apparently made no attempt to rule out the possibility that this "hidden observer" might be an ego state, or a "latent" multiple personality. Watkins, J.G. & Watkins, H.H. (1979-80) extended Hilgard's inquiry to a number of "hidden observers" located in good hypnotic subjects to such questions as: "What is your name?" "Where do you come from?" "How long have you been in the person?" "Under what circumstances were you born?" and "What is your function within 'George'?", etc. They found that these entities described themselves as having identity, content, specific functions within the psychological economy of the entire individual and could often indicate their origins— sometimes related to traumatic events. In other words, they acted like "covert multiple personalities." Further exploration of the hidden observer phenomena would seem to have significant implications to personality theory.

Federn's ego state theories appear to parallel and to predict the kind of findings reported by Hilgard except that they are couched in a psychoanalytic rather than a behavioral terminology. If this is true, "cognitive control systems" and "ego states" are simply two names for the same phenomena, hence, dissociated parts of the ego.

If hypnosis is to be considered as a modality for the manipulation of cathexes then it has the ability to change subject to object and vice-versa, that is, it can be used to change parts of "me" into an "it" and back again. Psychoanalysts have used the term "introjection" to represent the internalization of an object. However, once it has been internalized they then treat it as if it is now part of the self. Kubie and Margolin do that when they speak of the "incorporation" of the hypnotist into the subject's ego. There has been great confusion in many psychoanalytic writings because of failure to distinguish between subject and object.

An "introject" is presumed to be an internalized object—

like a piece of undigested food within the stomach. It is within the person but not a part of him. Once food has been metabolized, assimulated and incorporated into the protoplasmic structure of the individual it is no logner an object but truly part of the physical "me." This is analogous to identification wherein a mental object is incorporated into the self. Federn clearly distinguishes between subject and object in that a mental object is activated only by "object cathexis." When this has been replaced by ego or self energy, the previous "object" has now become "subject." Identification has taken place.

The use of the word "identification" to represent both a process and the entity created by that process is confusing. Since there is no noun term which represents the entity created by the process of identification (in the same way as "introject" is the entity created by the process of "introjection", we (Watkins, J.G. & Watkins, H.H., 1981) have proposed the term "identofact." Through identification (the investment of an internalized object with ego cathexis) the object has been changed into subject and is now termed an "identofact." This distinction is important in understanding various hypnotic manipulations.

Hypnosis makes it possible for us to change introjects into identofacts and vice-versa. Kubie and Margolin speak of the incorporation of the hypnotist into the ego of the subject so that the voice of the hypnotist now becomes the thoughts of the subject and is experienced by him as his own self. This means that an initial introjection during the induction process is followed by a change of that introject into an identofact through its investment with ego or self energy. This is accomplished through modified attention, concentration, and the directing of ego energies within the hypnotic relationship.

Watkins, J.G. and Watkins, H.H. (1979) have developed a therapeutic approach which they have called "Ego-State Therapy" based upon the concept that anxiety is caused by inner conflict between different ego states. Both with and without hypnosis they activate the different component states of the conflict in turn (make executive), ascertain the role each plays in the "family" of ego states, and attempt to resolve the conflict. Ego-state therapy involves the application of group and family therapy techniques to the treatment of conflict within the "family of ego states" which constitute a single person.

"Trance Logic" as the Essence of Hypnosis

Orne (1959, 1979a) holds that the "essence" of hypnosis, and that which distinguishes a truly hypnotized individual (a "real") from a simulator, is the ability of the hypnotized subject to freely mix his perceptions derived from reality with those that stem from his imagination. This characteristic of tolerance of logical inconsistencies he termed "trance logic."

Trance logic might be manifested as follows: A truly and deeply hypnotized subject (a "real") is given the hallucination that he will see a certain friend sitting in a chair in front of him. He is then brought out of trance. He sees his "friend" and may engage in conversation with him. He is then asked to look behind himself where the real friend is seated and is asked, "Well, then who is this?" The "reals" demonstrate logical inconsistency or "trance logic" by indicating that they see both the real friend and the hallucinated image of him. Subjects who are faking or simulating hypnosis, having already reported seeing the hallucinated image, tend to deny seeing the real friend. They feel the need to demonstrate logical consistency.

Trance logic is closely related to the concrete thinking or primary process which characterizes the reasoning of psychotics, dissociative reactions, primitive peoples, and children (See Kasanin, 1944). It will be discussed in greater detail in the chapter on "Forensic Hypnosis" in Vol. II of this work, since the distinction between whether a witness or defendant is truly hypnotized during an interview or only faking may be important in court decisions. Whether or not trance logic represents the "essence" of hypnosis there is substantial evidence (Blum and Graef, 1971; Sheehan, 1977) that it is a significant factor in hypnotic behavior.

Multi-Factor Theories of Hypnosis

It is obvious from our previous discussion that different theoreticians have emphasized more than one factor in their proposals. Thus, Kubie and Margolin stress dissociation, identification, regression, and transference. The Hilgards emphasize dissociation within a state concept. Barber talks about "task motivation" within a "hypnotic relationship."

Watkins has called hypnosis a unique "state-relationship" within which the manipulation of object and ego energies is facilitated.

Shor, however (1962), has specifically called for a three-factor approach to hypnosis. He hypothesized that the normal state of consciousness is characterized by the mobilization of a structured frame of reference in the background of attention which supports, interprets, and gives meaning to all experiences. He termed this the "generalized reality orientation." Active (although not conscious) mental effort is required to maintain this generalized reality orientation. It is developed slowly throughout the cycle. It is a flexible entity with many facets which is constantly growing and developing.

In normal waking life this generalized reality orientation constantly operates and is in close communication with all experience. Whenever this generalized reality orientation fades a trance state develops. Hypnosis is characterized by two aspects. In the first there is the construction of a special, temporary orientation (concrete-like) to a small range of preoccupations. The relative fading of the generalized reality orientation into nonfunctional awareness is the second process.

When the generalized reality orientation has faded, experiences do not have their normal meaning since this background is gone. Accordingly, they develop special meanings as determined by the hypnotist through his suggestions. As the generalized reality orientation fades, primary-process modes of thought (such as those exhibited by the psychotic patient) flow into the background of awareness.

Shor held that there were three main dimensions of hypnotic depth and that some combination of these three factors were involved in every hypnotic induction. The first was that of *trance*, hence the abdication of the generalized reality orientation. The second was *role-taking*. This involved the interpersonal reactions to the hypnotist in the present as they are defined by him. The third was *archaic involvement*. This was equivalent to the transference factor. Here, the subject behaves toward the hypnotist as if he were some early significant figure in the subject's life. This special hypnotic transference relationship involved the "core" of a subject's personality.

Shor believed that in certain inductions, or within certain relationships, the trance factor was predominant (such as in the sleep-relaxation approach to induction or the use of immobilization and monotony as suggested by Kubie and Margolin). In other inductions the role-taking factor would be most emphasized as the hypnotist suggested vivid fantasies of interaction to the subject. Finally, when the attempt is made by the hypnotist to revive child states and to encourage primitive, dependent roles in the subject, then the archaic involvement factor would constitute the essence of the induction. Any one or combination of the three might be used to induce hypnosis, but the nature of the state which was induced could very considerably depending upon which factor was emphasized.

Summary

No completely adequate theory of hypnosis has yet been developed, nor can we even establish whether it is a unitary phenomenon or not. Many theories have been proposed, most of them being primarily descriptive rather than explanatory. Each of the theories tends to focus on one or more of the various characteristics of hypnotic behavior and present relative inattention toward other hypnotic responses. Current controversy is centered about whether it constitutes an altered state of consciousness or is simply a special kind of motivated behavior. Although many research studies have demonstrated that most hypnotic behavior can be elicited without the usual induction process, the majority of workers in the field hold that we are dealing with a special alteration of consciousness which is best described as a "state." A number of investigators, especially those with psychoanalytic orientations, are attempting to integrate the state concept with the psychodynamics of interpersonal relationships. The relationship factor appears to be increasingly significant as one moves from the laboratory in which the attributes of "hypnosis" per se is the object of study and the clinical treatment office where hypnosis becomes an adjunct to various forms of psychotherapy. For a critique and comparison of the various theoretical models of hypnosis and an appraisal of the research methodologies used in investigating them the reader is referred to the significant work by Sheehan and Perry (1976).

Outline of Chapter 2. Theories of Hypnosis

1. Hypnosis as a "trance" or sleep-like state.
    a. Hypnosis as related to relaxation and sleep.
    b. Hypnosis as contemplative meditation (Naruse)
2. Physiological theories of hypnosis
    a. A partial cortical inhibition (Pavlov)
    b. A primitive psychophysiological state (Schneck)
    c. A neurological response involving the hippocampus (Crasilneck and Hall)
3. Hypnosis as an altered state of consciousness
    a. A state of hyper-suggestibility (Braid, Liebeault, Bernheim)
    b. A state of altered awareness characterized by lowered criticality (Kline)
    c. A state of hyper-suggestibility characterized by "homoaction," "heteroaction," and "dissociation" (Weitzenhoffer)
4. Behavioral theories of hypnosis
    a. The ideo-motor theory (cognitive-behavioral)
    b. Hypnosis as task motivation (Barber)
5. Role-playing theories of hypnosis
    a. Goal-directed striving (White)
    b. Hypnosis as role-playing (Sarbin)
6. Hypnosis as an Interpersonal Relationship Process
    a. Transference (Freud)
    b. Father-mother hypnosis (Ferenczi)
    c. Trance-transference (Watkins)
    d. State-relationship (Kline, Watkins)
7. Hypnosis as dissociation
    a. Hypnosis as a form of hysteria (Janet, Charcot)
    b. Neo-dissociation theory: A cognitive structural system (Hilgard)
8. Psychodynamic theories of hypnosis
    a. Hypnosis as unconscious process
    b. Hypnosis as regression.
        (1) Regression in the service of the ego, emphasis on the process (Brenman-Gill)
        (2) Atavistic regression, emphasis on the profoundly regressed state (Meares)
    c. Hypnosis as a loss of ego boundaries (Kubie-Margolin)
    d. Hypnosis as a modality for manipulating ego or object cathexes (Watkins-Federn)

Chapter 3

Hypnotic Phenomena

Although hypnotists have engaged in considerable controversy as to just what hypnosis is, there is greater agreement as to its phenomena—what behavioral and perceptual changes are possible during it. The ability of hypnotized subjects to exhibit unusual behaviors and to transcend normal limits of function has never ceased to amaze the average person who observes it for the first time. Experienced workers learn to expect certain responses to their suggestions, reactions which are normally not obtainable in unhypnotized individuals. Still, even they commonly re-experience a sense of awe at the remarkable possibilities in human functioning which become amenable to initiation and control through the hypnotic modality.

When a class of scientifically trained professionals, such as physicians or psychologists, first sees a demonstration of deep trance phenomena, including post-hypnotic hallucinations, hypermnesia or regression, the common reaction is one of shock and disbelief. With seeming ease the hypnotist accomplishes miracles. Subjects recall and relive details of their lives long ago forgotten. They evince disturbances of perception that are seen only in psychotic patients. They compulsively carry out actions which they would hardly perform if they were in complete control of themselves. It is no wonder that the objective observer who has been educated not to believe in miracles immediately finds his rational processes challenged to account for such weird happenings. Some simply say that it is not "really" occurring. It is a trick, or the subject is only acting to please the hypnotist and fool the viewers. The strange behavior flies in the face of common sense.

Some professionals retreat into mystical explanations by a kind of dissociative reaction. Hypnosis cannot be science; it belongs to the realm of fairies and goblins. Some with religious bent may think of it as work of the devil, and one can understand quite clearly why hypnotists during the middle ages were often burned at the stake for practicing witchcraft.

Here we have observable human behavior which is contrary to normal expectations, to normal limitations, and we have no adequate theory or rationale to account for it. Reasonableness promotes reasonableness. Likewise, irrational behavior stimulates irrational reactions. So beginners in the field find themselves experiencing strange feelings of awe, perplexity, disbelief, anxiety, or laughter. Primitive transference reactions stemming from early fantasies of power and omnipotence are frequently mobilized. The clinical teacher of hypnotherapy often views with concern the early experiments of some of his students who are suddenly imbued with the idea that they have acquired god-like powers which they can use to control others and build up their own prestige. Shortly after a workshop in hypnosis that this writer once taught, he was dismayed to hear about one of his students, a physician, who proceeded to hypnotize patients, anesthetize their arms, and then stick needles through them before colleagues to impress them with his newly acquired "powers." It is with difficulty that the serious instructor in hypnosis guides his students safely between the early Scylla of skepticism on the one hand, and the Charybdis of over-involvement on the other. Hypnosis is a phenomenon which can initiate strange behaviors in the hypnotist as well as in the subject. Those of you who are reading this book, or perhaps are studying it as part of a course, should be ever mindful of this factor and strive to keep an even emotional keel, even though you remain highy curious and motivated. The hypnotherapist who learns to utilize this modality for helping others is the one who has also learned to react to it constructively within his own self. A "therapeutic self" (Watkins, J.,1978) finds in hypnosis a powerful adjunct to his healing abilities; but a pathologic self may employ this modality for the release of his destructive tendencies.

Regardless of the controversy as to whether an altered "state" is necessary to elicit hypnotic behaviors, let us take

Fig. 3:1. Hand-Wagging Compulsion

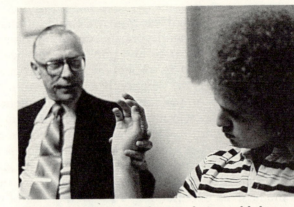

*Under hypnosis the subject is being told that
his right hand will wag up and down and that
he will be unable to stop this when he emerges
from hypnosis until the hand is touched by the
hypnotist. The suggestion is reinforced by the
hypnotist as he demonstrates the movement by
moving the hand up and down.*

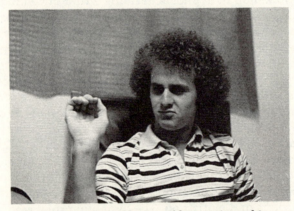

*The subject is brought out of hypnosis and is
greatly surprised to see his hand wagging
automatically.*

the position here held by the majority of hypnosis workers and
assume that such a state exists, has been induced and deepened (by one of the techniques to be described in later chapters), and that the hypnotist is now administering suggestions
aimed at influencing the subject's reactions. We shall also

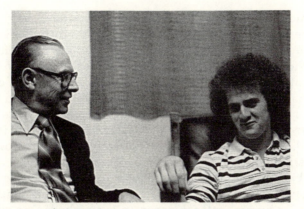

He is quite amused to find that he cannot control the hand and stop its' wagging.

assume that a moderately "deep" degree of such "trance" has been secured. What suggested behaviors are now possible?

Motor Behavior

It will be recalled (Chapter 2) that one of the characteristics of hypnosis is a loss in criticality. Hence, if the hypnotist were to say, "You will sit on the floor and cross your legs," the subject will act as if under a compulsion, that is as if he were no longer "critical" or able to resist carrying out such strange behavior, as he would be in the nonhypnotic state. Almost any motor behavior can be suggested and, if it is within his physical capabilities, the subject will probably carry it out as if he were a dutiful automaton. Sometimes he can even be induced to behave in ways which transcend normal functioning. Watkins and Showalter reported the case of a nineteen-year-old subject who was told that she was twenty-nine years old, a genius, and a doctoral graduate of a famous university. She could then read with amazing speed and facility, and increased her reading speed 63 percent with no loss in comprehension (see LeCron, 1968, p. 159). However, this increase was maintained for only a short period of time.

The subject who has been given a suggestion of an action to be carried out, such as walking across the room and examining a certain book, usually carries this through as if there were no other possibility. He may be unable to remember, after he has been removed from hypnosis, that he performed the action. Sometimes, when the hypnotic state is very light, or for certain inner dynamic reasons which may not be known to the hypnotist, the subject will sit motionless and refuse to carry through the action. If he does not respond in spite of the fact that he has actually been in a state of hypnosis, and it appears that the suggestion has been recorded and processed, his inhibition of the suggested action may have been achieved at the cost of anxiety and inner conflict. That is why the skilled and considerate hypnotist will either remove the suggestion which has not been executed, or simply instruct the subject during or after hypnosis to carry it through. An unresolved suggestion may leave the individual burdened with inner turmoil after the session is finished. One subject did not carry through a suggestion to pick up a teacup and put it down. He seemed pleased to mention that he had successfully resisted the suggestion. However, he reported the next day that he had been unable to sleep that night.

Accordingly, failure to carry through a suggestion may mean that the trance state was not deep enough to induce the lowered criticality, that some need to resist has been mobilized in the subject, or simply that it was not adequately heard and recorded. When in doubt be sure to remove all uncompleted suggestions. This is not always done by stage hypnotists who assume no therapeutic responsibility for their subjects, and who may move on to other communities leaving some of their volunteers with unresolved anxieties.

Not only compulsive behaviors can be suggested, but also compulsive inhibitions. The hypnotized subject who is told that he cannot rise from his seat may be quite unable to do so no matter how hard he tries. The subject who is told that he cannot speak his name may find himself unable to respond. Suggestions of inhibiting behavior have been used as part of the treatments aimed at stopping smoking, overeating, drinking, or other bad habits and addictions. There are complications which can occur when hypnotic suggestion is used to counter normal reactions or habitual responses. That is why hypnotists should be psychologically trained and sophisticated. Any suggestion is an intervention in a human system of equilibrium. Previous responses, even though unconstructive, may have been established for specific reasons. Intervening in them by either compulsions or inhibitions can change that equilibrium and release a train of subsequent reactions that may be worse than the ones which the suggestions aimed to supplant.

Sometimes the hypnotist tries to facilitate or improve behavior suggestively. During World War II, this writer, as an Army psychologist, suggested to a soldier that he would be exceptionally clear-sighted and steady while firing on the rifle range. On that particular day the soldier made an almost perfect score and qualified as "Expert," a level of behavior substantially above what he had previously achieved. That temporary improvement in behavior can be achieved through hypnotic suggestion has been so frequently demonstrated it no longer requires proof. However, much research needs to be done on the conditions which preceded or accompanied the administration of the successful suggestions and their potential duration. There is great variability. One report was made of a suggestion given a hypnotized subject which was carried out 30 years later.

It should be noted that sometimes suggestions are aimed directly at changing a specific behavior, "You will rise out of your seat and yawn." At other times a situation is suggested which results in a desired behavior as a consequence, e.g., "Your muscles will feel tired and stiff"—subject rises from seat, stretches and yawns.

Influencing Attitudes

Suggestions are sometimes intended to modify attitudes which underly behavior rather than the behavior itself. Thus, a suggestion directed toward improving morale, "You will begin to feel hopeful about getting well and will view your doctors as genuinely concerned in helping you," may have the effect of stimulating more cooperative behavior on the part of a hospitalized patient.

Not only is it possible to induce an individual to concentrate more highly when studying or to motivate him to a greater degree of interest, but he can often be programmed by suggestion so that he reasons selectively. Something of this nature was done by the North Koreans in "brain-washing" prisoners of war so that they perceived only data which was made available to them, anti-American and pro-communist. The same strategy was employed in the famous case of Cardinal Mindzenty in Budapest during the 1950s. Through hypnotic "brain-washing" he was induced to renounce his normal allegiances and accuse himself at a public trial staged by the communists. Hypnotic pressures can thus be used for malevolent as well as benevolent purposes.

Alteration of Perceptions

Since behaviors can be carried out under simple directions without hypnosis, or might be a consequence of the subject's need to please the hypnotist (role playing), the suggested disturbances to perception which are surprising (and sometimes alarming) to the subject are most convincing of the potency of hypnosis.

The most useful kinds of suggestions which influence perception are those directed against pain. It is quite amazing to the lay observer to hear a hypnotist say to his subject, "When I count up to five you will be wide awake, alert, and you will no longer have the headache which has been troubling you." The subject emerges smiling and reports that, "It doesn't hurt now." Has his pain really stopped, or is he merely saying this to please the hypnotist?

Fig. 3:2. Hand Anesthesia

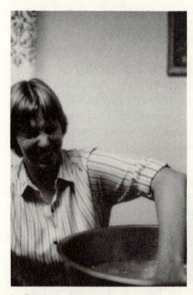 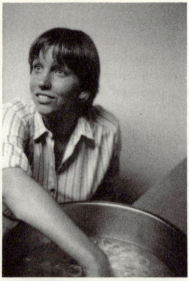

1. Prior to hypnosis left hand hurts in ice water.

2. Right hand, rendered pain-free posthypnotically, does not hurt in ice water.

The Hilgards (1975) have performed a number of studies which show quite conclusively that at the overt or conscious level the subject is indeed not experiencing pain. However, at a covert or unconscious level the pain is apparently being recorded. The football player who completes a game suffering from an undiscovered fractured clavicle demonstrates the same phenomenon. Even though a pain is initiated organically in some part of the body, the subject must "receive" it at a higher level brain function before he "suffers." If it is dissociated from perceptual centers he does not sense the pain. Such an ability to block off pain stimuli, as can be done under hypnosis, may be of great help to a suffering patient.

Furthermore, anesthesia or analgesia hypnotically induced in one part of the body may be transferred to other parts by the procedure of rubbing these other parts (or placing them in contact) with the anesthetized area.

The fact that such a manipulation of pain perception is possible under hypnosis does not mean that it can be achieved by all subjects. Differences in hypnotizability, the depth of trance which a subject can reach, the skill of the hypnotist and many other factors will determine just how much pain relief a given subject receives. There is tremendous variability.

Hallucinations can be induced in a good hypnotic subject. Thus he can be told that he will hear voices calling his name.

Fig. 3:3. Olfactory Hallucination

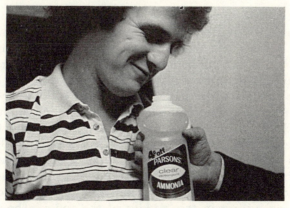

The subject has been hypnotized and told that he will smell some beautiful perfume. He is now enjoying "the perfume."

Fig. 3:4. Visual Hallucination

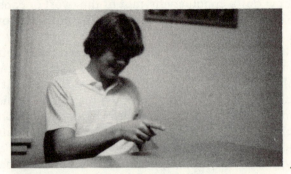

The subject has been hypnotized and given the posthypnotic suggestion that he will see a large, white rabbit. He opens his eyes, is amused, and points to "the rabbit."

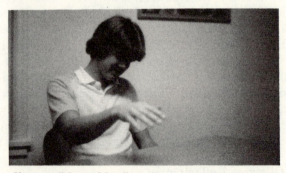

He pets "the rabbit."

Contrary-wise, total deafness can be suggested so that he does not flinch at a loud noise (Erickson, 1938). However, other studies (Kline, Guze and Haggarty, 1954) have shown that this deafness, while similar to that found in hysteria, cannot be equated with organic hearing impairment (See also Holombo, 1978; Kramer & Tucker, 1967; Malmo, Boag & Raginsky, 1954). Furthermore, demand characteristics placed on stimulators induced them to approximate the same behavior even though they were not hypnotized (Scheibe, Gray & Keim, 1968).

Even more dramatic are suggestions aimed at inducing visual hallucinations, either negative, "You will be unable to see anybody in this room," or positive, "You will see a large white dog sitting in the middle of the room." The deeply hypnotized subject responds so realistically that it is quite amazing to watch. He often demonstrates the hypnotic am-

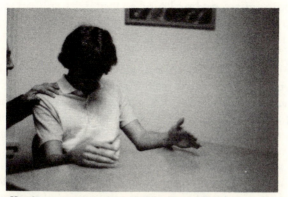

He demonstrates how long the rabbit is.

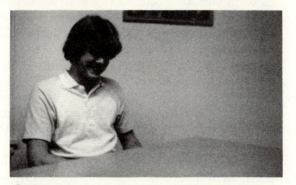

And is quite amused, after the hypnotist has removed "the rabbit" by touching his shoulder, to find that it has disappeared.

nesia which is commonly encountered in that upon emerging from the hypnotic state he disclaims any awareness of his hallucination. In fact, he may react with unbelieving dismay at being told about his behavior. It is also true that some subjects on coming out of hypnosis will report that, "There was an idea of a white dog in my mind, like a dream. I could see it even though I knew it wasn't really there."

A common demonstration of suggestion distortions in one olfactory sense is to tell a hypnotized subject that he will smell a most beautiful perfume. A bottle of ammonia is then held under his nose. If the trance state is deep he will smile and describe this "beautiful perfume." Later if told that he will smell some ammonia, and a bottle of water is placed under his nose, his reactions may involve grimacing and violent withdrawal just as if the liquid were truly ammonia.

The taste sense can be altered so that if the subject is told he will enjoy a "nice apple" and then given a piece of lemon, he will eat the lemon with much gusto and report how enjoyable was the "apple."

Every one of the senses is subject to influence under hypnosis. The degree can range from slight alterations to profound hallucinations, which are astonishing to observers and most baffling to the subjects. Little work seems to have been done investigating how long such severe distortions of reality perception can endure. It is obvious that to insist that a dog is present when one is not there, or to maintain that there is nobody in a room which is actually filled with people must require a great amount of energy in the denial of reality. There are limits in each situation related to the hypnotizability of the subject and the intensity of his relationship with the hypnotist. If the hypnotist pits his authority against reality, his closeness to his subject must be quite intense, or the subject will relinquish the hypnotist instead of the reality ("I know you told me to see a dog there, Doctor, but I don't see it").

Not only the temperature sense, but body temperatures themselves have been influenced hypnotically (Maslach, Marshall and Zimbardo, 1972; Reid and Curtsinger, 1969). If a subject is told that the furnace has been turned on very high, that it is becoming insufferable and that he feels like he is in an oven, he will fan himself, sweat, roll up his sleeves, etc. Or if the image of being in a wintry blizzard is suggested he will shiver, huddle for warmth, blow on his hands, and engage in other compatible behavior.

By suggesting to a subject that his hand was being placed in a basin of hot water, this writer raised the skin temperature of a subject's hand some four degrees as measured instrumentally. At first glance this seems miraculous, but if one considers that by suggesting to an individual a most frightening situation or showing him a gruesome film, the adrenal glands will increase their release of adrenaline into the blood stream, the phenomenon does not appear to be so unusual.

Influencing Autonomic Processes

Suggestions can be directly given for behaviors requiring activity of the striated muscles. Organ behavior usually has to be influenced indirectly by picturing to the subject emotional situations which will normally stimulate such activity

(Ikemi et al., 1963). Thus, suggestions of hunger combined with images of delectable food will result in an increase in gastric acidity (Eichhorn & Tracktir, 1955; Hall et al., 1967).

Pulse rate and blood pressure can be modified under hypnotic suggestion. Raginsky (1963b) even reported a complete cessation of heart functioning during the hypnotically-regressed reliving of a previous emotional situation. Salivation can be increased by suggesting that the subject visualize biting into a rich, juicy orange, or decreased when told that he has dry crackers in his mouth. This latter manipulation has been of value for some patients during dental treatment.

Influencing Mood and Affect

One of the most frequent symptoms for which patients consult psychiatrists and psychologists is depression. Since this is commonly based in some underlying guilt or inhibited anger, direct suggestive therapy is seldom successful in achieving a permanent resolution. However, temporary elevations of good mood may serve to provide the necessary lift and revival of hope which then can be used to therapeutic advantage. Manic individuals may also be temporarily quieted, thus increasing the likelihood of their cooperation in treatment programs. A continuous, but not severe, depression could accordingly be lifted for a day or so to permit a student to take and pass a crucial examination.

Influencing Cognition

It is quite obvious to everyone that the set, orientation, theory, or political position an individual has adopted materially influences the way he thinks. A piece of economic news will be evaluated quite differently by a conservative than by a liberal person. Not only perceptions, but also cognitions are filtered selectively through pre-established belief systems. It is accordingly not surprising that hypnotic suggestion does not easily nor quickly reverse those beliefs of which we are convinced. However, skillful suggestions implanted in a subject under hypnosis will quite often result in a modification of his selective cognitions. Specific instructions to him to concentrate and think about an interpretation given by his therapist may often result in his becoming convinced of a previous error in judgment and a willingness to modify his point of view much more quickly than would be the case if the argument were presented to him in the conscious, non-hypnotic state. Hypnosis does not provide magical change, instant reversal of previous sets, but it does offer a modality for strongly influencing thought processes. It is this ability which hypnosis presents to the psychotherapist who is trained to work with it, the opportunity to shorten the time for achieving constructive therapeutic change in many patients. Hypnoanalytic therapy, although not suitable for all patients, tends to progress more rapidly than traditional psychoanalytic therapy.

Post-Hypnotic Amnesia, Hypermnesia and Regression

A common characteristic of the deeply hypnotized individual is the appearance, spontaneously upon emerging from trance, of an apparent amnesia for that which had transpired while in the hypnotic state. It may be total or only partial. It may also be selective in that the subject sometimes reports to the hypnotist an inability to remember but does remember when questioned by others. This brings up the question as to whether the amnesia was real or only faking. At other times the suggestions given by the hypnotist not to remember may result in an amnesia for hypnotic events which otherwise the subject would normally recall. (For an extensive coverage of amnesia in general see Kihlstrom & Evans, 1979.)

Although there is considerable controversy over the theoretical rationale for this phenomenon there seems to be substantial agreement that it is not the same as simple forgetting (Hilgard, E., 1966; Orne, M., 1966). Thus, it has been viewed as a product of suggestion, direct or implicit, and also as a special form of dissociation. Kline (1966) has emphasized the psychodynamic needs of the subject as an initiating cause, while Wright (1966) has called attention to the unique interpersonal relationship between hypnotist and subject. Watkins (1966) views the selectiveness of the amnesia (specifically as related to the hypnotist versus others) as inhering in intra-personal gestalts or "ego states" which "forget" that which is cognitively inconsistent between the hypnotic and the post-hypnotic conditions. Often the subject will remember an item suggested during hypnosis but will manifest "source amnesia," that is, forget where he first learned it. Source amnesia has been suggested as a criterion to distinguish between genuinely hypnotized individuals and simulators. Its use in "forensic hypnosis" will be discussed further in the chapter on Forensic Hypnosis (vol. II).

Among the phenomena of hypnosis which are most surprising to the uninitiated is *hypermnesia* or the ability of many subjects to remember details of their earlier life which they were not normally able to recall. A deeply-hypnotized individual may be quite capable of naming every classmate in his first grade room and describe clearly all the features of the room. He may be able to recite poetry which he had learned early in school and had not repeated for many years. A 40-year-old school principal was asked if he had ever "spoken a piece" as a child in school. He stated that he had been valedictorian of his eighth grade class. No amount of conscious effort, however, could enable him to remember even the title of his address. When placed under hypnosis, "regressed" back to the eighth grade, and "introduced on the graduation platform," he delivered a fifteen-minute speech quite worthy of an intelligent fourteen-year-old. There were no hesitations in his delivery, and the nature of the speech was such that it was quite unthinkable that it could have been concocted on the spur of the moment merely to please the hypnotist. Afterwards, he confirmed that title and the content although he was still not able to reproduce it completely after he was removed from the hypnotic state. In another case a 30-year-old individual sat down at the piano and performed the number which she had played at her first recital about the age of thirteen. Prior to being hypnotized and subsequently, she was not able to execute it.

Hypermnesia is much easier to achieve than regression. In the latter a re-experiencing occurs with all the feeling and motor movements which are presumed to have accompanied the original incident. The phenomenon of hypermnesia seems to have been well substantiated experimentally (Hilgard, 1965). It is widely accepted and utilized in clinical practice. However, the accuracy of hypnotically-enhanced memories is controversial, especially in legal practice (Hilgard and Loftus, 1979; See also the chapter on *Forensic Hypnosis*, Vol. II) Early studies apparently verifying its reality have been reported (LeCron, 1968; Hibbard and Worring, 1981). Later findings, though, (Orne, 1951, 1979b) question the adequacy of

Fig. 3:5. Negative Hallucination, Posthypnotic

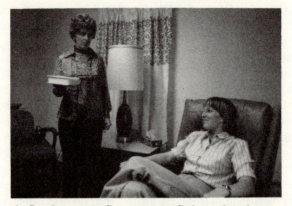

1. Posthypnotic Suggestion: Subject has been told under hypnosis Mrs. Watkins will be invisible. Hypnotist then hands a book to Mrs. W. It is perceived by the subject as floating in space.

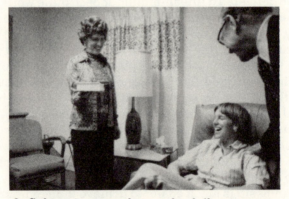

2. Subject is amused to see book floating up and down.

controls in these studies and have resulted in skepticism about this phenomenon.

The reality of hypnotic regression also remains controversial. Many hypnotherapists use it in clinical practice (Kline, 1960; Schneck, 1960; Watkins, 1949). A given subject may demonstrate a "true" or apparently real regression, another a partial regression, and another only a simulated one. Furthermore, various degrees of involvement in regression may be manifested by the same subject at different times. Experimen-

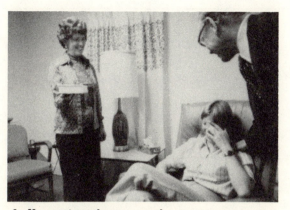

3. *Hypnotist releases posthypnotic suggestion by touching shoulder. Mrs. Watkins now becomes visible to the subject.*

talists have not always been able to achieve in the controlled laboratory studies the kind of regressed experience reported by clinicians with their patients. Accordingly, there are some workers who consider it as an artifact, an "acting-as-if."

This writer once hypnotized a nineteen-year-old college sophomore and regressed her to ages six, nine, twelve and fourteen. At each of these regressed ages she was administered standardized reading tests and her eye-movements photographed on an opthalmograph. When hypnotically regressed to six years and 10 months (June at the end of the first grade) she demonstrated a reading age of 6-10 in word recognition, 7-3 in sentence reading and 7-4 in paragraph reading as measured on the *Gates Primary Reading Tests*. When regressed to the age of 8-10, (June at the end of the third grade) she achieved reading levels of 9-6 in vocabulary, 9-10 in level of comprehension and 7-9 in speed of reading on the *Gates Reading Survey*. This averaged exactly to an age of 8-10 in general reading ability. Reading specialists judged her eye-movements as being typical for a first grader and third grader respectively (See Fig. 3:7, Photographs of Eye Movements). At the upper ages there seemed to be greater variance between her reading achievement scores and what would have been expected at those ages. A truly definitive study would involve comparing test scores and eye-movement photographs under regressed hypnosis with those which had been made years before when subjects were actually at the age to which later they had been hypnotically regressed. (Le Cron, 1968, P. 169).

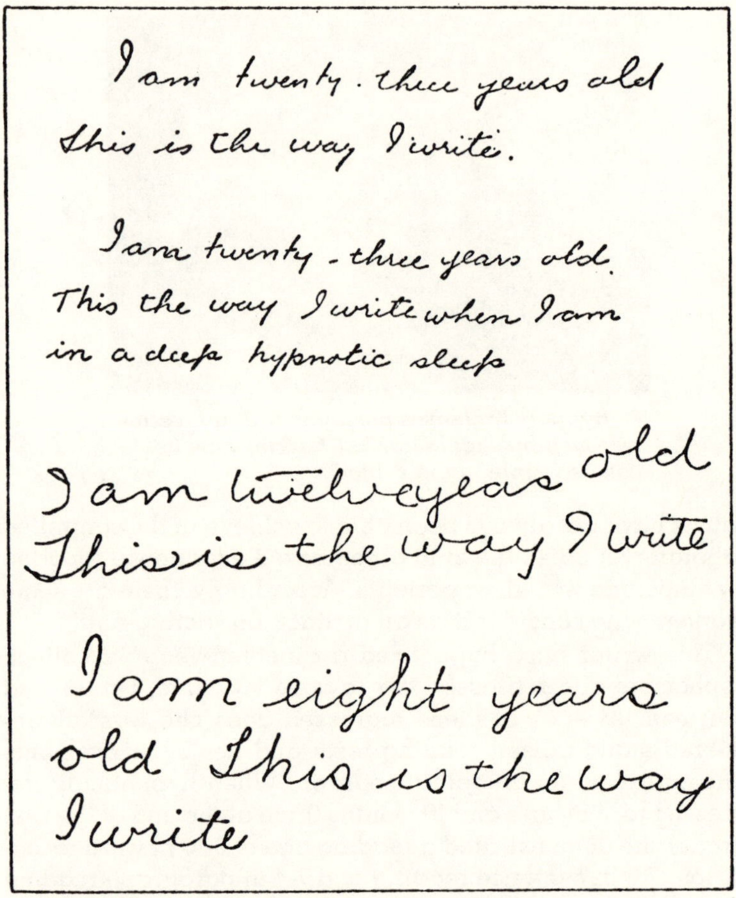

I am twenty-three years old
This is the way I write.

I am twenty-three years old.
This the way I write when I am
in a deep hypnotic sleep

I am twelve years old
This is the way I write

I am eight years
old This is the way
I write

Figure 3:6. *Samples of Handwriting of a Subject Regressed to Various Ages Under Hypnotic Trance*

Age regression is closely related to hypermnesia, and an increase in memory detail is usually found in hypnotically-regressed subjects or patients. However, the fact that the hypnotized individual is highly susceptible to suggestive influence throws doubt as to what extent the reenacting of the early experiences may have been initiated or altered by the hypnotist's influence. Both researchers and therapists must be careful to avoid suggesting happenings which did not occur. It is also possible that regressed subjects may relive fantasies rather than actual, historical occurrences. The experimental reliving by patients of such fantasized events can still be meaningful and constitute valid therapeutic material

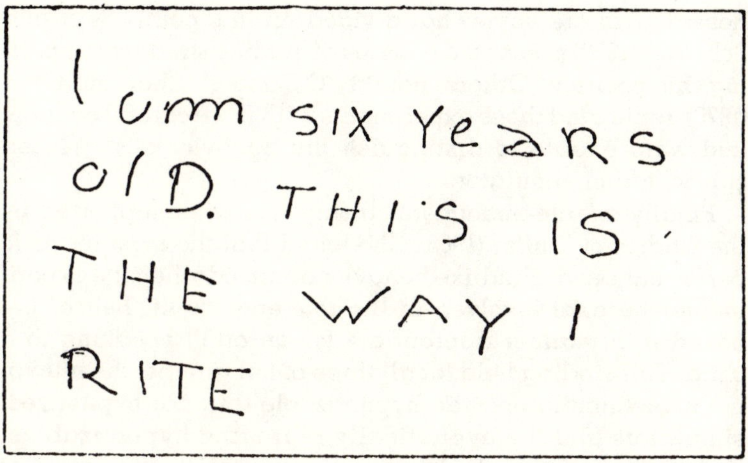

I am six years old. This is the way I rite

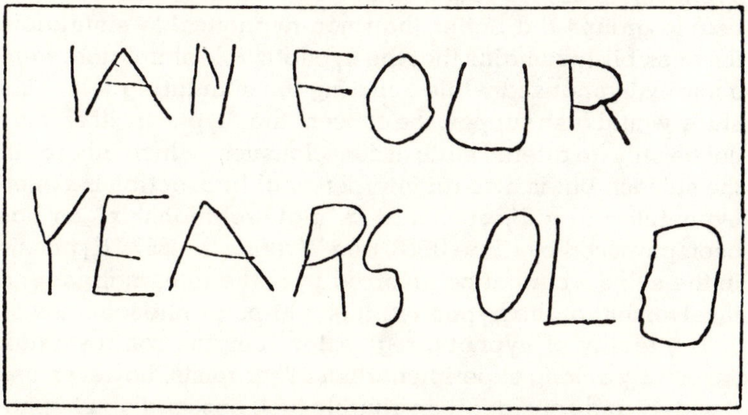

I am four years old

Figure 3:6. (Continued) *Regressed to Age Four: Subject could not spell but "drew" the single letters as words were spelled to her.*

since they generally have "personal" if not "historical" validity.

Hilgard (1977) has proposed three interpretations of hypnotic regression: one is the "ablation" theory, which holds that earlier experiences can be reactivated by hypnotically "ablating" away later ones. This rationale has been more accepted by clinicians and earlier workers (Erickson and Kubie, 1941) but is supported by rather sketchy experimental evidence.

A second conception, the "age-consistency" theory, proposes that subjects will behave in ways appropriate to their regressed age rather than simply relive actual experiences.

Researchers are somewhat divided on this point. Reiff and Scheerer (1959) presented a series of studies strongly supporting this position. Others, notably O'Connell, Shor and Orne (1970), replicated these experiments with more careful controls and were unable to distinguish the behavior of regressed subjects from simulators.

Finally a "role-enactment" theory has been supported by the studies of Troffer (1965). She found that the most realistic performances of childlike behavior occurred when the experimenter became involved in the role-enactment, hence, behaved in a manner appropriate for an adult speaking to a child. This finding held for all three of her groups, the unhypnotizable simulators, the hypnotizable (but not hypnotized) simulators and the hypnotically-regressed hypnotizables. Her study suggests doubt as to the necessity of a "state of hypnosis" to secure regression. However, since both hypnotizable groups did better than non-hypnotizable simulators the possibility remains that the hypnotizable simulators were actually hypnotized while enacting the simulating role. This study would also support the concept that hypnosis itself may not be only an altered state of consciousness which inheres in the subject, but is also an interpersonal transaction between hypnotist and subject, hence a "state-relationship" as has been proposed by Kline (1958) and Watkins, J. (1967). Hypnosis in the subject cannot be divorced from the role, manner and involvement of the hypnotist. It is a bi-polar phenomenon.

The reality of hypnotic regression remains controversial, especially among experimentalists. Therapists, however, use it widely and consider it a valuable tool, especially in hypnoanalysis. It is possible that the intensive, regressed hypnotic relationship which inheres in a therapist-patient interaction does not obtain in the more artificial laboratory setting. If so, clinicians and experimentalists may simply not be observing the same phenomena.

Dissociation

It will be recalled that hypnosis has been closely associated with the process of dissociation (Charcot, 1889, Janet, 1925; Hilgard, E., 1977). Whether or not hypnosis is itself a form of dissociation, there is little doubt that dissociation can be induced by hypnotic suggestion. Thus, subjects can be told that they are somebody else, perhaps a well-known celebrity, and they will act accordingly, often most convincingly. They can be given suggestions which they carry out and then show a complete amnesia about this behavior later. They can also be told under hypnosis that they will be unable to remember certain experiences which they have had while hypnotized, or that they will forget, for example, the pain which they had endured during an operation. Hypnosis, accordingly, is a modality in which dissociation can be established or re-solved. It is no wonder that some variation of hypnosis be-comes the therapy of choice in treating cases of amnesia and multiple personality. In the book *Sybil* (Schreiber, 1974), the analyst noted that the changes occurred much more rapidly when she was using hypnosis than during the more tradi-tional psychoanalysis.

This author and his colleague, Helen Watkins, have been systematically utilizing hypnotic dissociation in the develop-ment of a type of therapy which they have termed "Ego-State" Therapy (Watkins & Watkins, 1981). "Normal" individuals are dissociated into ego states, or "part persons," by hypnotic suggestion to evaluate intra-psychic conflicts, and "family therapy" techniques are employed to resolve them. This ap-proach will be described in more detail in Vol. II, *Hypnoanaly-tic Therapy.*

Altering Subject-Object Relationships

Closely associated with dissociation is the ability of hyp-nosis to *alter subject-object* relationships. Thus it is possible by hypnotic suggestions to create the feeling in an individual that a member of his body is no longer a part of him, hence, that it is "object" instead of "subject." This is similar to what occurs spontaneously without hypnosis in an hysterically paralyzed patient. By reversing this subject-object maneuver a part which has been experienced by the individual as "it" rather than "me" becomes once more incorporated into the self. Ideas, or entire patterns of behavior and thinking can be so altered as to subject and object. Through hypnotic manip-ulation an individual can be induced to throw himself into some "role" or to act-out and live-out a facet of his own self. He is then experiencing this role as "me." Later the entire role can be hypnotically changed over into an "object" and he will then experience it as "him," as if he were watching this behavior in another person, not himself. These complicated maneuvers are used in the sophisticated strategies of hypnoanalytic therapy.

Fig. 3:7. Photographs of Eye-Movements in an Experimental Subject

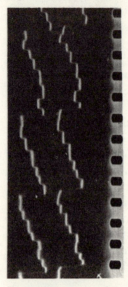

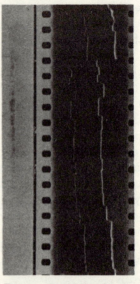

Eye-movements of a normal nineteen year old college student while reading.

Eye-movements of same subject reading when hypnotically regressed to the 3rd grade.

Eye-movements of same subject reading when hypnotically regressed to the first grade.

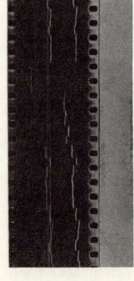

Time Distortion

A rather puzzling hypnotic phenomenon is the apparent ability of hypnotized subjects to experience greater or lesser amounts of experiential time within a given period of clock time. This should really not seem so unusual since most of us commonly experience time as passing rapidly when we are involved in interesting, meaningful activities, and to feel that time is "dragging" when our immediate environment is providing little stimulation, or we are assigned to boring tasks. The manipulation of time sense is spontaneous under such conditions.

A typical behavioral demonstration of time alteration under hypnosis involves setting a metronome at one beat to the second. The hypnotized subject is told that, "You will hear a tick each second, 60 to the minute. You will not consciously be aware of this ticking sound, but it will be recorded in you unconsciously, and you will know that a second passes between each of the ticks. Tick—tick—tick. One second—two seconds—three seconds," etc. Suggestions of this type are repeated until the ticking is built into the subject's time sense. The subject is then asked to write his name over and over again, either on paper or at a blackboard. After a norm is established for the number of times he normally writes his name within a one or two minute interval. The metronome is increased to 120 beats per minute. The subject responds by increasing his speed of writing, sometimes inscribing his name furiously. The metronome is then slowed to 30 beats to the minute. The subject now decelerates his writing speed, appears depressed, and writes his name in slow motion. His experiential and behavioral time seem to be tied to the ticking rate of the metronome. If questioned post-hypnotically he may maintain that he wrote at a constant rate.

Cooper and Erickson (1959) reported a series of studies involving the manipulation of time experience under hypnosis. They compared "world time" or "clock reading" with experiential time, which they termed "seeming duration." A typical experiment involved suggesting to hypnotized subjects that they would engage in the continuous activity of picking cotton for a "personal time" of one hour and twenty minutes. Actually the subjects were given only three seconds of actual time. They then signalled the number of cotton balls which they had picked—which generally were in the hundreds. Sutcliffe (1965) has criticized these studies in that no actual behavioral referrants were used. he argued that the subject was only conforming to suggested expectations and that we have no proof he actually experienced one hour and twenty minutes within a three second interval, which is true since one's internal, subjective experience is not perceptible to another person. Here again, the "skeptic" and the "credulous" worker can interpret the data differently.

Zimbardo, Marshall and Maslach (1971) found that hypnotic subjects given suggestions of "expanding the present" behaved differently from simulators, both in subjective reports and in behavior involving playing with clay. They were also able to distinguish between hypnotized subjects and simulators on the basis of their ability to translate the verbal suggestion of asychronicity between clock time and personal time into behavioral "reality" on a task involving the regulation of lights by pressing a telegraph key. Their carefully controlled studies added substantial experimental evidence to an acceptance of the reality of time distortion.

Therapeutic possibilities for the use of time distortion were demonstrated by Aaronson (1968) who found that when the present was "expanded" a state of euphoria ensued and that a schizophrenic-like state "followed removal of the present time sense." This entire area shows considerable promise for employment in therapeutic tactics but needs much further exploration.

The Problem of "Demand Characteristics"

A considerable controversy in the field exists over the problem of "demand characteristics." Rosenthal (1966) and Orne (1959) have shown that experimental subjects in research studies are very sensitive to the wishes of investigators. They tend to respond in ways desired by their experimenters, these ways being transmitted to them, sometimes directly and at other times indirectly or covertly. Hypnotized subjects appear to be especially susceptible to such influence. Accordingly, many "skeptics," who pride themselves on being scientifically objective, hold that hypnotic phenomena are simply acting behaviors engaged in by subjects who want to please their hypnotists. Some of them hold that a trance, or altered state of consciousness, is not a necessary prerequisite for eliciting such behaviors. Barber/1969, 1979) has been an especially strong exponent of this viewpoint. He has reported that most of the phenomena of hypnosis can be elicited by "task motivation" suggestions administered to subjects who are not hypnotized, or who, at least, have not had a traditional hypnotic "induction" procedure administered. Through the use of "simulators" Orne (1959) has demonstrated that unhypnotized subjects who are asked to act as if they were hypnotized are able to fool experienced hypnotists. However, in further studies (Orne, 1979a) subtle differences were discovered which differentiated those who had been told to act as if they were hypnotized and those who had actually been hypnotized.

Throughout our description of hypnotic phenomena we have used the word "can" rather than "will" simply to indicate that such behaviors and experiences may be initiated in hypnotic subjects. Not every subject will manifest all these phenomena. Furthermore, as Barber has shown, many of these phenomena have been produced in unhypnotized subjects by other methods of suggestion and motivation. However, Barber has not generally been able to establish that these phenomena can be as *easily* elicited in most subjects without some kind of hypnotic induction. Furthermore, critics of his studies have pointed out the fact that simply because a formal induction procedure was not used there is no assurance that the subject is unhypnotized. An hypnotic state may occur because of subtle factors in the experimental situation. Certainly demand characteristics operate both for and against the eliciting of hypnotic behaviors. The "believer" can be accused of getting his subject to behave the way he wants simply because of the subject's wish to please, not because it has anything to do with "hypnosis." On the other hand the "skeptic" may fail to initiate a hypnotic behavior of which the subject is capable because of subtle negative "demand characteristics" which suggest to the subject that the investigator wishes the subject to fail to elicit an hypnotic behavior and thus confirm the more skeptical beliefs of that particular experimenter.

Undoubtedly, this controversy will continue for a long time without any final resolution. Furthermore, if "hypnosis" is viewed as both an altered state of consciousness and an intensive inter-personal relationship (as does this writer), then how much of the behavior is due to the effect of "trance" and how much inheres in the interaction between hypnotist and subject? Fortunately, when we practice hypnotherapy we are interested in maximizing all factors which will facilitate the treatment. We will, therefore, normally employ techniques of hypnotic induction and deepening, and at the same time utilize all constructive inter-personal relationship aspects possible which exist in any good therapist-patient interaction. As therapists, we are interested in the outcome for the patient, not in the purity of each contributing factor.

Summary

In this chapter we have tried to describe the many different types of phenomena which can be elicited under hypnosis. By this is meant what is possible with some subjects or patients, not that every person is capable of exhibiting all of these. The more complex phenomena seem to require a greater hypnotic "depth." Because of the controversies in the field, research findings must be evaluated with the recognition that enthusiastic hypnotists often overevaluate their accomplishments[*] and overly-critical experimenters may simply have failed to elicit the phenomena. However, even the most critical and rigorous workers generally agree that, regardless of what hypnosis is, unusual alterations in behavior, perception, affect, and cognition can be achieved by means of it.

---

[*]For a review and critique of various studies on hypnotic phenomena from a "skeptical" viewpoint, see Sutcliffe, J. P. (1961, 1965).

Outline of Chapter 3.
HypnoticPhenomena

1. Motor Behavior
   Compulsions
   Inhibitions
2. Influencing Attitudes
3. Alteration of Perceptions
   Pain
   Hallucinations
   Deafness
   Temperature Sense
4. Influencing Autonomic Processes
5. Influencing Mood and Affect
6. Influencing Cognition
7. Post-hypnotic Amnesia, Hypermnesia and Regression
8. Dissociation
9. Altering Subject-Object Relationships
10. Time Distortion
11. The Problem of "Demand Characteristics"

Chapter 4

Hypnotic Susceptibility

.

If a patient walked into your office and requested hypnotherapy, how would you know whether or not he[1] was
hypnotizable? Would it be necessary for you to spend a long
and frustrating session with him only to conclude that he was
highly resistant to hypnosis?

Susceptibility to hypnosis has intrigued workers in the
field for many years, and frequent attempts have been made
to correlate it with some measurable psychological trait. If
only we could know in advance just who was hypnotizable
and who not, a great deal of wasted effort, humiliation, and
impaired status would be saved the practitioner. Many patients who had read about the "miracles" of hypnosis and
sought treatment with it could be spared subsequent disap-
pointment and disillusionment with the therapist.

Hypnosis as a Matter of Degree

Furthermore, the problem is not simply one of "either-or."
Hypnosis is a matter of degree. Some individuals apparently
can enter a deep state and exhibit very bizarre behavior such
as regression, time distortion, and hallucinations. Others
seem to reach a plateau where they will carry through simple
suggestions but not unusual ones involving severe distortions

Throughout the following chapters on "Hypnotic Suscepitibility," "Induction" and "Deepening" the masculine gender "he" or "him" is used to indicate
the subject or hypnotist, male or female, simply to avoid the repetitiousness
of frequent "him or her" or he/she." The author is completely in sympathy with
equal rights in all areas between men and women.

of perception. Still others relax but only slightly and with minimal involvement. We are, therefore, concerned not only with the question as to whether a given subject or patient is hypnotizable, but to what degree of "depth" he can be expected to respond. Some hypnotherapeutic techniques require a rather deep state; others can be effectively utilized with the patient only slightly hypnotized.

The Quantification of Hypnotic "Depth" and Susceptibility

A number of attempts to quantify hypnotic depth, or at least to indicate the characteristics of various levels of hypnotic involvement, have been published over the years. Charcot (1882) considered that there were three types of hypnosis: catalepsy, lethargy and somnambulism. Bernheim (1964) and Liebeault (1892) classified various levels of trance ranging from drowsiness through catalepsy (e.g. rigidity in the limbs achieved through suggestion) up to suggested hallucinations experienced post-hypnotically.

In 1931 Davis and Husband published a scale which suggested five levels of hypnosis, assigned a depth score, and indicated the percentage of subjects they found capable of reaching each level.

Davis and Husband Hypnotic Susceptibility Scale

Depth	Score	Objective symptoms	Number of cases	Percent of cases
Insusceptible	0		5	9
Hypnoidal	2	Relaxation	16	29
	3	Fluttering of lids		
	4	Closing of eyes		
	5	Complete physical relaxation		
Light trance	6	Catalepsy of eyes	10	18
	7	Limb catalepsies		
	10	Rigid catalepsy		
	11	Anesthesia (glove)		
Medium trance	13	Partial amnesia	8	15
	15	Posthypnotic - anesthesia		
	17	Personality changes		
	18	Simple posthypnotic suggestions		

	20	Kinesthetic delusions; complete amnesia		
Somnambulistic trance	21	Ability to open eyes without affecting trance	16	29
	23	Bizarre posthypnotic suggestions accepted		
	25	Complete somnambulism		
	26	Positive visual hallucinations, posthypnotic		
	27	Positive auditory hallucinations, posthypnotic		
	28	Systematized posthypnotic amnesias		
	29	Negative auditory hallucinations		
	30	Negative visual hallucinations; hyperesthesias		3
Total			55	100

Watkins (1949) published an expanded version of this scale which added the following items: 8 Hypermnesia slight, 16 Hypermnesia marked, 19 Regression and 32 Negative visual hallucinations, posthypnotic.

In recent years a number of standardized scales to measure hypnotic susceptibility have been developed. Perhaps the one which has been most extensively used, and which has served as a yardstick for other ones, is the *Stanford Hypnotic Susceptibility Scale* (SHSS) Forms A & B. It was developed by Weitzenhoffer and Hilgard (1959) and standardized originally on a sample of 124 Stanford University students. The scale consists of 12 items with exact verbalizations to be applied for each, and with objective criteria for scoring. The various items were selected from hypnotic suggestibility tests which have been published and used by various earlier workers and which showed the highest criteria of differentiating between good and poor hypnotic subjects.

Briefly the items on Form A are as follows:

1. *Postural sway.* The subject is requested to stand with his back to the hypnotist and to think of swaying backward. The operator assures him he will not be permitted to fall. Continued suggestions of "falling backward, falling backward" are administered for a certain number of repetitions. The item is scored plus if the subject falls backward within a certain period of time.

2. *Eye closure.* The subject is asked to fixate his eyes on a small bright object some six or more feet away and placed above, so that he must gaze upward. A standardized set of suggestions are given aimed at inducing a feeling of drowsiness and closure of the eyes. The item is scored plus if the eyes closed within the alotted time. If the subject's eyes have not closed within the prescribed period he is simply instructed to close them, and they remain closed during the remainder of the test.

3. *Hand lowering.* The subject is asked to extend his left arm straight out with the palm down. Suggestions are given to induce the feeling that it is getting heavier as if a weight were pulling on it. The item is scored plus if the arm drops at least six inches within the prescribed time.

4. *Immobilization of the right arm.* In this item suggestions are given that the arm has become heavy and that the subject will not be able to lift it. It ends with a challenge to him to "try." It is scored plus if the arm rises less than one inch within the alotted period.

5. *Finger lock.* The subject is instructed to interlock his fingers and press his hands tightly together. Suggestions are given aimed at creating difficulty in pulling them apart. A challenge is again made, and the item is scored plus if the fingers are incompletely separated within ten seconds.

6. *Arm rigidity.* In this item suggestions are given that the extended arm will become so stiff that it is not possible to bend it. After the suggestions are given the item is scored plus if the subject cannot bend his arm within ten seconds when requested to "try" to do so.

7. *Moving hands (together)*. The hands of the subject are placed about a foot apart facing one another. He is told to visualize a force pulling them together. If the hands are not over six inches apart after the prescribed period of suggestions, the item is scored plus.

8. *Verbal inhibition (name)*. It is suggested to the subject that he will have difficulty in saying his name. If he is unable to do so within ten seconds this item is then scored plus.

9. *Hallucination (fly)*. The subject's attention is called to an imaginary fly "buzzing about" him. The item is scored plus if there is any grimacing or other movement indicating his awareness of "the fly" or attempt to shoo it away.

10. *Eye catalepsy*. Suggestions are given that the eyes will be glued tightly shut and that the subject cannot open them. If he is unable to do so within ten seconds after instructed to try, this item is scored plus.

11. & 12. *Post-hypnotic suggestion (changing chairs); amnesia*. It is assumed by now that the good subject will be rather substantially involved in the hypnotic condition. Accordingly, suggestions are administered that the subject will become aroused while the investigator counts backward from twenty to one, and that shortly afterward when the hypnotist taps a pencil he will move into another chair in front of him. However, he is not to remember that he was told to do so. Item 11 is scored plus if there is some movement on the part of the subject to change chairs following the pencil tap.

The subject is now interrogated to determine how much of this last test he can remember. If he is unable to recall more than three items he is scored plus on Item 12.

The test is administered only after a rather thorough introduction given by the operator about the nature of hypnosis. This is designed both to allay fears and to prepare a favorable set. The above descriptions of the items are incomplete but are presented here to show the nature of tests of hypnotic susceptibility. For a complete picture of this instrument consult the Scale itself and the accompanying book which describes in detail the studies which culminated in the test's standardization (Hilgard, E., 1965). This work includes a great deal of the statistical data, norms, reliabilities, etc.

In 1962 Weitzenhoffer and Hilgard published a Form C of the *Stanford Hypnotic Susceptibility Scale* designed to fit the needs of the practicing clinician better. It contains more cognitive items relating to age regression, dream material and hallucinations, and less motor items than Form A. However, because its length was still discouraging to the clinician, Morgan and J.F. Hilgard published short forms (1978/1979) designed specifically for the clinical evaluation of adults and children. Hilgard & Hilgard (1979) proposed a set of criteria which should be ideally met by an adequate hypnotic clinical scale. They concluded that the Morgan-J.R. Hilgard Scales substantially met these criteria, and, since they correlated well with the original long forms (SHSS-A and SHSS-C), could be recommended for clinical practice.

The *Stanford Hypnotic Susceptibility Scale* is today the most thoroughly researched instrument for measuring potential response to hypnosis. Every serious investigator in the field should become familiar with it, and it is recommended that every student in the area of hypnosis, scientist or clinician, should at least have administered it one or more times. This scale occupies a position in the evaluation of hypnotic susceptibility comparable to that of the Stanford-Binet and the Wechler scales in the measurement of mental ability.

In 1967 the same authors published the *Stanford Profile Scales*, designed to discriminate in the higher levels of hypnotic susceptibility.

Because of the need to test the hypnotic susceptibility of groups of subjects, the *Harvard Group Scale of Hypnotic Susceptibility* (HGSHS) has been standardized and published by Ronald Shor and Emily Orne (1962). The items are similar but are modified so that they can be simultaneously administered to a group of subjects. Items are self-scored by the subjects.

London (1963) has standardized a *Children's Hypnotic Susceptibility Scale*. Again the Stanford items are used but are modified to accommodate the understanding and behavior of children. These instruments have made possible many research studies where it is desirable to screen for hypnotizable or nonhypnotizable subjects or to control this factor.

Informal Tests of Hypnotic Susceptibility

For the student who is new to the field of hypnosis, more informal tests may be desirable in screening suitable subjects for hypnosis practice and later in evaluating patients for possible hypnotherapy. Such tests not only serve to screen and evaluate, but their very administration can establish a set and make easier later induction of the hypnotic state.

Since it is the nature of hypnosis that things "happen" to the subject, apparently without his conscious control or "willing" it, the experience of an involuntary action can be administered by a simple situation known as the Kohnstamn phenomenon. It will give any subjects, including those who later prove to be resistant to hypnosis, the feel of having something "happen" to them which they had not consciously initiated. Students are advised to experience this phenomenon themselves if only to acquaint themselves more intimately with the kind of feeling the hypnotized subject has when he is responding to suggestions while under the trance state.

The Kohnstamn Phenomenon

The subject is instructed as follows:

"Stand near the wall, facing parallel to it, with your feet about a foot from the wall. Now, with your arm hanging at your side, push the back of your hand against the wall. That's it. Now harder. Do not lean your body toward the wall. Just push

Fig. 4:1. The Kohnstamm Phenomenon

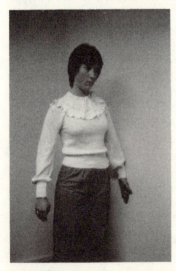 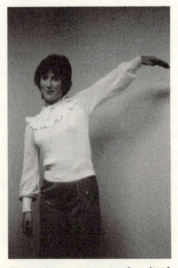

Initial Position. The subject is amused to find her arm rising involuntarily.

the back of your hand against the wall as if you were trying to push it down. Harder. Harder. Now I want you to continue this for an entire minute—and a minute will seem like a long time while you are doing this." (Operator may announce 15 second intervals but keeps on urging the subject to push harder with all his might and main against the wall with the back of his hand.) At the end of one minute the instruction is given, "Now turn and face me." In most subjects (and to their great astonishment) the arm will slowly rise as if automatically. Of course, the phenomenon is not hypnotic suggestion but is based on muscle fatigue. By tiring one set of muscles in the arm, the opposing muscles simply contract and lift the arm. While this is not hypnosis, the experience is akin to that felt by subjects who are responding to suggestions in the trance state. Something is happening to them; they are not doing it.[2]

The Chevreul Pendulum

This is an indicator of suggestibility which is highly correlated with hypnotizability. Although not particularly convenient for use with clinical patients, it makes a good demonstration of the effect of suggestion to a class and can also be used to screen research subjects.

A small object, such as a crystal ball, a plumb bob, or simply a bolt attached to the end of a string can be used. The subject is seated at a desk or table and is given instructions as follows:

"Put your elbow on the desk and hold this string between your fingers so that the weight at the end (bob, crystal, bolt) just misses touching the desk." (This means that the distance from the fingers to the desk will be about one foot.) The suggestions are now continued:

"Stare at the weight and concentrate all your attention on it. As you look at it you will notice that it has a tendency to move." (Movements, even though slight, are almost certain to appear. The operator watches carefully and when they begin to stabilize in one direction he capitalizes on this movement.)

---

[2]A qualification to this statement should be made. While most of the lifting tendency is based upon physiological fatigue in one set of arm muscles, there is also a non-verbal suggestive influence as the subject "feels" the lifting effect. Accordingly, there is probably some positive correlation, although small, with hypnotizability.

Fig. 4:2. Chevreul Pendulum

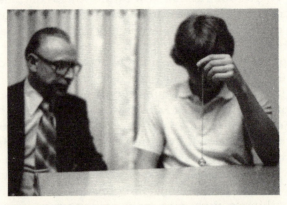

Initial position. Crystal ball suspended from chain just above table top.

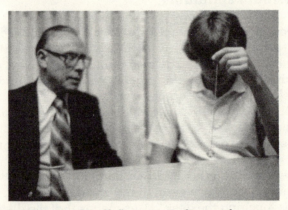

Bell "automatically" swings in line with suggestions of hypnotist.

"You notice that the weight is beginning to swing back and forth, back and forth, back and forth," (or whatever direction it is swinging).

(Permit this movement to continue and enhance it until it is clear to the subject and to all observers that this movement is indeed taking place. Then suggest a change in the direction of the movement.)

"Now, as you watch this weight you will notice that the direction of movement begins to change. There is now a tendency for it to move from side to side."

After the side-to-side movement has been established, one

may notice that the movement becomes a bit circular. The operator immediately takes advantage to suggest that, "The weight is now beginning to move round and round in a clockwise (or counter-clockwise) direction. Round and round it goes swinging in an ever increasing arc."

Finally, a change in the direction of rotation is suggested by indicating that, "It is now slowing down and beginning to turn in an opposite direction. Notice the tendency for it to move counter-clockwise (clockwise), round and round in an ever increasing arc.—That's fine. Now I'd like to ask you: Were you making that weight perform those movements—or were they just happening? Were you aware of any movements on your own part that caused it to swing back and forth, then side-to-side then clockwise and finally counter-clockwise?"

In almost all cases the subject will state that he was not aware of any voluntary action of his part to cause these movements to occur. Many will show considerable surprise, thus helping to condition them toward future positive responses. A few will even mention that they tried consciously to resist the movements, but that they occurred in spite of their efforts.

This test makes a good demonstration of the effect of suggestion to be presented before a class of initiates in the field of hypnosis. It is also tied in with movements on the Ouija board, and is probably closely related to the suggestive aspects of water-witching.

Many years ago when this writer was a high school science teacher, he lived in a community in which all the wells had been located by "witching." One of his students was the son of a local "witch" and volunteered to give a demonstration, since he "had been taught how to witch" by his father.

Louie came to class the next day bringing his forked peach branch, and all of us proceeded to the fields which surrounded this rural high school. As he came to one spot the branch turned downward. A peg was driven into the ground at that point, and Louie approached it from another angle, and then another. In each case, it turned down near the peg. Louie, with an air of considerable confidence, then stated that, "There's where the water is located."

No attempt was made to contradict him, but instead he was asked, "Louie, are you sure that you aren't doing this yourself with little muscle movements?" Louie assured us that it was the stick which had turned down by itself, that he had held it loosely, and had no part in its movement.

He was next asked, "If it is the stick that is doing the movement, you will not object to performing the experiment again blindfolded." Louie, in some surprise but still quite confident, indicated he was quite willing to submit to this control.

After he was blindfolded he was led all over the field, including several times by the point where the stake was driven. Never once did the stick turn down twice at the same location. Finally, Louie was led over an area where we knew that the water pipes entered the school building. Again the stick failed to turn down. When confronted with this evidence, Louie regretfully threw his peach branch away with the remark that, "It doesn't work, but I sure never could convince Dad of that."

At the end of the term the instructor asked a final (noncredit) question on the exam: "What do you think of water-witching?" Twenty-nine students indicated they no longer believed in it, but one wrote, "Louie just ain't a good witch."

The Arm-Drop Test

A simple and easily administered indicator of hypnotic susceptibility is needed for the clinical situation, in which the therapist wishes a rapid determination of his patient's probable response to hypnotherapeutic procedures.

The Arm-Drop test is the single, most valuable test in that it can be applied in a very short period of time, and has the advantage that the therapist need not even mention the word "hypnosis" to the patient. It is not a part of the Stanford Scale; however, based on the clinical experience of this writer, it is one of the most sensitive of the screening techniques. A positive response on this almost invariably means that the subject or patient is capable of responding favorably to the induction of a hypnotic state, at least to a significant degree. Furthermore, with a simple extension it can be turned into an actual induction procedure.

Perhaps one of its greatest advantages is that it permits the therapist, especially one who is relatively inexperienced and not secure in his ability to induce hypnosis, to determine the hypnotizability of his patient before committing himself to using hypnosis. When the hypnotist is uncertain of his chances for success in inducing hypnosis with a certain patient, this uncertainty is often initiated in the patient who

Fig. 4:3. Arm Drop Suggestibility Test

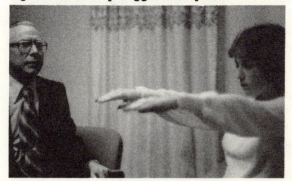

Initial position.

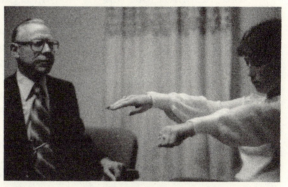

Holding "bucket." Beginning to feel "weight."

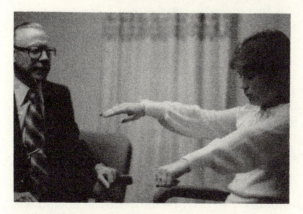

"Bucket" pulling arm down.

becomes resistant to the induction procedure, not because he is unhypnotizable, but because a lack of confidence in the hypnotist has been transmitted to him. When the test is favorable, the hypnotist, knowing that his subject is probably hypnotizable, begins his induction procedures with an air of confidence which then transmits itself to the subject and makes him more responsive. Accordingly, I recommend that the student of hypnosis learn this procedure and practice it on his first patients.

The subject is simply told that, "I would like to test your reflexes. Would you please sit up straight in your chair and extend both arms straight out in front of you, palms down. Don't let them touch each other. That's right. Now close your eyes and imagine that I am giving you a galvanized pail to hold in your right (or left) hand. Please close your fingers around the handle of the bucket." (Note that the imagined "bucket" is now treated by the hypnotist as a reality by asking the subject to close his fingers around the handle.)

"Now I want you to visualize what it would be like if I were standing in front of you pouring water into your bucket from a pail of water which I am holding. Your bucket can hold over two gallons, and I am now pouring one quart into the bucket. Observe the stream of water flowing into your bucket. Now, I'm pouring more and more water into your pail. There are now two quarts in it, and you can feel the increase in weight. Three quarts. More and more water going into it.———Four quarts———now five quarts, and your bucket is half filled. You are becoming increasingly aware that more and more water is being poured into your bucket.

"I shall continue to pour water into it. Six quarts——— seven quarts———eight quarts, and the bucket is beginning to fill up. Notice how heavy two gallons of water are?——— Now nine quarts and the bucket is almost full, almost full. There now. I shall pour the tenth quart into it, and the bucket is full right up to the brim. Two and a half gallons of water and the bucket is completely full.———."

Allow another ten to twenty seconds and carefully observe the movements in the subject's arm. Hypnotizability is indicated by the following movements:

1. The hand *gradually* lowers while the therapist is suggesting that more quarts are being poured into "the bucket." The degree of lowering of the arm is significantly related to the hypnotizability. That is, if the hand goes all the way down

until it rests on the lap, or on a desk or table in front of the subject, then it is quite probable that the patient is highly hypnotizable and can either enter hypnosis rapidly or is capable of entering a deep trance as will make possible the initiating of such phenomena as regression and hallucinations.

2. If during the period of the test the hand lowers somewhat but does not go all the way down the inference is that the patient is responsive to hypnotic suggestions, but may either be resistant, a slow responder, or capable of reaching only a light or medium trance, not a deep one. However, in our experience the individual who responds in this way initially may become a very good hypnotic subject after his initial doubts and anxieties have been resolved, and he has established a better relationship with his therapist. The slowness of response may only be his way of saying, "I don't completely trust you yet, and this situation is disturbing to me."

The extent of his response is related to his hypnotizability at this time. Thus, if his right hand is some six or more inches below the left at the end of the test, then he shows a very substantial degree of hypnotizability even if it has not come all the way down. If it has slowly moved downward for at least three inches he is manifesting a positive response to the suggestions even if it is not strong. Such a patient indicates to his therapist that he is at least able to become hypnotically involved to some degree and with proper handling may be able to achieve an even more significant response level. Since it is not necessary that a deep degree of hypnosis be induced in a client for the effective utilization of many hypnotherapeutic techniques, this individual should certainly not be rejected as a possible candidate for hypnotherapy.

Occasionally a subject's right hand will not drop downward at all, but he will manifest a considerable struggle to keep it level with the left one. There may even be slight tendencies for it to drop followed by slight corrective movements designed to pull it up level with the left hand again. This might be interpreted that the subject is responsive to hypnotic suggestion, but doesn't think that he should be, that he is fearful of "losing control," or that he perceives the situation as one in which he is in competition with the hypnotist, one in which he must demonstrate that he has strong "will power" and cannot be pushed around.

When this occurs the therapist should not let it deteriorate into a struggle for "control." The subject might be approached as follows: "I noticed that you seemed to have some difficulty. It was as if your arm felt like dropping down as the bucket became heavier, but you did not want it to do so and wished to show that you were capable of resisting this tendency. You obviously are quite capable of resisting it, but it might be interesting to see what would happen if you did not fight such tendencies; simply let happen whatever occurs naturally."

3. Perhaps the response which is most related to unhypnotizability is no response whatsoever. The hand does not go down; it does not rise, and its position parallel to the other hand seems to be maintained without any effort. In this case it is often useful to ask the subject about his response and his feelings concerning it with such questions as:

"Could you visualize the bucket when I described it to you?"

"Could you experience the water being poured into it?"

Often the non-response subject will say, "I was not able to imagine the bucket." or "I could see the bucket, but I didn't feel as if any water was being poured into it."

Further questioning might be continued as follows:

"Did the bucket feel heavy?"

"Did you notice any difference in the feel of your two arms?"

"Do your arms feel tired now?" (This often elicits a positive response even in the resistant subject. Holding one's arms out for a minute or more naturally creates physiological fatigue. The normal person admits it. A complete denial of feeling any fatigue suggests an individual who is very fearful of hypnosis and determined to show that he can be "the Rock of Gibraltar."

If the subject admits that his arms feel tired he may then be asked:

"Which arm feels the most tired?"

The response that they both feel equally tired usually indicates considerable resistance to hypnosis, either because the individual does not possess the "trait," or because of fear and a strong determination not to be "controlled." When there has been no overt movement of the hand downward, but the subject states that the right arm feels more tired than the left one, he is showing that at least to some extent he is responding to the suggestions, that they are influencing him at a perceptual level if not at the motor level. With such patients the possibility of using hypnotherapy is still open.

In case the matter of employing hypnotic treatment techniques has already been explored, and the patient is not completely ignorant of this possibility, then the two of them might discuss the matter. If the patient says,

"Doctor, does this mean that I am not hypnotizable?"

A good response would be, "Not necessarily. Some people respond easily to hypnosis. Others have more difficulty and are slower to react. This simply means that it might take a little longer to teach you how to respond. If hypnosis seems to be a possible treatment for your problem we can work on it more intensively. It may well be that you are a bit nervous, tense, or that you have some fears about hypnosis. Tell me how you feel about the matter."

This may lead into an airing of the patient's fears, doubts, and preconceptions. However, let us leave a fuller discussion of how to handle them in later chapters on induction procedures.

There are a number of other suggestibility tests which can be administered, and these will be described shortly. Nonetheless, the Arm Drop appears to be the single most sensitive one, and is the technique of choice if only one can be given.

The Postural Sway Test

This test is also positively correlated with hypnotizability and has the advantage that in the case of a strong favorable response it can be turned into an actual induction technique. The subject is asked to stand up straight with his heels and toes together. This distributes his weight over the smallest area and maximizes minor signs of unsteadiness. A chair is placed about six inches behind him. Preferably this should be a large, cushioned easy-chair with arms and a high back. He may then be given the following instructions:

"Close your eyes and take several deep breaths. That's good. Now I want you to imagine that your feet are hinged to the floor and that your body extends upward. You may feel a bit unsteady, but don't worry. If you should fall I will catch you." (If you think that the subject is highly hypnotizable a little more suggestive leverage can be gained by saying, "When you fall I will catch you," instead of if you fall. In the first case the suggestion of a possible fall is implanted; in the second, a conviction that this will happen is inculcated.) Since the therapist's conviction that a suggestion he gives will be carried out is an important part of its success, the choice of wording may depend upon his own certainty regarding the particular subject with whom he is working. If the second suggestion is given, but by an insecure and doubting hypnotist, it may well fail.

In all hypnotic work, whether it be suggestibility tests, induction techniques, deepening procedures, or therapeutic suggestions, the manner, confidence, and precise communications of the hypnotist are paramount and determine why one operator is successful with a given subject while another is not.

The hypnotist should now position himself at the side of the subject so that he can sight along the subject's nose or the back of his head so as to detect slight movements in relation to the opposite wall. Successful hypnotizing requires that we align our suggestions as closely as possible to reality during the initial stages of a susceptibility test or an induction. Accordingly, it is wise to wait for a brief period while observing any signs of swaying movement by the subject. This can be enhanced by saying, "The longer you stand there, the more unsteady you may feel yourself becoming. Don't worry. Just remember that I will not allow you to fall and hurt yourself. I am here to catch you. This unsteadiness will increase, and you may develop a swaying feeling."

Wait a little while longer while observing carefully signs of movement as determined by a sighting on the nose or back of head of the subject projected onto the further wall. Time and the implementation of the above suggestions will tend to increase the feeling of unsteadiness. By having the feet placed together, heel to heel and toe to toe, slight swaying motions and adjustments of posture are almost certain to appear in any individual. The hypnotist then builds upon these as follows:

"You notice that you are now drifting————forward." After the word "drifting" the hypnotist pauses and observes the movement. As soon as it has been ascertained as forward he then labels it, "forward." If it were backward he would describe it accordingly. The point is that some swaying has almost certainly been initiated. The hypnotist then calls it correctly immediately after he has determined its direction. This may continue for some time as the hypnotist reports the natural movements of the subject.

"You are now drifting————backward. Now you are floating————forward. Forward————backward," etc. Floating and/or drifting are good words to use at first. Later as the movement becomes more pronounced, and more obviously in response to the hypnotist's suggestions, the wording can be changed to "swaying."

It will be noticed in most cases that the subject's back and forth movement soon tends, like the swinging of a pendulum, to become rhythmical and evenly spaced. He sways through a specific arc which may be three or four inches forward, then two or three inches backward. During this time the hypnotist has been following these movements and reporting them in a firm and confident voice. His credibility rises in the mind of the subject. It is almost as if the patient were thinking, "The doctor says I am swaying forward, and I am. Then when I am swaying backward he calls that correctly also. He knows what he is saying, and he is right. I can believe him."

At this point the hypnotist moves from following the movement to leading them. If he has been following and correctly reporting the area of movement he might be saying, "Swaying forward, swaying forward, swaying forward——now swaying backward, swaying backward," etc. He can now attempt to interrupt this cycle in mid-point. When the subject is swaying forward, and has reached the center of his arc, hence before he has completed all of his normal forward swaying motion, the hypnotist in the same confident voice reverses his suggestion to, "Swaying backward, swaying backward," etc.

If the subject has by this time become hypnotically involved he will interrupt his normal pattern of forward movement in mid-stream and reverse the sway. After this the hypnotist can lead the swaying movements rather than simply follow them. The subject is then following suggestions at a hypnotic level. At this point, the hypnotist can conclude that the test has been positive and that the subject will be hypnotizable at least to some degree. (See photographs, Chap. 6, pp. 134-135)

What we have done so far constitutes another "test" of hypnotic susceptibility. In a later chapter on Advanced Induction Techniques we will return to this point and describe how this Postural Sway Procedure can be continued on into an induction of an actual hypnotic state, sometimes a very deep one, in which various hypnotherapeutic techniques become possible. A slightly different form of this procedure is found in the *Stanford Hypnotic Susceptibility Scale*, in which the hypnotist stands behind the subject and suggestions are given to induce him to fall backwards where he is then caught by the operator.

The Hand-Clasp Test

This is a somewhat more aggressive procedure which culminates in an actual challenge to the subject. It is useful as part of a group screening procedure but may have less value in the clinical situation where the object is to work therapeutically with a patient. It relies to some extent on suggested intimidation of the subject, hence pulling on his transference relationships to a dominating parent figure, if that had characterized his childhood. It is like what Ferenczi (1926) called "father hypnosis."

The subject or group of subjects are instructed as follows: "Clasp your hands tightly in front of you and stare at my clasped hands at the same time." The hypnotist demonstrates by interlacing his own fingers so that the hands grip each other very tightly. The suggestions to the subject are now being given both verbally by the commands of the hypnotist and visually as he focuses on the clasped hands of the operator.

"Now make those hands tighter and tighter. Imagine they are like fingers of steel encased in a block of concrete which is shrinking. They get tighter and tighter and tighter." The voice of the hypnotist is raised and becomes ever more strong and firm. At the same time his own fingers dig into each other so that the muscles and blood vessels stand out.

"That's it. Make them tighter, tighter, tighter. In fact, so tight that it doesn't seem as if they could come apart. It seems as if the more you try to take them apart the tighter they stick together. The more you try to take them apart the tighter they stick. They are sticking so tightly they will not come apart. They will not come apart. They are tightly stuck together. Try to pull them apart. Try to pull them apart.———You see, they are so tightly stuck together they cannot come apart. The harder you try to pull them apart the tighter they stick together," etc.

At this point a challenge has been issued, and it will be found that a substantial number of subjects will be unable to pull their hands apart. The subject or subjects are now observed as they struggle to pull their hands apart. The hypnotist is still holding his hands tightly clasped together. He may then pull his own hands apart, as if with difficulty, and say,

"Now you can pull them apart. See! They will come apart now."

Fig. 4:4. Hand Clasp Suggestibility Test

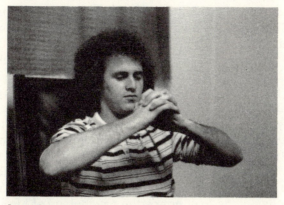

Initial position.

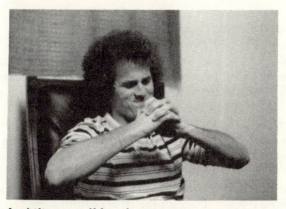

Inability to pull hands apart.

If only one subject is being tested, and he seems to be succeeding in pulling his hands apart, hence, they show signs of loosening, the hypnotist intervenes before the hands are apart with a cessation of the challenge and permission to pull them apart. The subject is then left with the recognition of how tightly they were stuck together and with doubt as to whether he would have been successful in pulling them apart if he had continued to try. The test is considered to be successful if the subject, after several seconds of struggling, is unable to separate the hands.

It will be noticed that toward the end of the test the *principle of reversed effect* was used. It was suggested that, "The harder you try to pull them apart the tighter they will stick together." Hence, trying itself becomes the stimulus cue for being unable to separate the hands. This principle can be used in many different ways as a part of induction and therapeutic procedures which will be described later.

Some subjects will resist this test by not making the grip tight to begin with. Others will respond to the challenge by pulling their fingers apart easily. The amount of hypnotic susceptibility of any subject may be inferred by the degree of difficulty he experiences in pulling the hands apart at the time of the challenge. In this test we are, of course, enlisting normal physiology on our side. By "freezing" the tightly clasped hands together we make it much more difficult physically to draw them apart. The good hypnotist uses normal muscle physiology to enhance the psychology of his suggestive procedures.

Arm Levitation

This particular procedure is especially good in screening the more susceptible subjects from a group of volunteers. It is not to be confused with the induction technique of the same name which will be described in the next chapter.

Subjects are asked to sit up straight, close their eyes, and hold out one arm. The following visualization is then given:

"I want you to imagine that a balloon filled with helium gas has just been connected to your wrist with a cord. It is large and of your favorite color. It is floating above your wrist. As you observe it you will notice that it is pulling strongly upward on your wrist. Watch it as it floats higher, higher, higher. With each passing moment the lifting sensation becomes stronger and stronger, and the balloon is floating up, up, up, higher, higher and higher."

Notice that the suggestion is not given that "your hand" is moving higher. Rather, attention is centered on observing the balloon as it floats upward. The rising of "the hand" then becomes a consequence of the balloon's upward movement and is suggested indirectly. By indicating that the balloon is "of your favorite color," the feeling of participation is encouraged. As the subject visualizes it in his favorite color he becomes more personally involved, exercises his "free will" in the choice, and what happens afterward can then occur on a more involuntary basis. Again repetition is used, a technique which is commonly a part of all induction procedures and often effective to intensify therapeutic suggestions. The above wording is continued and repeated for a minute or so until a number of the subjects show substantial lifting of the arm. Very good subjects may finally have their arms lifted almost straight up. In a large group they are easy to spot. Hence, your "volunteers" for further hypnotic study now have raised their hands.

Head-Nod Forward

Although the experienced hypnotherapist usually becomes sensitive to many slight signs of hypnotic involvement, for the beginner in the field it is desirable that susceptibility tests show some overt movement as a positive signal. Accordingly, if the eyes have become closed during one of the foregoing procedures, the following test is useful. A positive response confirms the suggestibility which the subject has demonstrated so far. And in line with the principle that the carrying out of hypnotic suggestions is itself hypnotizing, its successful accomplishment by a subject will tend to deepen whatever hypnotic state is now present. If an eye-closure was part of a group screening, but not all of the subjects have yet closed their eyes, they are now all simply instructed to do so. Then the operator proceeds as follows:

"Now that your eyes are closed you will notice a tendency for your head to nod forward as if some force were pushing on the back of it. The head will tend to move forward and the chin to drop down toward your chest. The head is becoming heavier, and heavier——and heavier."

Notice that the hypnotist said, "*the* head" not "*your* head". This has a tendency to remove the head from voluntary control so that "it" is responding. "You" are not bringing your head down. The head is removed from "subject" and designated as "object." Objects are elements outside the self over which we have no voluntary control. They are controlled by outside forces for which we have no responsibility. They just happen to us.

Inability to Push Hands Together

This test can now be conveniently administered to subjects whose eyes are closed and who may have indicated some nodding forward of the head. It is similar to one of the items in the *Stanford Hypnotic Susceptibility Scale*. The subjects may be given the following suggestions:

"Hold both hands in front of you facing one another about a foot apart. You will notice if you try to bring your hands closer together that there is a force which seems to push them apart. It is like trying to push in on the two sides of a pillow. The harder you try to bring them together the stronger becomes the force holding them apart. It is almost impossible to bring them together so closely that they touch each other. Try to bring them together."

This test, like the finger lock, consists of a "challenge." However, if the subject has responded favorably to the previous ones, such as eye-closure and the head nodding forward, he is probably already considerably involved hypnotically. Accordingly, he may manifest a positive response by struggling to bring his hands together and finding himself unable to get them closer than about six inches.

By now, in this series of suggestibility tests, many subjects will be quite hypnotically involved. In fact, a true hypnotic state has been induced in them. As we proceed in hypnotic technique, it will be noted that suggestibility tests with a little extension turn into trance-induction procedures, and induction techniques when continued become methods for deepening the hypnotic state. They are all part of the psychological process of restricting attention, concentrating on minor movements first, and then spreading the involvement to larger areas of the person, psychological and physiological. They include the elements of narrowing the perceptual field and regression to earlier modes of response which characterize the hypnotic condition. Many of our subjects may now be capable of responding to suggestions of an hallucination.

Hallucinations of Warmth

Those subjects whose eyes spontaneously closed, whose heads nodded forward, and who were unable to push their hands together in the previous tests, may now evidence an actual perceptual hallucination when suggestions such as the following are administered:

"I wonder what is wrong with the furnace. The thermostat must be stuck because it's getting hotter and hotter in this room. The air is becoming stifling. It's getting so warm that it's very hard to breathe. What wouldn't I give for a breath of fresh, cool air. It certainly is getting warmer and warmer. Makes one sweat. What can we do in the face of all this heat?"

At this point the good subjects, those who are rather deeply involved hypnotically, will make some movements indicating they are experiencing the intense "heat." These may include heavy breathing, fanning themselves, wiping the forehead, etc.

As the hypnotic involvement becomes greater we approach that stage which has been called somnambulism. The subject has now passed beyond the point of perceptual restriction and the performance of minor motor movements. He is capable of walking about and behaving in many complicated ways while still remaining in a deep hypnotic state, one which is often so dissociated from his normal condition that he manifests a complete amnesia for it on being removed from hypnosis; that is, he cannot even remember what he did while in the hypnotic state.

The earlier tests of suggestibility should have indicated to us that a subject was or was not likely to be able to respond to hypnosis. The initiation of hallucinations and the following test, which involves decisive motor action, may indicate those subjects who are capable of entering a fairly deep hypnotic state.

Compulsive Rising

Let us continue to assume that we are screening good subjects from a group (although the following suggestions similar to those given previously can just as well be applied to a single individual). The subjects are now told:

"As you sit there you begin to be aware of a strong need to stand up, to rise from your seat. This tendency is becoming stronger and stronger. Feel that need to stand up. The need is becoming so powerful that if you remain seated you will feel increasingly uncomfortable. Your inner tension gets stronger and stronger, and you know that if you could stand up you would immediately feel relieved. It seems that only by rising from your seat could you get rid of this uncomfortable tension and feel at ease."

Such suggestions are continued until some members of the group rise from their chairs. It will be noted that others may put up quite a struggle while some sit passively and manifest no tendency to stand up. After several have risen, a number of those who had been struggling may also rise. They have wanted to rise for some time but felt embarrassed to be the first ones to do so. As those who are still seated (with their eyes closed) hear the sound of others standing up there is a strong group suggestibility effect. Finally, all or almost all of the subjects will rise, even though some of them are not really hypnotically responsive, but feel the need to conform. Accordingly, the early risers tend to be better subjects. This, too, involves a kind of challenge. It is, therefore, better adapted to the selection of good hypnotic subjects for research, demonstration or practice purposes than for the evaluation of the hypnotizability of patients with whom one may wish to develop a sensitive, therapeutic relationship later.

Spiegel's Eye-Roll Technique

Spiegel has published two procedures for testing hypnotic susceptibility; the Eye-Roll Test (1972) and the Hypnotic Induction Profile (See Spiegel & Spiegel, 1978) which includes the first as one of its sub-measures. He reports a high correlation between the two based on 2,000 cases.

The Eye-Roll Test consists of three rather simple procedures. In the first, called the "Up-Gaze," the subject is instructed to look upward toward first his eyebrows and then toward the top of his head. Spiegel presents diagram pictures of five levels of response graded 0, 1, 2, 3, and 4, depending on "the amount of sclera visible between the lower eyelid and the lower edge of the cornea." In the second stage of this test called simply "Roll," the subject is instructed to continue to look upward and simultaneously close his eyelids slowly. Again the amount of sclera visible is used to determine whether the response is at the 0, 1, 2, 3, or 4 level. In this test the 4 level is achieved when no part of the cornea remains visible. Finally, a "Squint" test is described which is scored at three levels.

Spiegel's Hypnotic Induction Profile begins with the Eye-Roll tests and then follows with a series of suggestions related to floating and cataleptic positions of the left arm. Approximately twelve different movements are scored and arranged on a scoring sheet in such a way that a response profile can be drawn and a final score of hypnotic susceptibility computed with ranges from 0 to 5. Spiegel holds that Grade 5 individuals represent highly responsive subjects such as are commonly associated with hysterical reactions. The Eye-Roll procedure requires less than a minute to administer and the Hypnotic Induction Profile five to ten minutes. His method of screening suggestible subjects, therefore, is quite rapid. However, there has been some controversy among workers in the field concerning the adequacy of controls in the standardization of his procedures.

Efforts to correlate hypnotizability with other personality traits have in general been unsuccessful. However, J.R. Hilgard (1979) has shown that the ability to respond hypnotically is related to "keeping alive the imaginative involvements of childhood." Those individuals who enjoy fantasies through reading or identification seem to respond better than average.

In the Thematic Apperception Test subjects are asked to imagine stories about the pictures that are presented to them. One of those shows a boy lying, apparently asleep, on a couch with an older man leaning over him. This is often perceived as a picture of hypnosis. There is some evidence that the relationship between this boy and the older man as described by the subject may tell something about whether the individual regards the therapist (hypnotist) favorably and trusts him or is suspicious of his motives and feels a need to resist. Response to this picture may be of help to a therapist (who practices either hypnotherapy or other types of psychotherapy) in assessing the therapeutic relationship and the possibility of favorable response from his patient.

For successful therapeutic intervention, theory must be translated into practice. Clinical hypnosis cannot be learned from reading books alone. The ability to employ the hypnotic modality in effective treatment of patients requires that the learner spend considerable time in practice, working with real, live subjects. Accordingly, practicum exercises, which include some of the preceding suggestibility tests, should enable a researcher or clinician to develop his skill at selecting suitable subjects for hypnotic work. A program will be described which employs some of the suggestibility tests presented in this chapter. This can be applied to a group of volunteers and should result in the selection of a number of subjects of known hypnotizability on whom the student of hypnosis (with proper supervision) can practice. It is also a way of getting acquainted with hypnosis and desensitizing one's self to the strangeness of working in this modality. See Instructor's Manual, pp 9–21.

Outline of Chapter 4.   Hypnotic Susceptibility

1. Hypnosis as a Matter of Degree
2. The quantification of hypnotic "depth" and susceptibility
   a. Charcot: Catalepsy, lethergy, somnambulism
   b. Bernheim and Liebeault: Levels of trance ranging from drowsiness through catalepsy
   c. The Davis and Husband Susceptibility Scale
   d. The Stanford Hypnotic Susceptibility Scales (SHSS, Forms A, B and C)
   e. The Morgan-Hilgard short form of SHSS for clinicians
   f. The Stanford Profile Scales, Forms I and II
   g. London's Childrens Hypnotic Susceptibility Scale
   h. Harvard Group Scale of Hypnotic Susceptibility
3. Informal tests of hypnotic susceptibility
   a. Kohnstamn phenomenon
   b. Chevreul pendulum
 * c. Arm-drop
 * d. Postural-sway
   e. Hand-clasp
 * f. Arm-levitation
   g. Head-nod
   h. Inability to push hands together (pillow test)
   i. Hallucinations of warmth
   j. Compulsive rising
   k. Spiegel's Eye-roll Technique
   l. Spiegel's Hypnotic Induction Profile

*Not to be confused with induction techniques of the same name. These latter are described in Chapters 5 and 6 and often represent extensions of the susceptibility tests.

Chapter 5

Introductory Techniques of Hypnotic Induction

Assuming that hypnosis is an altered state of consciousness, there are innumerable ways by which this hypnotic state, or trance, can be initiated. They differ widely in the relative emphasis on motor, perceptual, or ideational processes, but you will notice that each contains some of the following elements.

Elementary Principles of Induction

1. A narrowing or restriction of the perceptual field. The subject is asked to concentrate on some aspect of his physical or psychological functioning. To concentrate on one means to remove attention from other aspects of his being. Thus, he may be told to gaze at an eye-fixation object, to sense the feelings in his hand, or to visualize a certain scene.

2. Suggestions are aimed at minimizing conscious, volitional effort. The patient may be told that he need not attend to the words of the hypnotist; these will enter his mind without any focusing of his listening. He may be asked not to *try* to do anything, merely to *let happen* whatever does.

3. The hypnotist may use words aimed at turning normal self or "subject" movements into not-self or "object" actions. For example, he may say, "*The* hand is moving toward *the* face," not "*Your* hand is moving toward *your* face."

*An audio tape recording of some actual inductions by John G. Watkins and Helen H. Watkins (designed for Chapters 4, 5, and 6) is available $10.00. Irvington Publishers, 740 Broadway at Astor Place, New York, NY 10003.

4. He may try to by-pass voluntary or ego participation by such statements as, "You are not really concerned about the fact that you can achieve many things without having to think about them." Statements of this type have been highly developed by Erickson. They constitute a "confusion" technique. (See Erickson, M.H., Rossi, E.L. & Rossi, S.I., 1976).

5. The hypnotist may attempt to induce a regression by stressing comfort, relaxation, passivity, even infantile dependency ("You are in a soft, warm place where all your needs are taken care of, and you can enjoy this experience with every fibre of your being"), hence, a womb fantasy.

6. He may tie together hypnotic reactions with ordinary suggested behaviors like, "As you sit there relaxed in the chair you begin to notice a sensation of lightness coming into your hand."

7. He may use repetition ("You are becoming sleepier and sleepier and sleepier").

8. He will call attention to tiny normal movements and expand them into behaviors with larger segments of the body. ("You are blinking and your eyes are getting heavier and wanting to come down, down, down, down").

9. He may establish a set for entry into trance such as, "I will count up to twenty. Your arm, which I am holding, will get heavier and heavier. At the count of twenty, when I drop it, you will drop rapidly with it into a deep state of relaxation." This is like "on your mark, get set, go!" A readiness for hypnotic response is suggested. The subject waits and anticipates its occurrence.

10. The hypnotist may ask the patient to imagine a kind of fantasy or dream. As he becomes involved in it he slips naturally into a trance state.

In this chapter we will describe several of the more customary and traditional approaches to trance induction in considerable detail so that through practice sessions with suitable subjects the beginner can learn how to hypnotize. In the next chapter additional techniques will be considered which involve greater complexity and skill for their successful execution or which deal with specialized problems. In Vol. II we will consider advanced theory of trance behavior and aspects of technique which are related to psychodynamic processes, considerations important to the analytically oriented hypnotherapist.

Introductory Induction Techniques

The Relaxation Technique

As noted in the chapter on history, earlier workers, such as Liebeault, perceived the hypnotic state as akin to sleep and used the word frequently as part of their induction verbalizations. Since research has shown that the condition of hypnosis is both physiologically and psychologically different from that of sleep, workers in the field now tend to avoid this term. However, in its place there is a great deal of utilization of the term "relaxation," both in orienting patients into the meaning of hypnosis and in providing a set for the more effective inculcation of suggestions.

There seems to be some difference of opinion as to the necessity of "relaxation" as a significant factor in hypnotic induction. Meares (1961) devotes almost an entire chapter to describing a relaxation approach and specifically tells his patients that, "It is easier to attain the mental state of hypnotic sleep if one lies flat on one's back." On the other hand the Hilgards (1975) found no difference in the response to hypnotizing suggestions depending on whether the subjects were seated or standing. Several techniques, such as the postural-sway and certain rapid approaches utilize an initial standing posture. The fact that individuals can be hypnotized who are standing, sitting, or lying down is indicative of the point that hypnosis is not the same as simple relaxation.

However, most induction and deepening techniques do employ some variation of relaxation, both as a process and as verbalized to the subjects, and its use seems to make the induction process develop in a more gradual and natural manner. Furthermore, when hypnosis is described to patients as a form of "natural relaxation" they may lose any fears of involving themselves in it. It becomes, then, no longer a weird, mysterious experience in which their "will" can be overpowered, but simply a natural and pleasant physiological state to which they are already accustomed.

A form of treatment for tension has been developed by Jacobson (1934) called "progressive relaxation." He did not consider this to be hypnosis. However, the utilization of progressive relaxation techniques often results in an easier entry into hypnosis by a patient. These same procedures can also be employed as a pre-conditioning preparation for hypnosis when patients are initially very tense and resistant. As they relax they tend to relinquish rigid postures of opposition to suggestions.

The progressive relaxation suggestions are aimed at making the patient highly aware of the difference between a state of tension and a state of relaxation progressively in different members of the body. An example might be as follows:

"Lift your right foot off the floor and extend your leg straight out. Now imagine that there is a heavy weight placed on your ankle. Be keenly aware of the tensions throughout your entire leg. Think about them. Notice the pulling and the fatigue. Concentrate on all the feelings in that leg. That's it. Now let go. Let your leg drop down loose and limp until it is completely relaxed. Let all the tension and control go out of it."

The procedure is now repeated with the left leg. Similar suggestions may now be moved to the abdominal region.

"Tighten the muscles across your abdomen. Make them like a tight band. Tighter, tighter, tighter. That's it. Hold that tension. Concentrate on it. Be keenly aware of every feeling in it. Good. Now let go. Let all the stiffness and tension go out of the abdominal muscles. Let them become completely relaxed."

Similar suggestions are now administered to the chest muscles, each arm, the hands, the facial muscles, the eyes and the forehead. Each in turn is tensed, sensed and then relaxed. The patient becomes very conscious of the difference between tension and relaxation and learns how to achieve relaxation first in each part of the body and then finally throughout the entire body. The exercises have been found to be very beneficial in treating many kinds of anxiety reactions and psychosomatic conditions in this day where the demands of our complex society are significantly related to ulcers, arthritis, migraines, etc. If they have been employed in treating such conditions it is an easy step to incorporate them into an initial stage of hypnotic induction.

The hypnotist using such techniques talks in a slow and soft voice, thus modelling the state of relaxation. Meares repeats phrases such as, "Calm, easy, comfortable, let yourself go, drowsy, drifting, feel the heaviness, let the muscles loose, all your body relaxed, it's all through you," etc.

Each hypnotist will modify the exact wording, but the general principles involved in this induction will be the same, namely, continuous suggestions of relaxation, letting tensions go, drifting, relaxing imagery and the modelling by the hypnotist of a state of relaxation. Although the skilled operator always observes movements of his subject and attempts to coordinate his suggestions with them, this approach probably calls for less attention to this factor than many others. The monotonous voice and the suggestions of ever greater involvement in relaxation have a cumulative effect which ultimately results in the subject slipping into a trance state to a depth of which he is hypnotically capable.

The Eye-Fixation Technique

The induction method which has been practiced most frequently was one originally described by James Braid (1960).

The subject or patient is seated in an easy chair, preferably with arms and a high back, and asked to rest comfortably. A pencil (or other object) is held just above the bridge of the nose, perhaps 6 - 8 inches away, and sufficiently close as to induce ocular fatigue. To focus on it the subject has to look upward and direct his eyes inward. We wish to build on the eye fatigue so that it ultimately becomes natural to eliminate it by closing the eyes. The good hypnotist is extremely attentive to all tiny muscular responses and uses each to build upon for the administration of suggestions aimed at inducing reactions in greater segments of the body.

Eye-closure may be rapid or it may take a considerable period of time in the resistant subject. Accordingly, the arm of the hypnotist may become quite tired after holding it for a long time above the subject's eyes. Furthermore, in this approach it is better to stand at the side of the subject's chair rather than in front. This position is easier to maintain. If the hypnotist stands in front of the subject and holds his arm high it will become fatigued more rapidly, and slow reactors might require 15 or more minutes before the eyes close. In the preferable position the hypnotist's arm is resting against his side and the pencil is held by his fingers which are below the subject's eyes.

The hypnotist should observe the subject's reactions carefully and time his suggestions very closely with them. For example, the remark, "Occasionally, they are going to blink," might be made immediately after he perceives a blink. What is important is that his suggestions must be very close to reality. In the early stages of the induction they *follow* movements of the subject. Later, as the hypnotic involvement becomes greater, he can *lead* or initiate such movements by his suggestions. Knowing just when to change from a following to a leading is important and requires the closest attention. There are a number of variations to this approach, but a typical set of verbalized suggestions might be as follows:

"Stare at the shiny part of this pencil. Fix your eyes on it. Take a few deep breaths. Just keep breathing deeply. Listen to the sound of my voice. You will find that your eyelids have a tendency to get heavy. Almost as if they had a heavy weight attached to them. And the longer you stare at this, the more your eyelids get heavy, and you blink, and they have a feeling like something is pulling them down, as if they wanted to slowly close, and get drowsier and sleepier and heavier. And you have a feeling as if they were slowly closing, slowly closing, getting drowsier and more tired, and when they finally do close, how good you'll feel. Drowsy, heavy, pulling down, down, down, slowly closing, getting harder and harder to see, and you feel good. Very, very hard to keep them open, feel that very soon they will close tightly, almost tightly closing, almost tightly closing, tightly closing. Your eyes are tightly closed; you feel good; you feel comfortable; you're relaxed all over; just let yourself drift and enjoy this comfortable relaxed state. You will find that your head will get heavier, tends to nod forward some, and you just let yourself drift in an easy, calm, relaxed state."

The *feeling* of heaviness and the *feeling* of the eyes "wanting to close" are suggested first, perceptions first which cannot be challenged as can actual behaviors. If the hypnotist said at first, "Your eyes are closing," when in reality they were staring wide open, then his credibility would be lowered. Often in such a case the subject structures this into a challenge. Then he and the hypnotist engage in a kind of battle where the hypnotist is insisting, "Your eyes are closing," while the subject is fiercely resisting the eye closure. In such cases the hypnotist often loses. Even if the eyes finally do close the effort on his part to induce the closure and that of the patient to resist has initiated a confrontive type of relationship, not at all what a therapist may want. There are some cases where verbal force and pressure are the only way to induce a trance state, but these should be employed minimally in therapeutic hypnosis.

Sometimes the heaviness in the eyes and the tendency for them to close can be enhanced by the hypnotist passing his hand, perhaps with fingers apart, slowly downward several times between the subject's eyes and the pencil.

The induction proper is considered completed when the subject's eyes are completely and firmly closed. This may be tested by a challenge as follows:

"Your eyes are tightly closed, and you will find that they want to remain closed. They are tightly stuck together, so tight that it seems as if the heavier you might try to pull them apart, the tighter they would stick. The harder you try to pull them apart the tighter they stick together. They stick so tightly together they will not come apart no matter how hard you try.————Try to pull them apart."

After the subject has tried for a moment or two the hypnotist may then say, "That's all right. You don't have to try any more. Now you can go down into a very deep state of relaxation, deep, deep, deep."

Experienced hypnotists tend to avoid challenges. Furthermore, if the subject is a patient for whom hypnotherapeutic treatment is to be administered, challenges may have an impairing effect on the relationship. At least, they tend to establish a dominant-dependent type of relationship which may be contrary to the aims of the therapist. However, in some cases the hypnotist may feel it necessary to test the extent of hypnotic involvement before proceeding further. At this point deepening procedures are usually employed, or if the doctor feels that the patient is sufficiently involved in hypnosis, therapeutic suggestions or other treatment procedures may be applied.

Variations of the Eye-Fixation Technique

It may be inconvenient to hold an eye-fixation object, such as the pencil, in front of the subject's eyes. Accordingly, he can be asked to fix his gaze on some object across the room, preferably one that requires him to look upward. Some practitioners, such as those who use an analytic couch, may place a thumb tack in the ceiling at which the patient is asked to look. By having subjects fixate on an object across the room, this eye-fixation procedure can be used to hypnotize simultaneously a number of members of a group. Group hypnosis is quite feasible (as in the group suggestibility tests), and hypnosis is also being employed by some group therapists.

However, the difficulty is that the suggestions cannot be timed as precisely to subject's eye movements or other postural indicators of hypnotic involvement. Accordingly, some subjects will have achieved eye-closure in a few minutes while others are still staring with wide open eyes at the fixation object. The group hypnotist obviously has to adapt his verbalizations to such a general situation.

Some hypnotists place the fingers of their hand on the subject's forehead and ask him to fixate on the end of the thumb. This, too, can be tiring and may also create other matters for consideration since it involves touching.

Patients who wear contact lenses should be asked to remove them before beginning an eye fixation induction.

The Eye-Blink Method

This is an eye-closure method which has the advantage of requiring little vocal effort on the part of the hypnotist and might be desirable when he is suffering from a cold or sore throat. It is also quite easily administered to a group. The subject or subjects are asked to sit back comfortably in their chairs, to close their eyes and to take a few deep breaths. This, of course, is fairly standard procedure for many different inductions and simply establishes a responsive set and a feeling of security. Instructions may then be given as follows:

"I am going to count some numbers starting with 'one.' Each time I say a number I want you to blink your eyes open for just a fraction of a second and then immediately close them. Continue doing this, responding to each number I speak by a rapid and momentary opening and closing of the eyes until such time as your eyes become so tired and heavy that they no longer wish to open. You may then just keep them closed and relax deeply."

The hypnotist then begins counting at five second intervals, "one———two———three, etc." The eyes of the subjects are closely observed to see that they are carrying out the instructions, making only a very quick blink open and instantly closing again each five seconds.

After about twenty counts the hypnotist begins to put longer spaces between each count, perhaps a transitional period of 7 - 8 second intervals while counting from twenty-one to thirty. After that the intervals are systematically increased by about five seconds each for ten to twenty counts.

Hence, from thirty to forty or fifty each number may be separated by a ten-second interval. From fifty to sixty or seventy by a fifteen-second interval. By the time twenty-second intervals are reached as much as fifteen minutes or more has been spent in the induction. It is recommended that the early numbers be spoken in a strong, firm voice, and that as they proceed the voice of the hypnotist becomes softer and more gentle, until by the time he is counting with twenty-second intervals he is speaking in almost a whisper.

This procedure pulls on natural physiological tendencies. As the subject becomes increasingly relaxed he finds it less and less desirable to open his eyes. Each time he does he is confronted with a visual perception of reality to which he must adjust, but which is so momentary that he really does not have time to reaccustom himself to the normal, unrelaxed, unhypnotized state. The hypnosis is then induced by the learning principle of negative reinforcement, which holds that we tend to repeat behaviors which result in the cessation of feelings of unpleasantness. We also avoid behaviors which bring about unpleasantness or punishment. Opening the eyes creates a feeling of unpleasantness; closing them reinstates the pleasant state of relaxation. So, in time, it is much easier simply to keep the eyes closed and continue on into a "deep state of relaxation" which the hypnotist has not only given permission to enjoy, but has also suggested would occur.

The Direct Stare

This technique was used widely by Bernheim and is described in much greater detail by Meares (1961, pp. 195-204) than we will here. It is an extremely aggressive approach which relies for its success on the domination by the operator of a subject or patient who is submissive or somewhat disorganized. It may work rather rapidly.

Since it is quite forceful in manner there are certain specific indications for its most effective use and certain precautions and contra-indications. It establishes the rather traditional dominance-submission relationship described in the Svengali-Trilby story (du Maurier, 1941) and thus is not advised for a long-term treatment situation which may involve analytic or other similar types of psychotherapy. This does not create the type of relationship which is normally considered to be therapeutic.

However, when it is essential that a trance state be rapidly induced, especially for the purpose of relieving an acute pain (such as might occur on a battlefield or following a severe accident), it can well be the method of choice. The hypnotist must initiate it only with the greatest air of confidence, boldness and in a firm, commanding voice. It is an approach which would be infrequently used. The presence of paranoid trends in the patient are contraindicative, since such patients may well incorporate the hypnotist into their delusional system as a possessor of "the evil eye." There is also the possibility of traumatizing a timid subject and developing in him a conditioned fear of hypnosis or to that specific hypnotist. Still, when it is necessary that immediate, firm action be taken to quiet an hysterical individual or to administer immediate and effective hypno-anesthesia (perhaps when chemo-anesthesias or analgesias are not available) the practitioner should be prepared to utilize this procedure.

With the patient lying down or sitting and facing the hypnotist directly, the eyes of the hypnotist are fixated on a point between the patient's eyes and at the bridge of his nose. The face and eyes of the hypnotist should be quite close, in fact may well be so close that the hypnotist's eyes cannot actually focus on the nose bridge; rather they stare through it as if fixed on some distant point on the other side of the patient's head. This staring through the bridge of the patient's nose rather than at it will greatly relieve feelings of eye tension in the hypnotist, but will be just as effective to the patient. Grasping the shoulders of the patient the hypnotist might then give suggestions such as the following in a commanding voice:

"Stare into my eyes. Look, don't take them away. You have to look into my eyes even though you would like to turn them away. Your eyes are becoming very, very heavy. They cannot stay open. There is an irresistable force pulling them down. Down! Down! Down! Heavier. They blink (spoken immediately after the patient has blinked). They are closing, closing tightly shut. The eyelids are sticky. Struggle how you like. You cannot keep them open. The harder you try to keep them open the more irresistible is the force pulling them down. Your eyes are tightly closed, and your body is growing numb."

Suggestions of this type are continued for two or three minutes by which time those subjects who can respond favorably to this approach will have achieved a firm eye-closure. Occasionally a subject will enter a deep hypnotic state with his eyes staring, wide open. This will be noted because hands passed in front of the eyes will evince no response. The eyes will not adjust to fixate on them, and the subject will react as if he were not seeing the hypnotist's passes. Such an "awake" trance state can often be very deep. It involves a catalepsy of the eyes but with them wide open rather than tightly closed. It may be useful then simply to close the lids by pulling them down saying, "There, they are now tightly closed and will not open. You will now go down into a very, very deep state."

This technique is often used by stage hypnotists. It typifies that manner described by Ferenczi (1926) as "father hypnosis" in which transference reactions involving fear of early authority figures are mobilized as a motivation for entering the hypnotic state. One must decide whether the covert fear which is engendered toward the hypnotist by this procedure is offset by the advantages of rapid induction and immediate receptivity of the patient to powerful suggestions—such as might be necessary to counteract acute pain.

The Arm-Drop Induction Method

This approach in some ways resembles the Arm-Drop test for susceptibility. However, it is different and begins with a variation of eye-fixation. The subject is asked to raise an arm so that the hand is slightly above the head and given suggestions as follows:

"Stare at one of the fingers, either the index or the middle finger. You may continue to look at it, or, if you wish, close your eyes and visualize it in your mind's eye. As you fixate your gaze on it you will notice that the other fingers tend to fade out of focus and that your entire arm begins to feel heavier and heavier. The longer you concentrate on that finger the heavier and heavier your arm becomes. But you will not go into a deep state of relaxation until the arm has come all the way down. Keep concentrating on that finger while the arm gets heavier and heavier and heavier." (When downward movement becomes apparent.) "Notice that as the arm is getting heavier it is slowly coming down, down, down. But you will not relax into a deep and profound state of relaxation until the arm is all the way down and touching. Going down, down, down, deeper, deeper, deeper," etc. The suggestions must be timed with the actual movement of the arm.

There are a number of aspects of this induction which are worthy of special notice. First, the arm is placed in such a position that fatigue will eventually bring it down. The downward movement is tied into going "down" into a "deep state of relaxation." The harder the individual keeps fighting to hold it up, the more he is committed to the proposition implied by the statement that, "You will not go into a deep state of relaxation until the arm is all the way down." This means, of course, that, "You will go into such a state when the arm comes all the way down."

Quite often the eyes also come down with the arm and close when the arm is all the way down, unless the individual has chosen to close them at the first. Notice that the subject is given a number of choices in which he feels that he is exercising conscious volition. However, none of these choices imply the freedom to avoid going into a "deep state of relaxation." He can choose which one of his fingers to fixate on. He can decide whether to stare at it or visualize it in his mind's eye, and he is given the option of not going into a deep state simply by preventing the hand from coming down. But normal physiology is against him. Sooner or later the fatigue and sense of discomfort will be so great that the arm must come down. His resistive energies have been spent fighting himself rather than the hypnotist.

This is somewhat of a pressure technique. Trance can be avoided only by a complete refusal on the part of the subject to be drawn into the dilemma with which he is confronted. Sometimes the subject will simply lower his arm rapidly and voluntarily, then open his eyes and decline to "play the game."

Fig. 5:1. Arm Drop Induction

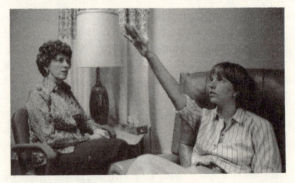

1. Initial position

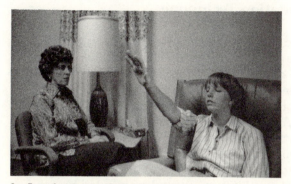

2. *Arm begins to lower*

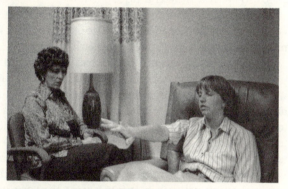

3. *Arm continues to lower*

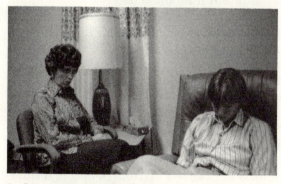

4. *Arm is all the way down.*

No technique will hypnotize all subjects, but this one is frequently effective, combining as it does the principles of eye-fixation, physiological fatigue, "apparent choice," restriction of perception, reversed-effect, and repetition.

The Arm-Levitation Technique

In this approach the reverse movement is suggested, so it does not utilize the physiological fatigue factor. In fact, it operates in the opposite direction and must overcome such fatigue. However, it does start with focused attention, directed perception, and tiny movements which are then spread to larger ones. At each stage of the induction there are overt movements which indicate the extent of hypnotic involvement so that the hypnotist is continually receiving cues from the subject. This makes it possible to continue each step with further repetition until it is successfully executed before proceeding with the next stage.

So that we can analyze each step and the principles involved, the following verbalizations have been numbered (the numbers are not part of the verbalization):

"(1) Put your right hand on the table. (2) I want you to concentrate all your attention on that hand. You can look at it and I want you to be aware of all the sensations and feelings in the hand. (3) For example, you are aware that it is sitting on the table. There is weight there. You are aware of the texture of the table; you can keenly sense the position every finger has toward every other finger. (4) You're thinking about the temperature of that hand, and as you look at that hand with this concentration you are going to notice that one of the fingers in that hand will feel different from the others. (5) Now it might be the thumb or the little finger or perhaps the index finger or the big finger or the ring finger, but one of them will feel distinctly different from the others. (6) And that feeling may be that it's a little more warm or that it's a little cold. It could be that it kind of stings a little or that it's numb. It could feel lighter or heavier, (7) but if you concentrate well, you will be able to know which finger it is that has the different sensation from the others (8) and as you pay close attention that particular finger will lift itself a little bit from the table over the others. Now concentrate on that, and you will notice that one of the fingers will tend to lift itself up from the table a little. (9) It's that (little?) finger. (10) Now I want you to concentrate and you will find that finger becoming kind of numb; it's sticking straight out; it's almost as if it were made out of wood (11) and that wooden feeling will start spreading to the other fingers around close to it, and they too will begin to lift

Fig. 5:2. Arm Levitation Induction

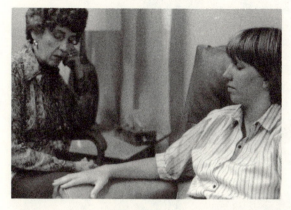

1. Initial position

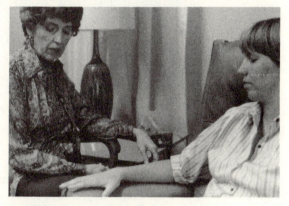

2. First finger movement

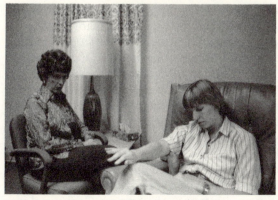

3. Hand begins to levitate

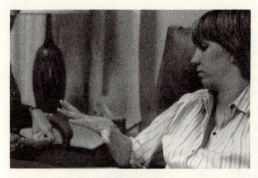

4. *Hand continues rising*

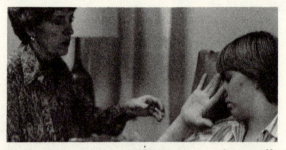

5. *Hand touching face. Hypnotist ready to pull hand down.*

themselves and straighten. And you will find that next the ring finger will come up. And you will find that same lifting feeling coming into the (big) finger, and it sort of stiffens and straightens itself. And there is a light feeling, a wooden-like feeling, and then it moves into the (little) finger, and that, too, gets light and feels like it's floating, and then it gradually spreads into the hand. (12) And the hand begins to feel like it is made out of wood or cork and like cork it sort of wants to float as if it were in water and wants to come up. (13) Or perhaps you can imagine there is a balloon attached to the wrist and this hand keeps wanting to float up (14) in the direction of your face and it gets higher and higher and higher. (15) And you feel a drowsy sensation as it comes closer to the face. (16) It's about twelve inches away, then it's about eleven inches, (17) and the higher the hand comes, the drowsier you feel, (18) and you begin to think that when the hand touches the face you will go into a deep and profound relaxed state. (19) Now it's only five inches away. And now, it's four inches away. Coming closer and closer. It's going to touch pretty soon. Three inches away. (20) And when it touches you will go into a very deep state. (21) Almost touching, almost touching, almost touching. An inch away. Coming closer and closer. (22) Touching, touching. (23) And you just feel a sense of relaxation, (24) and as your hand goes down, you go down, too, into a deep, deep, deep relaxed state. And you feel yourself go down to a deep, comfortable, relaxed state.

Let us go through this induction again, indicating the purpose and principle involved in each suggestion or set of suggestions.

(1) "Put your right hand on the table."

A specific, directed instruction, not contestable.

(2) "I want you to concentrate all your attention on that hand. You can look at it, and I want you to be aware of all the sensations and feelings in that hand."

Concentration and directed attention.

(3) "For example, you are aware that it is sitting on the table. There is weight there. You are aware of the texture of the table; you can keenly sense the position every finger has toward every other finger."

Highly specified perceptions, one after the other. There is no time to think and criticize each.

(4) "You're thinking about the temperature of that hand, and as you look at that hand with this concentration you are going to notice that one of the fingers in that hand will feel different from the others."

Concentration on one part of the body. Tying together the act of attention to first perception of an unusual, and hence suggested feeling. No specification as to the nature of that "different" feeling.

(5) "Now it might be the thumb or the little finger or perhaps the index finger or the big finger, or the ring finger, but one of them will feel distinctly different from the others."

The subject is given a choice of fingers, but no choice of not having this "different" feeling.

(6) "And that feeling may be that it's a little more warm or that it's a little cold. It could be that it kind of stings a little or that it's numb. It could feel heavier or lighter."

Again a choice of feelings but not a choice to have no such unusual feeling. Subject feels that procedure is extremely permissive, which it is, in the manner in which subject goes into hypnosis.

(7) "but if you concentrate well,

The difference in feeling is pre-

you will be able to know which finger it is that has the different sensation from the other."

(8) "and as you pay close attention, that particular finger will tend to lift itself up from the table a little."

(9) "It's that (little?) finger."

(10) "Now I want you to concentrate and you will find that finger becoming kind of numb; it's sticking straight out; it's almost as if it were made out of wood."

(11) "and that wooden feeling will start spreading to the other fingers around close to it and they, too, will begin to lift themselves and straighten. And you will find that next the (ring) finger will come up. And you will find that same lifting feeling coming into the (big) finger and it sort of stiffens and straightens itself. And there is a light feeling, a wooden-like feeling and then it moves into the (index) finger and that, too, gets light and feels like it's floating, and then it gradually is the (thumb) that straightens itself and this wooden-like feeling gradually spreads into the hand."

(12) "And the hand beings to feel like it is made out of wood or cork, and like cork it sort of wants to float as if it were in water and wants to come up."

(13) "Or perhaps you can imagine there is a balloon attached to the wrist and this hand keeps wanting to float up."

sented as a fact. It is the subject's responsibility to perceive this by demonstrating his ability to concentrate.

If it doesn't lift it is because you have not paid close enough attention. A tendency to lift is suggested first, not that it is lifting.

Slight movement is seized upon by the hypnotist and verified, thus increasing his credibility.

Suggestion from movement back to perception, this time of anesthesia and rigidity. Comparison is made to the insensibility of wood.

The paraesthetic feelings, the stiffness, the rigidity and the lifting movement is spread from one finger progressively through all fingers and the entire hand. More and more of the body of the subject becomes hypnotically involved. By using such a phrase as "you will find," he is placed in the position of being a passive observer of finger behavior which is happening to him. He is not doing it; it is perceived as "object," not within voluntary self action. "It" happens; he is not doing it. A dissociation between his hand movements and his perception of his own voluntary processes is being established.

Wooden feeling is spread to entire hand and then comparison is made from wood to cork so that the next suggestions of floating in water will be facilitated.

Another image which may be suggested in order to facilitate floating upward tendency. Notice "the" wrist, not "your" wrist—treating it as object, not part of the self. Note also that it "keeps wanting" to float up, hence, "it," independent of self, is making the choice of movement.

(14) "in the direction of your face, and it gets higher and higher and higher."

Specific direction of movement suggested with repetition.

(15) "And you feel a drowsy sensation as it comes closer to the face."

Involvement in hypnotic "sleep" being tied to upward movement toward "the," not "your" face.

(16) "It's about twelve inches away, then it's about eleven inches"

Hypnotist suggests approaching movement of hand toward face but keeps close to actual position of hand. Don't lead too much.

(17) "and the higher the hand comes, the drowsier you feel."

Increased sensations of hypnotic "sleep" tied directly to hand movement.

(18) "and you begin to think that when the hand touches the face you will go into a deep and profound relaxed state."

Anticipation of subject that he will enter profound hypnosis at the moment of touching.

(19) "Now, it's only five inches away. And now, it's four inches away. Coming closer and closer. It's going to touch pretty soon. Three inches away."

Further suggestions of movement and anticipation of touching.

(20) "And when it touches you will go into a very deep state."

Repetition of anticipated touching and tying it again to entry into "a very deep state."

(21) "Almost touching, almost touching, almost touching. An inch away. Coming closer and closer."

Repetition and urging of movement.

(22) "Touching, touching."

Confirmation at moment of touching.

(23) "And you just feel a sense of relaxation."

Make this a moment of personal achievement for subject and rewarded by pleasurable positive reinforcement.

(24) "and as your hand goes *down*, you go *down*, too, into a deep, deep, deep relaxed state. And you feel yourself go down to a deep, comfortable relaxed state."

Subject has achieved touching; now the consequence of entry into a "deep relaxed state" can take place. Repetition with firmness. Subject verifies this by his own "comfortable" feelings. Note repei-

tion of word "down" with more
than one meaning.

To awaken an hypnotized individual a suggestion may be given
such as, "When I count up to five you will be wide awake, refreshed
and feeling good. Coming up now. One, two, three, four, five." At this
point the subject can be questioned about his feelings, behavior and
his sensations as to how deep a state he had entered.

Repetitive Movement

A much simpler induction technique involving hand movement is that of *repetitive movement*, sometimes facetiously
called "hand wagging." It combines eye-fixation and concentration on a moving object, repetition, a gradual change of
the movement from subject to object and a tying of this action
to eye closure. Less skill is required of the hypnotist than in
the arm-levitation approach. It is one of the best techniques
for a beginner to use.

Meares (1961) described this approach in considerable detail and reported that it was especially effective in working
with resisting subjects who were unable or unwilling to relax
completely. Suggestions to be given the patient are as follows:

Repetitive Movement

"Place your elbow on the table with your forearm up like this. Now I want you to stare at that hand while I move it up and down. Up—down, up—down, up—down. As you stare at that hand you will notice a tendency for your eyes to become heavier and heavier, as if they might want to close. Keep staring while the hand continues to go up—down, up—down, up—down."

The hypnotist positions subject's elbow on the table with his own fingers on the back of the subject's hand and his thumb on subject's palm just above wrist.

"You will also notice that the movement in this hand is becoming more and more automatic. It is as if the hand itself wants to move up and down without your doing anything about it. Up—down, up—down, up—down. Your eyes are getting so very heavy that they are gradually closing. It doesn't seem as if they could be held open."

The subject's hand is wagged up and down in time with the verbal suggestion of "up—down." The hand is increasingly dissociated by referring to it as "the" hand, not "your" hand. The hand is becoming an "it."

"You are relaxing deeply all over

The hypnotist now gradu-

while the hand is moving more and more by itself. Up—down, up—down, up—down. Now, the movement of the hand is so automatic that it keeps going up—down, up—down, up—down all by itself and it doesn't need any more help from me to continue its movement. Up—down, up—down, up—down."

"It is now becoming so automatic that it continues to move all by itself without any control by you. Up—down, up—down, up—down. It seems to be almost outside you with a will to move up—down independently of you. It controls its own actions. You do not control them."

"As it goes automatically up and down it seems to be saying to you, "Deep—relax, deep—relax, deep—relax. Up—down, deep—relax, up—down, deep—relax. You are going more and more into a deep and profound state of relaxation. Your eyes are closed. Your head is heavy. It is nodding forward, and you are going deeper and deeper and deeper."

"I will take the hand now and stop its movement. As I bring the hand *down* you will go *down* with it, deeper and deeper."

"Deep, deep, deep, deep, deep."

ally loosens his hold of the subject's hand until he is only lightly touching it by the thumb and forefingers. As soon as he is convinced that its movement will continue automatically he removes his hand entirely.

The hypnotist continues to reinforce the movement with "Up—down" as long as necessary to assure automatic action.

The "up—down" movement is now tied to the suggestion of "deep—relax," keeping the same timing and coordination.

The hypnotist now stops the movement and brings the hand down to the table emphasizing both "Downs." The "deeps" are said strongly and rapidly as the hand comes down. For emphasis, press subject's near shoulder down slightly.

Summary

The methods of induction described in this chapter represent those which probably have the widest use. They are well validated and will show a high percent of success when employed skillfully with susceptible subjects or patients. Many of the principles of hypnotic suggestion are utilized although no single technique will exemplify all aspects of the modality. The prestige of the hypnotist and his sense of confidence are most important for successful induction. At one time when this writer was first hypnotizing, a group of student volunteers were waiting (in a colleague's office) to be screened for susceptibility. Buzzing with curiosity they inquired of him, "Can Dr. Watkins really hypnotize us?" My associate replied, "Of course, I have seen him hypnotize dozens of people. You'll be in a deep trance state in no time at all." This was a gross misstatement of fact. However, the effect of my friend's "recommendation" was that almost all the volunteers became quickly and easily hypnotizable. It is no wonder that professional hypnotherapists display their qualifying certificates and stage hypnotists assume mysterious and awe-inspiring titles. Yes, hypnosis is both an altered state of consciousness and an intensive interpersonal relationship experience.

There is nothing wrong with professional prestige as long as it is used in the service of the patient's needs, not for personal aggrandizement and the satisfaction of power needs in the hypnotist.

Outline of Chapter 5. Introductory Techniques of Hypnotic Induction

1. Elemental principles of induction
   a. Narrowing of perceptual field
   b. Minimizing conscious, volitional effort
   c. Turning "subject" (self) actions into "object" (non-self) actions
   d. By-passing ego participation
   e. Inducing regression
   f. Tying suggestions together
   g. Repetition
   h. Focusing on tiny movements initially and expanding into larger behaviors
   i. Establishing set
   j. Involving in fantasy

2. Introductory induction techniques
   a. Relaxation
   b. Eye-fixation
      1. Variations of eye-fixation
   c. Eye-blink
   d. Direct stare
   e. Arm-drop
   f. Arm-levitation
   g. Repetitive movement

Chapter 6

Advanced Techniques of Hypnotic Induction

Controversy Over Hypnotizability as a Fixed Trait of Subject to Variability

The number of techniques and their variations by which hypnotic states can be induced are almost infinite. Each tends to emphasize certain principles of suggestion more than others. Although there have been many studies concerning the trait of hypnotizability almost no empirical evidence seems to be available directly comparing one induction procedure with another upon the same or comparable populations. Some research, especially certain earlier studies published by Hilgard, E. (1965), implied that hypnotizability was a fixed trait inhering in the subject. Accordingly, little variability would be expected between different hypnotists and different induction techniques. If a subject was hypnotizable almost any technique applied by any hypnotist would be successful. Most clinical workers, however, are convinced that there is a great deal of difference between the effectiveness of different techniques and between the skills with which they are applied by different practitioners. The hypothesis of hypnotizability as a constant state denies psychodynamic aspects of the hypnotic relationship as being significant. Much more research is needed in this area. However, since most practitioners believe that induction techniques are an important part of their modes of operation, and since there are so many different approaches, we will describe in this chapter a number of additional ones, particularly some which differ from

134

those discussed so far in being rather unusual, more complex, requiring greater skill or being better adapted to certain specialized cases or problem patients.

Advanced Techniques of Induction

The Postural-Sway Technique

In Chapter 4 a suggestibility test was described called "postural sway." It was noted then that this approach could not only serve as a test of hypnotic susceptibility, but that it could also be extended into an actual induction. This procedure has the merit that it is very different from the types of eye-fixation which are frequently characterized in movies involving the swinging of a watch or other object before the subject's eyes—often depicted as the unwilling victim of some villain. Individuals who have observed such films may have developed anxieties about eye-fixation and accordingly are able to respond with less fear to something entirely different such as this postural-sway method.

Fig 6:1. Postural Sway: Suggestibility Test and Induction Technique

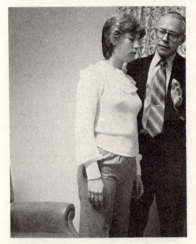 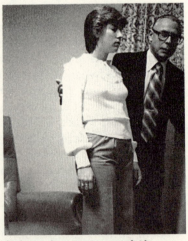

Initial position. Hypnotist sighting along bridge of subject's nose.

Subject beginning to drift backward. Hypnotist reassures her he will not let her fall by hand behind shoulders.

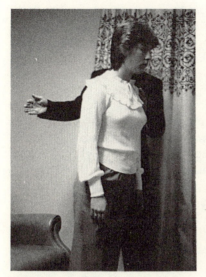

Subject swaying forward. Hypnotist prevents her from falling
by his left hand on her left
shoulder.

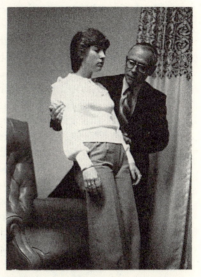

Subject falling back. Hypnotist
shifting his position back and
catching her.

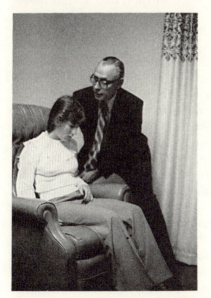

Hypnotist eases subject slowly
back into chair.

Since the induction is simply an extension of the suggestibility test, it will not be necessary here to repeat the
initial stages of the procedure. The reader is referred back to
Ch. 4, pgs. 99-101 in which the verbalizations for taking the

subject or patient up to the point of some significant hypnotic involvement have already been presented. Continuing from this point, the amplitude of the swaying arc is increased and swaying suggestions are further repeated so as to allow time for the subject to shut out opposing stimuli and become increasingly caught up in the hypnotic process.

To induce deeper trance the voice tone is now made much firmer, and the swaying suggestions are given somewhat more rapidly. "Swaying forward, swaying backward, forward, backward," the volume of the voice growing stronger and stronger. Finally, an attempt is made to induce the patient to fall over backward into a deep trance. The emphasis on the "backward" is increased and on the "forward" diminished, and the verb is changed from "drifting" or "swaying" to "falling, *falling backward*, falling forward, *falling backward*, falling forward, *falling over backward*, falling, falling, *falling, falling*," rather rapidly and in a higher pitched and more emotional tone. If a deep trance has been induced, the patient will increase the amplitude of his sway until he can no longer stand erect. He will then fall over backward in a deep trance state where he is caught by the therapist and eased into a waiting chair.

If the patient is in a light trance only, he may start to fall backward, but catch himself by placing one of his feet back, or attempt to sway sideways or steady himself voluntarily in some manner. This indicates to the therapist that a deep trance has not yet been induced. He can then do one of two things: he may either continue the monotonous repetition of "falling forward, falling backward," etc., to induce a deeper degree of trance; or he may reassure the patient that he will not fall by placing a hand lightly behind his shoulder. This allays fears which might arise and interrupt the hypnotic process. After the patient realizes that he will not be permitted to fall and hurt himself, he tends to lose the signs of anxiety which may have begun to appear. He may then allow himself to fall back against the therapist's arm, whereupon the therapist continues the suggestions, "falling over backward, falling backward, falling back into a deep sleep, back into a deep sleep, deep sleep, deep sleep," and then eases the patient gradually over into a chair. This, preferably an arm chair, should have been placed behind the patient. He can also be gradually lowered back upon a couch which has been located conveniently near.

If the patient is either completely limp or in a stiff cataleptic posture when he is placed back on the chair or cot, it is evidence that a fairly deep degree of trance has been induced. If, however, he is able to help himself either by taking steps backward or by putting his hands on the armchair and guiding himself into it, then only a light or hypnoidal trance has been induced.

Several very important postural reactions on the part of the hypnotist will enhance the effectiveness of the procedure. Since the subject is standing with his eyes closed, he must rely entirely on his kinesthetic sense to verify that he is indeed swaying backward and forward. This feedback can be enhanced by the hypnotist if he will hold one of his hands behind the subject's back just below the neck and one on the subject's near shoulder blade in front. The hands of the hypnotist will be about eighteen inches apart, leaving room for the swaying of the subject back and forth between them such that when he has reached the forward part of the arc his shoulder blade just barely touches the hand of the hypnotist. Likewise, when he reaches the back part of the swaying arc his back just touches the hypnotist's hand. Such touching at each extreme of the arc gives him a tactual cue which validates his swaying in addition to the kinesthetic feel. When the subject is female it is appropriate to hold the hand in front sufficiently high that it is the shoulder and not the breast which is touched.

After the subject's body has touched either hand, a slight push is given to suggest that he sway in the reverse direction, but the hand does *not* follow the contrary movement of the body and continue the touching. To do this would simply mean that the swaying would be caused by the hypnotist's hands pushing him back and forth, not by the effect of the suggestions.

There is another value to this touching. The hypnotist has already assured the subject that, "I will not let you fall." The touching, since it involves the entire flat of the hand on the back and on the shoulder blades gives further validity to that assurance. In fact, as the swaying increases in amplitude, the point will be reached where if the hypnotist's hand were not restraining the subject, he would fall over. As this point is approached it is wise for the hypnotist to extend the arm around the back until, when the subject is falling back, he will be supported by the hypnotist's arm curved around his entire upper back region. It will be noted that restraint from falling forward does not require that the forward arm be extended further than just enough to place the hand on the near shoulder. If both arms had to be all the way around, the hypnotist would have to be standing very close and embracing the subject.

Since the terminal point in this induction is assumed to be reached when the subject falls back (often in a cataleptic condition) into the easy chair placed behind him, it is imperative that he be gently lowered into that chair, not dropped into it—which could jar him out of his hypnotic state. He must have no fear of letting himself go and sinking back into the chair, hence no anxiety that he will be permitted to fall and hurt himself.

Therefore, it is important that as the swaying backward increases in amplitude, the hypnotist gradually work his feet farther back so that one foot is about level with the patient's feet and the other two or three feet back, perhaps behind the front legs of the easy chair. This makes it possible for the hypnotist to support the subject who is falling backward and gradually, very gradually ease him into the chair. Sometimes patients will become so cataleptic throughout their entire body that they fall backward completely rigid, like a board, and their hips even have to be pushed down to conform to the chair. If the subject is either rigid or completely limp the induction proper is considered to have been completed at this point. Deepening techniques may be applied, or perhaps he is ready now for research or therapeutic procedures. Some subjects react to this Postural-Sway method with entry into a profound trance; others may be resistant or unresponsive to the procedure.

A variation in the technique can be employed with the resistant subject who manifests very little sway. When the hypnotist is saying, "You are drifting forward, forward, over forward, etc.," he lets his own body sway further to the rear of the patient, putting his weight on the leg which is behind the subject. Thus, as he starts the suggestions of swaying forward, the mouth (and hence the voice) of the hypnotist might normally be about level with the subject's ear. But as the subject sways slightly forward, the hypnotist has swayed in the opposite direction so that the subject hears the hypnotist's voice as it emanates from a position one or more feet behind him.

Then, when the hypnotist changes his suggestions to, "You are now swaying backward, backward, over backward, etc.," he moves himself in the counter-direction. As the subject drifts backward, the hypnotist's mouth (and hence the source of his voice) is a foot or so forward of the subject. The hypnotist's weight is now on his forward foot. Since we orient ourselves in space and determine direction by the angles at which sounds enter our respective two ears, the subject's illusion of swaying backward and forward is substantially enhanced. In fact, sometimes an unresponsive subject, who is standing quite still and not drifting at all, will get the feeling of a great arc of swaying because of the changing locus of the hypnotist's voice. Hypnosis relies on credibility. The illusion of much greater sway, therefore, operates to increase the subject's suggestibility.

Contra-indications for use of the Postural Sway procedure are that the patient is an invalid, weak or bedridden, suffers pain on standing, or is much larger than the hypnotist. A heavy person is very difficult to control when falling backwards, especially by a small hypnotist. Women wearing high heels should be asked to remove their shoes. In Volume II we will consider some of the underlying psychodynamic processes which may be initiated by this approach.

A Rapid Induction

The following method probably is not suited to clinical work. However, it may be used to demonstrate to a class that the trance state can often be initiated in a good subject in a very short period of time. Lengthiness of the induction process is not necessarily related to depth of involvement.

In this procedure the subject is asked to stand. To protect him, and to establish a set, two assistants are stationed at his side and told to "catch him when he falls." This method should not be attempted unless the hypnotist is certain that it will be successful as suggested by the subject's previous strong positive responses on susceptibility tests. The subject is then instructed in a firm, confident voice as follows:

"I am going to count 'one,' and you will remain wide awake and free from any hypnotic trance. Then I will count 'two,' and you will continue to remain awake. When I count 'three' you will still stay awake, but the moment afterward when I clap my hands you will *fall* instantly, in a fraction of a second, into a deep hypnotic state. Don't worry because my assistants will catch you when you fall."

The hypnotist counts "one" and then asks the subject, "Are you awake?" The affirmative reply is frequently accompanied by smiling. The count of "two" is given, and then the count of "three," after each of which the same question is asked. The hypnotist then claps his hands, and the good responder usually slumps immediately. As an additional precaution a chair should be put behind the standing subject, and the assistants can ease the slumping and deeply hypnotized person back into it.

Rapid Re-Hypnotization

If the subject has already been hypnotized at least once by the hypnotist and has clearly demonstrated the ability to enter a deep trance state, a long induction procedure may be quite unnecessary. This is especially true if a patient has been brought out of hypnosis to inquire about his reactions while in the state, and the period of conscious interview was brief—five minutes or less. The rapid re-hypnotization may be accomplished as follows:

"Extend your arm upward and out. Focus your eyes on the hand while I take your wrist. I am going to bring your arm down, and as I do you will go back into a deep state of relaxation like that from which you have just emerged." The hypnotist takes hold of the subject's wrist and brings the arm down gradually until it is all the way down, usually on the lap or leg. While doing this he says in a strong, commanding voice, "Here we go. Down—down—down. Deep—deep—deep," etc. If the subject is highly hypnotizable, has been hypnotized before by this hypnotist, and has recently been brought out of hypnosis, he usually sinks rapidly back into a hypnotic state. This is due to a condition called "the aura" which probably is simply the fact that when first brought out of hypnosis vestiges of the trance state continue. In fact, it may take five or more minutes until the patient is fully "out" of hypnosis and therefore requires a more lengthy induction to reenter trance.

Fig. 6:2. Rapid Re-hypnotization

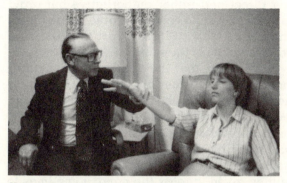

Hypnotist grasps wrist of subject and informs her of what will happen when he lowers her arm.

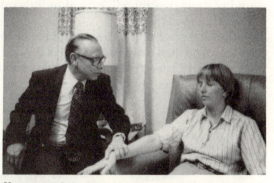

Hypnotist brings subject's arm down while simultaneously instructing her to go "deep-deep-deep."

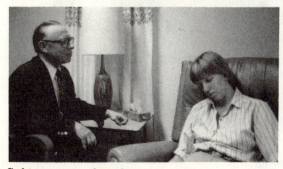

Subject enters deep hypnotic state.

The Coin Technique

This is another direct and rather authoritative but rapid approach. Different variations are advocated by different writers. Crasilneck and Hall (1975) suggest that the coin should be placed in the palm of the subject's hand. As suggestions are given to the effect that the hand will slowly turn there comes a moment at which the coin falls off. The subject has been told that when he hears the clink of the coin striking the floor his eyes will close and he will be deeply relaxed.

Kroger (1977) is most detailed in his instructions and begins the induction with the subject's eyes closed. In his approach the subject is instructed to clasp the coin tightly in his hand. Suggestions are then given to relax the hand, sometimes to the point of a count for each finger which then comes unclasped. The goal is the same, that when the coin falls the sound of its striking the floor will induce an immediate, deep hypnotic response.

In the Coin Technique the principles of set and expectation are employed, just as in the previous Rapid Induction method. It should be remembered that such approaches are quite directive and have both the advantages and limitations which inhere in an authoritative manner towards subjects or patients.

Fig. 6:3. The Coin Technique

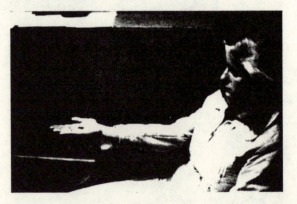

Subject stares at coin which has been placed on her hand.

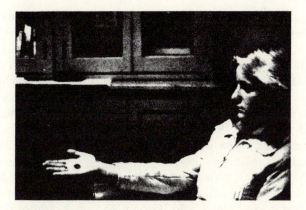

The hand gradually tips until coin falls off and subject enters hypnotic state.

Opposed Hand Levitation

This approach is designed for the subject who shows a great deal of overt resistance to the induction of hypnosis. Occasionally, one will have a patient who obviously perceives the hypnotic situation as one of confrontation between himself and the hypnotist. This may be manifested by such remarks as, "You can't hypnotize me because I have too strong a will power." Sometimes this tendency will be demonstrated in the arm-drop suggestibility test by a rising instead of lowering of the arm which is carrying the suggested weight. This phenomena has been described as "countercontrol" and represents a kind of reverse reaction to the "demand characteristics" of the situation.

The procedure involves the acceptance by the hypnotist of the subject's interpretation of the induction as a contest. In fact, the hypnotist specifically builds it up as a conflict situation between them. However, he then subtly restructures the suggestions until they imply that he, the hypnotist, is actively opposing the subject's efforts to achieve a "deep relaxed state," hence that the subject's "natural" desire to enter a hypnotic state is being deliberately counteracted by a physical conflict between the hypnotist's hand and the subject's hand. After a considerable struggle the subject finally "achieves" a state of hypnosis by overpowering the hypnotist. His needs to triumph over the doctor are mobilized and enlisted in the induction process.

The technique starts out the same as the traditional "hand-levitation" procedure described in Chapter 5. (See pages 124-131). However, instead of suggesting a differential sensation in one finger (Pg. 124, Item No. 4) the suggestion is given immediately that the hand is getting lighter and lighter and wants to float up off the desk or chair arm. This is continued for some time, and the amount of resistance to bringing the hand up noted. At a certain point the hypnotist abruptly changes his voice into a more demanding and challenging manner as follows:

"Even though your hand is getting lighter and wants to lift up into the air, I will not permit it to do so. I am putting my hand on it, and I will hold it down so that it cannot rise."

The hypnotist then places his hand firmly on top of the hand of the subject and presses down. The subject's reaction at this point is usually one of surprise and sometimes one of anger. His freedom of movement is now being specifically and physically restricted. This acts as a challenge and tends to mobilize his will to resist the hypnotist's suggestions. Accordingly, the hypnotist continues:

"I am holding your hand so strongly that even though your hand wants to rise up it cannot do so. My hand is stronger than yours, and yours is too weak to push back against mine."

The hypnotist then alternates slightly between pushing down on the back of the subject's hand and relaxing that pushing. If the will to resist is being stimulated in the subject, one will soon feel a tendency for his hand to push back. This will become evident as his hand slightly rises and maintains contact with the hypnotist's hand each time the doctor has raised his slightly.

The hypnotist continues with strong challenging remarks to the effect that the subject's hand is not as strong as the hypnotist's, that it must accept being held down and that it will not be able to rise. Notice that the "contact" is described as being "my hand" vs. "your hand," not between you and me. Of course, the subject inwardly interprets it as between himself and the hypnotist. However, by describing it as a conflict of the hands the subject feels freer to engage in the "battle." Moreover, the hands are being treated as "object," hence outside the self, not as "subject" or within one's volition. The rising of the subject's hand, therefore, constitutes a victory over the hypnotist for which he has no control and so no responsibility. ("Look what my hand does to yours. It can beat yours.")

While continuing the challenging remarks the hypnotist relaxes his downward pushing from time to time, permitting the hand of the subject to push back and begin to rise. When this occurs the hypnotist changes his remarks to take notice of the progress of the patient's hand as it rises against his.

"I shall push down against your hand with all my might, and even though yours seems to be pushing back a little it cannot be strong enough to overcome my hand."————"Your hand seems to be rising a bit, so I shall redouble my efforts to hold it down. It must be held down; it must not be permitted to

Fig. 6:4. Opposed Hand-Levitation Technique

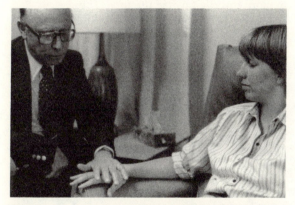

The hypnotist has just changed his voice to the more demanding and challenging manner, and he is pressing down firmly on the subject's hand.

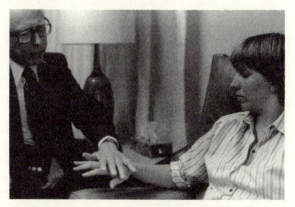

The subject's hand is pushing back against his and beginning to lift itself upward.

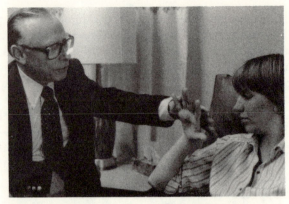

Subject's hand is gaining "strength" and is moving up more rapidly toward the face. The hypnotist's hand, although still resisting the upward movement is becoming "weaker."

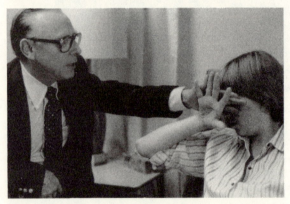

Subject's hand triumphally achieves its goal of touching face in spite of opposition from hypnotist. Subject enters hypnotic state with feeling of success.

rise any higher."————"Your hand is getting closer and closer to your face. It seems as if some very strong magnetic attraction between the hand and the face is drawing it closer. So I will push it back down all the harder," etc.

Of course, the hypnotist is slowly giving way. Whenever the subject's hand slows in its rise upward the hypnotist pushes down again. This is usually sufficient to cause it to resume its pushing back again and consequent further rise. Finally, when the two hands are getting close to the face, and the "struggle" is quite intense, the hypnotist begins to include such suggestions as the following:

"Your hand seems determined to reach your face in spite of my strongest opposition. And if it achieves a victory over my hand you can reach your goal of a wonderful state of relaxation in spite of all my opposition. I know you are thinking that you can reach this goal and enter a very deep comfortable state by proving that your hand is stronger than mine, and by it finally succeeding in touching your face in spite of my best efforts to stop it.————Now it's getting closer, closer, closer. It's almost touching, almost touching, *touching*. The hand has been able to reach your face in spite of my best efforts to prevent it from doing so. It won out, and you can now go into the deep state of relaxation feeling completely triumphant in that my best efforts were not strong enough to prevent you from achieving this comfortable state."

Obviously this procedure involves a certain measure of deception as the entire situation is restructured into a contest between hypnotist and subject whereby the subject triumphs over the hypnotist by entering a hypnotic state in spite of the hypnotist's "strong opposition." The technique is not frequently used; however, I have found it successful with certain hostile, paranoid patients who could not be hypnotized by any of the other methods.

The Progressive Anesthesia Technique

This method is much more gentle. It lacks the aggressiveness of the Opposed Hand-Levitation. It does involve touching and stroking the patient with all the meanings related to such contact, positive and negative (see Vol. II, Chapter 2).

The subject is asked to sit at a desk or table and to place both arms on the table in front of him. His attention is directed to one finger on one hand (the hypnotic narrowing of the field of perception) as follows:

"Focus all your attention on this finger. As I stroke it you will notice that it begins to feel numb." (Hypnotist strokes finger.) "As the numbness increases the finger gets stiffer. It tends to lift and become stiff, and it feels like a wooden peg." (Lifting and straightening of the finger is a motor sign of its involvement.) "Now I will stroke the next finger and it, too, will become numb and stiff like the first one. Both of them become numb and stiff.————Now the numb stiffness flows into still another finger," etc., until all the fingers are straight, stiff and slightly lifted. The numbness is then suggested into the whole hand. Each time the part of the body to become numb is lightly touched and stroked by the hypnotist. Gradually the numbness is moved up into the wrist, the forearm, through the elbow, into the upper arm and into the shoulder. While this is being suggested the entire arm, like each finger before, should become stiff and straight to signify the movement of the numbness through it.

Since the entire induction takes a few minutes it is well to support the stiff arm by letting the hand rest on the table. This avoids the undue fatigue which can result from holding the arm straight out for a considerable period of time.

From the shoulder, the numbness is passed over to the other shoulder by stroking across the back of the neck. It is then transferred down the other arm as the hypnotist continues the stroking while simultaneously describing the movement of the numb feeling, first into the other upper arm, through the elbow, the lower arm, the wrist, the hand, and each of the fingers. Both arms are now stiff and numb with the hands resting on the table.

At this point it seems wise not to continue the physical stroking on other parts of the body because of the sexual suggestiveness which it would entail. Accordingly, we simply desribe the continued flow of numbness:

"Down from your shoulders into your chest, then into your abdomen. Now your right (left) leg is beginning to get numb" (usually on the same side as the first arm which became numb). "The leg is getting straight and stiff down through the knee, the lower leg, your ankle, your feet and your toes," etc. The entire leg may at this point be sticking straight out and

Fig. 6:5. Progressive Anesthesia Procedure

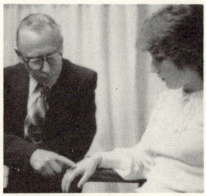

Initial position. Subject focusing on one finger which is being stroked by hypnotist. Finger is becoming stiff and numb.

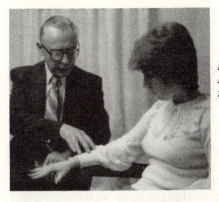

Hand is now stiff and numb. Hypnotist by stroking is transferring numbness up arm.

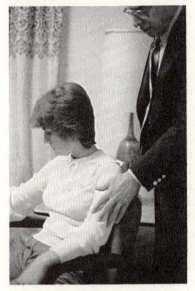

Hypnotist transferring numbness from right arm through right shoulder, back of neck and left shoulder to right arm.

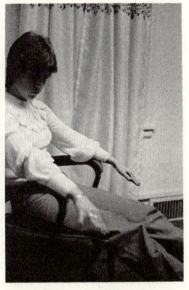

Numbness and stiffness now moved down trunk of body to legs.

suspended off the floor, a posture which will result in fatigue if continued too long.

The same suggestions are now implanted as relating to the numbness flowing down into the other leg. At this point all the body below the shoulders should be stiff and numb. Of course, it is essential that the suggestions closely follow the responses of the subject. Do not be rushed and permit plenty of time and repetition to occur, so that each member of the body is clearly affected before proceeding to the next one.

Finally, the numbness is suggested as moving up through the neck, through the face, the lips, up through the forehead, and last of all (if it is still necessary) closure of the eyes is suggested followed by suggestions of entering a deep comfortable "sleep" or state of relaxation. The stiffness may be removed, and the muscles told to relax, but retain the loss of feeling.

Depth of trance will be related to the extent and depth of the numbness. This can be tested by pricking the skin. This induction may be useful in preparing a patient for some painful surgical procedure in which some other anesthetic is to be further applied, or if hypno-analgesia is to be the only pain suppressant.

Non-Verbal Method

On rare occasions communication problems may make difficult, if not impossible, other standardized induction procedures. Perhaps the patient is deaf or speaks a foreign language unknown to the therapist. This technique may also be indicated with child subjects who are more responsive to postural suggestions than to verbal ones.

The subject is seated in a chair and instructed to hold both arms out in front of him and upward so that the hands are above the eye level. They should be parallel, the hands being about two feet apart. The hypnotist now moves back and forth in front of the subject from one side to the other, making a small postural change in the patient's right arm first, then over to the other side to make a similar change in the left arm.

First the right arm is bent at the elbow so that the hand comes a bit inward and downward (the right elbow simultaneously extending more outward). The hypnotist then moves over to the left side and repeats the movement of the patient's left arm in the same way. After each movement he pauses a few seconds and observes the posture. This permits him both to observe the patient's reaction and to allow time for adjustment to the new change in posture.

Once again he moves to the patient's right side and adjusts the right arm again slightly downward. This is then matched in a few seconds with a similar adjustment in the left hand. The postural adjustments of the arms and hands are constantly transmitting the message of "inward and downward," inward into one's self, downward toward a more unconscious level of awareness.

Finally, when the hands are almost together and are barely above the lap the hypnotist grasps both of them firmly by the wrist and forcibly lowers them rapidly all the way down. At this point the subject's eyes will usually close and his head slump forward on his chest. If this does not happen the hypnotist can pull the eyelids down, and by a push on the back of the head, administer this final forceful suggestion which implies, "Go inward and downward, close your eyes and enter a deep, relaxed, hypnotic state!"

No words have been spoken, but the induction has been accomplished by the series of progressively spaced changes in posture. To remove the hypnotic state which has been so achieved the hypnotist simply reverses the movements. First, he lifts up the head. Then he lifts up both arms to the position they held just prior to the forcible lowering of them. Next, one arm and hand at a time the movements are reversed. The movements are now outward and upward, "Come up out of yourself and back into the conscious state," is the message. Finally, the arms are back in their original position; the patient's eyes are fully open, his head is up. The hypnotist smiles at him and gently brings the arms down to his side from which he had originally raised them.

Fig. 6:6. Non-verbal Induction

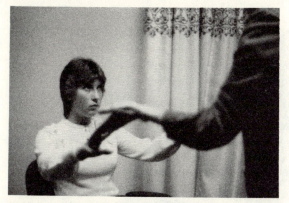

Initial position. Hypnotist lifting subject's hands into position with her own hands then gently withdrawing them and providing non-verbal communication to subject to keep arms extended.

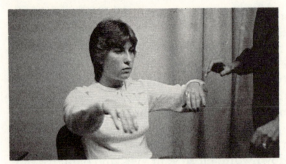

Subject has received message. Maintains arms extended.

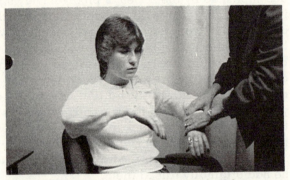

Hypnotist moves an arm downward and inward. Message to subject is, "Go down deeper and into your self."

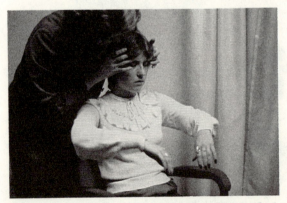

Hypnotist puts downward pressure above subject's eyelids. Non-verbal message is, "Close your eyes."

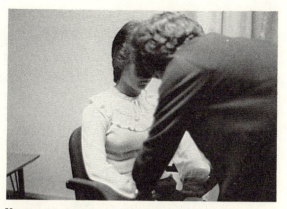

Hypnotist presses subject's hands all the way
down. Non-verbal message is a very forceful,
"Down!"

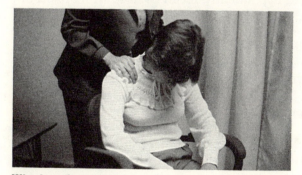

Which is then reinforced by pressing the shoulders down. Subject lowers head and slumps
into a hypnotic position.

The Rehearsal Technique

A simple way to hypnotize a patient who has experienced
hypnosis from some previous practitioner is to repeat or "rehearse" exactly the procedure used earlier. One inquires of
the subject what his other therapist did in hypnotizing him
and precisely in what order the suggestions were administered. For example: "You say that when your dentist, Doctor
X, hypnotized you he had you lie back in the dental chair and
relax?—All right. Please lie back on the couch and relax in the
same way.—Now what did he tell you to do first?—He said to

hold up your hand and focus your eyes on it? O.K. Do that. Hold up your hand and focus your eyes on it just like you did in the dental chair.—Then what did the doctor say?—He said to take three deep breaths.—O.K. Take three deep breaths. One—two—three. Good. Now what did the doctor say?—He told you to focus your eyes on the index finger and let yourself relax all over.—All right, then focus your eyes on the index finger and start relaxing all over. What came next?—He told you that your arm would get very heavy.—Let your arm get very heavy now.—Then what?—He told you that as your arm slowly came down, you come down with it into a deep state of relaxation.—Good. Now as your arm comes slowly down you will experience it just as before. You will come down with it into the same state of relaxation."

This procedure is then continued until the subject is completely involved hypnotically. It can be used with almost any technique and has the advantage that the patient is simply repeating step by step a procedure which has already been found to be effective for inducing in him a state of hypnosis. We assume that the subject's relationship with the previous hypnotist was constructive, and that he left at that time with a good feeling. Some inquiry might be undertaken before beginning this procedure, since if he had felt angry at his previous hypnotist, or the practitioner had not helped him, his underlying resentment can operate as a resistance making difficult or impossible his re-hypnotization by the same technique.

Sleep Variation of Rehearsal Technique

An interesting variation of the rehearsal approach can be used to hypnotize a subject for the first time utilizing his customary behavior in going to bed. The patient is simply asked to re-live the steps he goes through in retiring for the night. He is told to imagine that it is bedtime and he is ready for bed. It may be best to avoid suggesting the steps in removing his clothes since this could be interpreted by the patient as a sexually seductive move by the doctor or provoke erotic transference reactions. However, it can be suggested to him that he visualize himself as turning out the lights, pulling the bed covers back, crawling between the sheets, snuggling down, and then feeling the warm, relaxed feelings pouring through his muscles, his eyes getting heavier and heavier, his thoughts becoming less and less—and his final involvement in a "deep, relaxing, sleepy feeling." The procedure is the same as in the typical rehearsal of a previous induction, except here we must rely on the patient's report of his customary retiring behavior. It is possible to make errors in this approach since the hypnotist might say, "You feel your head sinking back into the comfortable pillow," when the subject does not generally sleep on a pillow. Suggestions which are contrary to reality tend to alert the patient and operate in the reverse direction from hypnotizing him.

Fantasy Techniques[1]

These are methods which employ suggestions aimed at getting the subject involved in rich imagination. They usually begin by asking him to close his eyes and then visualize something like the following:

"Just imagine that you are going to take a trip to Hawaii. You have your luggage in your hand and are in the airport getting ready to board the plane. You have your tickets, and you can see yourself now going through the hand luggage inspection. Everything is O.K., and you walk toward the boarding area. You can see many of the other passengers around you, some older people and a few children. You are now boarding the plane and finding your seat. You sit down, buckle on the safety strap, and relax back. The plane's motors start—you can hear their hum and feel the vibration. Now the plane begins to taxi out to the beginning of the runway from which it will take off. The sound of the motor increases, and you feel the thrust back into your seat as the plane roars down the runway and lifts off the ground. How exhilarated you feel about this wonderful vacation. You look down from the plane's window and see the tiny houses and cars way below you. You settle back in your seat. Perhaps the stewardess brings you some coffee or a drink. Now you reach the ocean shore. The beaches slip behind you, and all you can see is the great blue sea with a few tiny, white-capped waves below. It is so pleasant, and you are relaxing deeper and deeper, perhaps into a drowsy nap. Hours pass, and as you look out the window

[1]For specific verbalizations of a number of fantasies see Chap. 12. Guided Fantasy Techniques, in Gibbons (1979).

again, you see ahead some little dots of islands. You are coming in over Hawaii. Soon the features of Diamond Head with the beaches surrounded by many palm trees become visible below. You are feeling very excited about reaching your destination and getting to do all the interesting things you have been dreaming you would do when you got to Hawaii."

The fantasy can be made short or long. However, the important point is that the hypnotist must picture each step in the most vivid language possible, using descriptive adjectives. In this way he induces the subject to halt his own inner, distracting thoughts and to exclude his contact with outer reality other than that in the relationship with the hypnotist. The hypnotist and the fantasy he is elaborating become the universe of experience for the subject. Once this has been established he is most likely to follow other suggestions, such as therapeutic ones. Fantasy techniques like this one can serve both as an induction method and as a deepening procedure once initial induction has been completed. In fact, suggestibility tests, induction techniques, and deepening procedures (to be discussed in the next chapter) are all on a continuum. The extension of one leads on into the other.

Other fantasies might involve going to see a movie, descending in a diving sphere to the bottom of the ocean, traveling on a train, going to a department store, or participating in an archeological expedition. The numbers, of course, are unlimited and restricted only by the hypnotist's ingenuity at providing the kind of fantasies with which the subject can identify. Occasionally, a fantasy will cue off a resistance or negative response in the subject, perhaps manifested by his suddenly shaking off the state and alerting himself. Simply inquire what it was that induced this reaction, and then start again by deleting the negative item in the fantasy which disturbed the patient, initiating another fantasy, or trying an entirely different induction technique.

Subject-Object or Indirect Technique

This is a rather unusual approach since it involves a manipulation of the locus of the patient's self perception. There seems to be considerable variation in individuals' ability to respond to it. Some enter rapidly into a very deep state with this procedure; others find that they cannot throw themselves into the alterations of psychological position which it requires. It might go like this:

"Imagine that you are coming to my office like you did today. You are in your car and driving from your house along the streets you need to pass to get here. You can visualize the various buildings, the people walking on the sidewalk, the other cars. You experience yourself in the driver's seat with your hands on the steering wheel and making all the little turns required to manuever your car in the traffic. You turn into the driveway and stop your car in this building's parking lot. You turn the keys to the engine off and open the car door, preparing to get out.

"At this moment a change seems to occur in you. You are now standing a few feet behind your car in the parking lot and watching a person get out of your car. She (he) is wearing your clothes and has your color of hair. You follow her as she walks to my office and opens the door of the waiting room. She sits down for a few minutes and then is ushered into this office sitting down in the easy chair beside mine. You are standing just inside the doorway watching her. You notice that she is wearing a brown suit with a green scarf just like yours, that she has your red hair, and that her face looks just like what you see when you look into a mirror.

"Notice how she is reacting to my talking to her. I am starting to give her some hypnotically inducing suggestions, and it occurs to you as you watch her, the one who looks like you and is wearing your clothes, that she is beginning to get rather drowsy. Her eyes look very heavy. They blink and are beginning to close. You keep watching and observe a deep relaxation passing through all her body. Her arms relax. Her chest relaxes. Her legs relax, and you think to yourself 'My, that person who looks like me is relaxing into a very deep state of relaxation. Notice how deeply she is going.' You keep observing her as she sinks deeper and deeper, and as you hear my voice droning on you think that you, too, would like to achieve the same deep relaxation as she has. You decide that you would like to join her, and accordingly you walk across the room and stand just in front of her chair. You turn around and back down into her seat merging your body with hers until your head coincides with hers. Your arms and hers are the same. Your body fuses with hers, and your legs and hers are the same. As you take on her entire body you are aware that you are also taking on her feelings. You sense the deep relaxation she had achieved pouring through your own self, and you enjoy the profound sense of security and warmth which she had reached. You and she are now one and the same, and you are involved in a most deep and comfortable state of relaxation."

Notice how subject and object have been manipulated in this procedure. The patient first involves herself in rehearsing her trip to your office. This is vivified with many suggestions as to the buildings, people and cars she has encountered along the way. They should be described as specifically as possible but not so specifically that they do not represent reality. Hence, don't tell her she is driving along 9th Street if she actually came to the office along 10th Street. Up to the point of parking the car the suggestions must coincide with reality.

Ego states have boundaries, and so we use boundaries to shift from one to another. Walls can symbolically represent boundaries, and doors are passages from one state to another, hence, passing from one room in one's "ego-house" to another. Accordingly, we used the moment of leaving the car to make a change of self perspective. The self (subject) is now moved to a position behind the car. And the "driving ego-state" is changed from subject to object. She now "sees" the driver of the car emerging from it, while before she experienced herself as the driver. The state of being the driver of the car is now no longer subject. It has become object ("her" instead of "me"), and the patient perceives her body as a "not-me." To keep the identity clear, the person who is emerging from the car is described as having the patient's clothes and hair, and later as having the same features which the subject sees when she looks in the mirror. When we look into a mirror we see ourselves as "object," hence, as others see us.

This change, which is really a kind of temporary dissociation, is continued as the woman who looks like her enters the office and sits down in the chair next to the doctor. It is that image (object) which is then hypnotized, while the subject's self views the process from a different location near the office door. Finally, the observing ego-state is fused again with the experiencing ego-state, and the person resumes the experiencing of her own body again. However, as she takes on the body she must also take on all the feelings which that body has. Accordingly, if her "body over there" has been hypnotized, and she returns to it, she must also assume the hypnotic state which it includes.

This is an intricate and sophisticated induction technique, but is often effective when other more direct approaches have failed. The subject-object manipulations which are involved can also be utilized in a number of therapeutic techniques which will be described in later chapters.

Self-Induction Procedure

Many of the techniques which have been described can be adapted to self-hypnosis if this is indicated. This writer has some reservations about teaching individuals self-hypnosis. Many people request it, and there is no doubt that at times it is a valuable approach. The doctor may not always be available; the patient may suffer from intractable pain and is in need of immediate relief. People can use self-hypnosis to improve study habits, teach themselves to go to sleep, improve their golf games, etc.

However, there are many individuals who seek hypnosis as a new kind of thrill. They wish to experiment with their own states of consciousness. Some have tried various drugs; they want a new and cheap way of "turning on." Still others are already given to too much dissociating. These include borderline psychotics or others who are increasingly living their lives in fantasy rather than facing up to the realities of adapting to a world of people and challenges. Such individuals may be more harmed by hypnosis, especially of the self-induced type, than helped by it. They employ it as a way of avoiding life's problems rather than solving them. Also, some people will use self-induced hypnotic analgesia to suppress every pain, even those which should serve as warnings to consult their doctor or dentist. For these reasons one should be conservative about teaching self-hypnosis, and consider carefully both the purposes to which the individual intends to put the hypnotic modality, his inner motivations, and the condition of his own inner integration, ego strength, and maturity.

For those for whom such a procedure is indicated, either for self treatment, or as an adjunct to be used between sessions with their doctor, Helen Watkins has developed an adaptation of the arm drop approach which can be easily taught and practiced. She proposes the following steps:

SELF-HYPNOSIS

1. Finger concentration with hand drop to relaxation. (Initial induction by hypnotherapist involves staring at index or middle finger with eyes either open or closed, suggesting that the other fingers will fade into periphery of their vision and that as they continue to stare the hand and arm become heavy; the more they stare the heavier the arm becomes. The suggestion continues that as the arm and hand become heavier, the hand begins to move down and as the hand moves down they begin to move down into a state of relaxation but they will not enter a deep state of relaxation until the hand is all the way down.)
2. Muscular relaxation—head to toe.
3. Internalize distractions—"With every bit of noise I hear I can go deeper and deeper."
4. Concentrate on breathing—"With every breath I exhale I will become more and more relaxed."

Down 10 steps to room with couch.

6. Repeat mentally: (Spoken by hypnotherapist during initial induction.)

Relax deeply ... relax deeply ... As I relax deeply ... I can go to a deep state of concentration ... I won't be asleep, I can be alert ... and I can learn to use these procedures in my own style and my own way ... so that I can become the kind of person I wish to be, the kind of person I can be ... I can learn to use this technique to rest and relax more deeply ... I can use it to go to sleep at night ... I can use it to study or to concentrate more ... or to gain more self-understanding and more self-control.

7. Meditation for a minute using personalized sentences that state positive ideas about yourself, or use for whatever purpose self-hypnosis is initiated.
8. Self-arousal by counting from 1 to 5.

Self-hypnosis has received increasing interest among both experimental and clinical workers. The entire July 1981 issue of the *International Journal of Clinical and Experimental Hypnosis* is devoted to this topic. Fromm, Brown, Hurt, Oberlander, Boxer and Pfeifer (1981) have pointed out that the experience of "absorption" and the facing of the general reality orientation is found in both hetero-hypnosis and self-hypnosis. However, age regression seems to be easier in hetero-hypnosis. Self-hypnosis is much richer in imagery. Johnson (1981) analyzes the findings of the Chicago group (Fromm et al.) and points out that self-hypnosis opens a new and rich field which has as yet been relatively unexplored. Benson, Arns and Hoffman (1981) argue that the chief value in self-hypnosis is in establishing a physiological state related to relaxation. Sacerdote (1981) holds that there is no "pure" self-hypnosis and describes a number of difficulties encountered by subjects during self-hypnosis. While finally, Orne and McConkey (1981) compare research and theoretical viewpoints relating self- and hetero-hypnosis. Shor (1978) has published an *Inventory of Self-Hypnosis* designed to evaluate self-hypnotic performance (see also Gardner, 1981, who discusses self-hypnosis with children). In general, the area has been much less researched than hetero-hypnosis but promises to open new approaches to effective clinical treatment.

The Approaches of Milton Erickson[2]

Milton Erickson (Haley, 1967, 1973; Zeig, 1982) was a widely known practitioner in the field of clinical hypnosis who contributed broadly to its literature. His approach to the hypnotic modality was so unique and substantially different from other workers in the field that specific analyses have been published which aim at a theoretical explanation of his techniques (Erickson, Rossi & Rossi, 1976).

He apparently had considerable success in hypnotizing relatively resistant subjects and in developing innovative therapeutic strategies within the hypnotic modality. We will not attempt here to present a detailed description of his procedures, and readers so interested are referred to his original publications (see Haley, 1967) for a compilation of many of these. However, a brief coverage of some of his basic concepts and illustrations of how he translated these into hypnotherapeutic manipulations is in order.

Erickson believed that hypnosis is primarily an intra-psychic process and hence, induction techniques should not rely on apparatus, such as crystal balls, metronomes, etc. Rather, the subject should be induced to image the crystal balls, to "hear" imagined music or to sense the touch of a hypnotist's hand which is visualized in his "mind's eye." This movement

---

[2]For a complete bibliography of Erickson's publications from 1929 to 1977 see Gravitz and Gravitz (1977).

from attention to outer stimuli into concentration with inner images has a profound influence in drawing the subject into an hypnotic state.*

Erickson held that many failures in hypnotic induction are the result of the hypnotist's spending too little time with the patient. He stated (1952) that he often devoted several hours conditioning a patient before securing a trance state. When it is suggested to the patient that he hallucinate, he may report visual images. However, if these are readily accepted by the hypnotist as real they may remain simply at a conscious image level. The time and continued suggestion, that which began as an "as if" becomes real. The subject becomes deeply involved in the experience.

Another principle which Erickson emphasized is that of "pacing." By that he meant assuring that each suggestion given to the subject is within his ability to execute and is fully carried out before the next and more challenging one is administered. Amateur hypnotists attempt to jump rapidly from a simple suggestion, perhaps the lifting of a hand, into an extremely demanding one, such as distorting perception into a positive or negative hallucination. The induction process must proceed stepwise with ample time for the subject to become increasingly involved in the hypnotic state.

Perhaps one of the most important principles emphasized by Erickson is the protection of the integrity of the subject. In one case he described an incident involving automatic handwriting in which the subject agreed to permit the reading of that which she would write, but Erickson continued to protect her right to secrecy, even after her apparent permission to break it. The result was her involvement shortly in a very profound trance. Similarly, he would suggest to a subject who was in a light trance that he can dream a dream then forget it, that he will not recall it until it is so desired. Or he would instruct the patient to withhold some item of information from the hypnotist. Strong appreciation of all of a subject's responses are given. In Erickson's approach he emphasized what was happening experientially within the patient rather than what the hypnotist was doing to the patient. Erickson often issued his induction suggestions in the form of a challenge. For example, when a subject asked if hypnosis could be

---

*It is interesting to note that present-day cognitive-behaviorists such as Cautella (1975) are rediscovering the value of visualization techniques for the facilitation of such behavioral therapy techniques as desensitization.

induced while standing, Erickson's response was, "Why not demonstrate that it can be?" He held that one should accept resistance that is offered and work with it rather than trying to overcome it. When resistance shows that a subject is ambivalent about entering hypnosis, a suggestion might be given which fails. The subject is pleased at defeating the hypnotist and becomes less resistant to future suggestions. Erickson often employed a technique suggesting the repetition of dreams with different content but the same meaning. He reported that the trance is deepened with each dream.

A perceptual approach suggested by Erickson which seems to be effective involves having the subject move his attention from one object to another in the room and then close his eyes and visualize them again.

A trance may be induced or deepened by asking the subject to speculate and describe what his behavior and experience would be like if he were hypnotized. This is a variation of the rehearsal technique.

Erickson would often make a series of requests which could hardly be avoided, but compliance would gradually induce the subject to enter hypnosis. The following is an example. "Are you willing to cooperate with me by continuing to pace the floor—as you are now doing? Will you please turn toward the chair in which you can sit. Now please turn away from the chair in which you can sit. Now please turn again toward the chair in which you will shortly find yourself comfortably seated." (Note the implication here of involuntary activity, e.g., "in which you will shortly find yourself comfortably seated.") Finally, "Now you can sit in the chair and go deeply as you relate your history." By complying with each request the subject has committed himself gradually to sitting in the chair, and has further committed himself to "going deeply" as he relates his history once seated there.

Summary

The number of approaches to hypnosis are legion. Each practitioner has developed specific techniques which he finds effective. Furthermore, many of those which we have described may have different results depending on whether the hypnotist has used an authoritative or permissive manner in administering them. Most of them, however, will be found similar to one or more of the foregoing. It is advised that you learn certain ones well. Practice them a great deal, with volunteer subjects if possible, before using them on patients. The professional hypnotherapist will usually find that a few approaches in which he is sensitive and highly skilled will serve the needs of most of his patients. Familiarity with some of the other, more advanced approaches may be found valuable in specialized instances. Confidence and skill are probably more important for the induction of hypnotic states than the techniques themselves. Hypnosis may be an altered state of consciousness, but for clinical practice it is equally an intensive inter-personal relationship experience between the therapist and the patient.

Outline of Chapter 6. Advanced Techniques of Hypnotic Induction

1. Controversy over hypnotizability as a fixed trait or subject to variability
2. Advanced techniques of induction
   a. Postural-sway
   b. Rapid inductions
   c. The coin technique
   d. Opposed hand-levitation
   e. Progressive anesthesia
   f. Non-verbal approach
   g. Rehearsal
      1. Sleep variation
   h. Fantasy techniques
   i. Subject-object or indirect technique
   j. Self-hypnosis
   k. The approaches of Milton Erickson

Chapter 7

Deepening Techniques

Hypnotic "Depth" as One of Degree

If hypnosis were simply an either-or we could at this point proceed directly to treatment. However, its induction appears to be a continuous process, starting with the first responses to suggestion and gradually developing into an increasingly profound involvement in the hypnotic modality. Although some techniques bring an almost instantaneous immersion in hypnosis, in most cases time is required for the subject to adjust to the hypnotic mode of perception and behavior. Suggestibility tests which elicit hypnotic responses merge into an induction process with no demarcating line, except one we have arbitrarily defined. Induction techniques, when prolonged, tend to carry the subject even further into the trance state. Accordingly, we can conceptualize that state as one of degree. A person is not either in or out of a hypnotic state; he is in such a state lightly, significantly, or deeply. Thus the hypnotic susceptibility tests, described in Chapter Four, appear to measure, not only the ability of an individual to be hypnotized, but also the "depth" to which it is possible to hypnotize him.

There is a misconception among lay people and many professionals that unless one is deeply involved one has not truly been hypnotized. Therapists often hear a new patient react to his first hypnotic induction with a statement like, "But doctor, I wasn't hypnotized. I could hear you all the time." Being "under hypnosis" seems to mean to many being in an unconscious condition, one in which the voice of the hypnotist is not heard and his suggestions not remembered upon "awakening." There is further the implicit feeling that unless such a state was achieved, therapeutic suggestions will be ineffective and hypnotherapy contraindicated.

The Therapeutic Value of Light and Medium States

It was pointed out in Chapter Three that certain phenomena, such as regression and post-hypnotic hallucinations, require a rather deep state to be elicited. Such phenomena represent the more striking aspects of hypnosis and tend to establish the conviction of its reality to the observer. It is also true that suggestions planted in the deeper trance states have an increased probability of being carried out and of lasting longer. Since we know that less than one-quarter of unselected subjects are usually capable of reaching deep hypnotic levels, this would tend to discourage practitioners on the grounds that they could hope for effective results only with a minority of their patients.

Fortunately, the picture is not that discouraging. Not only do many therapeutic suggestions hold when implanted during light and medium states of hypnotic involvement, but some practitioners have argued that in certain types of therapy the condition of a light hypnosis is to be preferred (Conn, 1959). For example, if our goal, as in the analytic therapies, is both to lift into consciousness material of which the patient has previously been aware, and also assure that this new awareness has been consciously assimilated and integrated to the fullest degree, then material which has been discovered while the patient has been only lightly hypnotized may bring about greater therapeutic change. Deeply repressed material may, as maintained by Anna Freud (1946), come temporarily to consciousness, but in by-passing ego-integration be soon forgotten and re-repressed. Nothing happens and the patient does not change.

The Relationship Between Depth of Hypnosis and Ego Participation

At this point perhaps we might formulate the relation of trance depth to various therapies, psychoanalytic and hypnoanalytic, as follows (See Figure 7:1):

Figure 7:1.

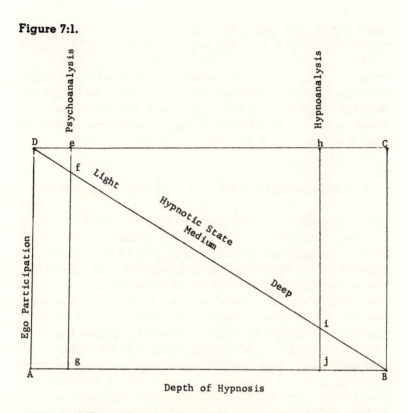

DAB: Conscious Awareness.
DBC: Pre-conscious and Unconscious Material.

In the rectangle in Figure 7:1 let the dimension AB represent the depth of trance, extending from A, a completely alert condition, to B, the deepest possible hypnosis. This might represent what Erickson (1952) has termed a "plenary trance." At right angles might be designated the degree of ego participation, correlated at least, if not theoretically identical, with the factor of conscious awareness. As the state of hypnosis (represented by the area DBC) increases, the condition of conscious, egotized experience (represented by the area DBA) lessens. At the AD position an individual is completely alert, fully in contact with his outer world, and retaining all critical faculties. As he moves along the diagonal line DB through induction and deepening procedures his behavior and experiencing take on increasingly the characteristics typical of hypnosis. His contact with the external world (except that with his hypnotist) is gradually withdrawn. His sense of criticality is lowered. He regresses into more primitive behavior and thought. First pre-conscious then unconscious and primary process ideation become more evident. Theoretically, at point B the ego ceases participation, and he would lapse into a coma-like state, which if it were ever completely reached, would result even in breaking off contact with the hypnotist. We might hypothesize that under such a circumstance we would have to wait for natural forces within the subject to change and bring him back into contact with reality.

Characteristics of Very Deep Hypnosis

Sherman (1971) studied subjects who had been placed in very deep hypnotic states, much more profound than are secured in therapeutic hypnosis. They described their experiences as "being everything, feeling oneness with everything, loss of knowledge of individual identity, no 'self', absolute mental quiet, no thoughts or images." According to Sherman, the subject had "passed beyond all those cognitive patterns that define him as a specific person and separate him from other people and his environment. What is left is undifferentiated awareness—the awareness of purely 'being' through which the person is identical to everything in the universe." Such a state seems to be similar to the condition of "satori," the goal of Zen meditation (Watts, 1957). Satori aims at a loss of individual identity and a complete merging with the universe.

It is interesting to speculate that this is the condition of experiencing reached by subjects at point B on our scale in Figure 7:1. However, the achievement of such levels of depth is extremely rare and accomplished with only a few individuals after extremely protracted and skillful induction. We simply do not see such states in the general practices of clinical hypnosis. At no time in the experience of this practitioner has any patient ever passed beyond the limits of communication.

Handling the Subject Who Resists Coming Out of Hypnosis

We need have no fear that our patient will go into a hypnosis so deeply that we cannot bring him out. Occasionally a subject will so much enjoy the tranquility of the hypnotic state that he will be somewhat slow to emerge. For example, suppose we have informed him that he will be completely alert at the count of five. We have counted to five, and he has either not opened his eyes, or does so slowly. All that is necessary is to suggest to him something as follows:

"It really is enjoyable to relax in this comfortable state— and I wish it was possible to stay in this position. Unfortunately, I have someone coming whom I must see this next hour. However, I promise you that we can repeat this experience if you wish at your next session. Why don't you bring yourself out of hypnosis in your own way and at your own speed. By simply suggesting to yourself that you will continue to feel very good and counting up to five you can become quite awake and yet retain the pleasure of the present moment. I will be quiet while you do this."

I have never found a subject or patient who did not respond to such an approach. There is no cause for alarm or fright simply because a subject is somewhat slow in responding to suggestions for terminating hypnosis.

Returning to our consideration of Figure 7:1 it will be noted that line "efg" is drawn at the left hand side of the figure to represent the condition typical of psychoanalysis where the patient is reclining on the couch, hence probably in a light hypnoidal state. He is told to preoccupy himself with inner associations and to ignore external stimuli. This has moved him inward from the AD axis and permits the release (line segment "ef") of preconscious material and unconscious derivatives as described by Freud (1953). There is still a large part of his "self" egotized as represented by line segment "fg."

In the deeper states of hypnosis, such as are sometimes employed in hypnoanalysis, the reverse is true. A great deal of unconscious and possibly primary process material becomes accessible as represented by line segment "hi." However, there is present at that time only minimal conscious ego participation in the process as measured by the short line segment "ij."

Without wishing at this point to proceed too far along hypothetical lines we might ask whether the greatest therapeutic movement in an analytic treatment would occur at stage "efg" or at level "hij." Would the greatest production occur where there is a small amount of raw material (ef) and a large processing factory (fg) or where there is a large quantity of raw material (hi) and a relative small factory to integrate and process it (ij)? From such speculation we might arrive at the position that, either in an alternation of hypnotic depth or in the intermediate trance states, would be found the optimal conditions for lifting repressions and integrating newly discovered insights into a significant personality change. From such a viewpoint neither the state in which traditional psychoanalysis is conducted nor that in deep hypnoanalysis would represent the most efficient condition for therapeutic movement. But let us leave further speculation along these lines to later chapters on hypnoanalytic therapy and return to a consideration of procedures for measuring and altering hypnotic depth.

Measuring Trance Depth

While the depth of the state can be inferred by trying out the subject's ability to execute various phenomena (see the Davis and Husband Scale, Chapter 4, pp. 85-86), this involves interrupting the deepening procedure. A more subjective approach can be tried using an informal number scale whose coordinates have been set by the hypnotist.[1] This can be especially valuable when a patient has been once hypnotized and we want to know whether he is as deeply involved as he was during the previous session, less deeply so, or has achieved an even deeper state. He may be instructed somewhat as follows:

"Let us use the number zero to represent your state of mind when you are unhypnotized, completely alert and not hypnotically involved at all. Levels 1 and 2 would indicate a light hypnotic relaxation. Let 10 represent the deepest stage you have ever achieved under hypnosis. Now tell me, what number would represent your present level of involvement." Perhaps the subject says, "seven." One can then continue the deepening procedure if he wishes to get the patient at least to the same depth as previously. As one works further with that patient he may sink into new levels of depth and report that he is now at levels 12, 15, etc. Such a scale, or course, is not validated; it is subjective, and it varies with every subject. However, it does provide a useful yardstick to the therapist in estimating just where his patient is during the induction-deepening procedure. It seems to have an internal validity to the subject.

[1]Self-report scales have been found to correlate well with objective measures of suceptibility such as the SHSS. For a review of these see Tart (1978/79).

Deepening Techniques

Hypnotic movement, itself, seems to deepen the state. By that we mean that each suggestion which is carried through intensifies the subject's involvement in the process. On the other hand, suggestions which are administered but not executed by the subject may have the effect of lightening his trance. It is important, therefore, that suggestions be timed and proceed in a systematic way from the simple to the more complex. One does not suggest a post-hypnotic hallucination before one has achieved such easier responses as eye-closure or arm-drop. As in many other life situations nothing succeeds like success. When one moves through a hierarchy of suggestions ranging from simple movements to complex alterations of perception and thought, the state of hypnosis progressively deepens. Each suggestion successfully executed makes easier the accomplishment of the next one. This phenomenon has been termed "homoaction" by Weitzenhoffer (1953). Therefore, as long as we continue to administer suggestions, especially of a difficulty and complexity which increase by small degrees, we will be deepening the state.

Fractionation

The principle of deepening through hypnotic movement has been termed "fractionation" by Vogt (1896). In its simplest form the subject is hypnotized, awakened, re-hypnotized, re-awakened, etc. As the in and out of trance movement is continued the individual tends to sink deeper and deeper into involvement in the hypnotic state.

A more systematic use of this principle that can be used after an initial induction would be as follows:

"When I say an odd number, like, 'one,' let yourself relax more deeply. Go down into a more profound state. However, when I say an even number, like 'two,' alert yourself slightly. Let yourself come up a little. But then as soon as I say the next odd number, 'three,' go down even deeper than before. Go down and down and continue to relax more profoundly until I say the next even number, 'four.'" (Continue this way.) "Go down on five. Then up a bit on six. Down again further on 'seven.' And up, 'eight.' Down, 'nine.' Up, 'ten.'" (At this point emphasize the word "down" strongly and wait a few seconds after each "down" suggestion. Speak "Up, ten," much more lightly and go almost immediately into, "Down, eleven." Now continue as follows: "Twelve-*thirteen*"———"fourteen-*fifteen*"———"Sixteen-*seventeen*"———"Eighteen-*nineteen*," etc. The even number is spoken lightly and rapidly. The odd number is articulated almost immediately afterward, drawled out, and there is a pause after speaking it before going to the next pair, "Twenty-*twenty-one*." This procedure can be continued as long as it is felt desirable to deepen the state further.

The Summer Day (a freedom from distraction scene)

Inducing the subject to visualize a very pleasant, relaxing scene is often effective in achieving greater hypnotic depth. The writer has found the following one typical of this approach:

"Just imagine that it is a warm summer afternoon and you are lying on a green, grassy slope on a hillside miles away from where anybody or anything could disturb you. It is extremely peaceful. The grass is very soft and thick. There are a few trees in the distance but the landscape is like a meadow, covered with thick, green grass and a few wild flowers. It is quiet and the sky overhead is a deep, rich blue with only a few soft, fluffy clouds floating in it. The sun is beating down, and you feel so peaceful, so relaxed, so safe and so comfortable that you are allowing yourself to drowse more and more. It is as if the only thought you have is one which goes round and round in your head and says, "deeper relax, deeper relax, deeper relax."

The therapist may continue to describe this scene as the patient becomes increasingly involved in the pleasurable fantasy.

Progressive Warm, Heavy Feeling Procedure

Another deepening technique can be added onto this summer scene if one wishes, as follows:

"There is a warm, numb feeling beginning to form in your forehead just above the eyes. Now it starts to spread over the top of your head, into your face and all through your head. Your head feels warm and heavy. This is like a numb wave of warmness that is sweeping down through your body. It brings the most pleasant sensation of heaviness and relaxation. Now it moves down through your neck, and your neck becomes heavy. You make it heavy. Heavy, heavy, heavy. This warm, numb, heavy feeling now goes through your shoulders and down into your arms and hands. They feel like the limbs on the trunk of a tree.

"And now this warm, heavy feeling moves into the trunk of your body, down through your chest and your abdomen, and the trunk of your body feels warm and heavy. This feeling now drifts down into your legs, your thighs, the calves of your legs and into your feet, and they, too, feel warm and numb and heavy."

This pattern may be repeated several times. Some hypnotists prefer to have the "warm, numb, heavy" feeling or a "relaxed" feeling start in the feet and move up the body instead. The subject's report of the way that causes him to respond best should be the one of choice after it has been tried.

Descending Stairs Technique

This procedure combines visualization with implicit motor movement. It also brings in tactile and kinesthetic imagination, the concept of going "down," and is open-ended in the sense that it can be continued as long as necessary. The verbalization might go somewhat as follows:

"Imagine that you and I are standing at the top of a staircase looking down. The steps are covered with a soft, plush carpet of your favorite color." (Note opportunity for choice by subject.) "As you look farther down, the stairs seem to fade out into a soft, warm darkness. We will walk down these stairs as you slide your hand along the smooth, hardwood bannister. I will walk with you and count steps. Each count is another step down the soft, plush-carpeted stairs. Here we go, stepping down, one—two—three—four—five—six—seven—eight—nine—ten. Warm, heavy feelings spread over your entire body as your feet sink into the soft carpet, and the gentle darkness floats around you more and more with each step. Let us walk down more stairs together, plush-carpeted stairs as you slide your hand along the smooth bannister, eleven—twelve—thirteen—fourteen—fifteen—sixteen—seventeen—eighteen—nineteen—twenty."

This deepening process is open-ended, and one can continue to count the descending stairs with a reinforcing repetition of the image of the plush carpet, the smooth, hardwood bannister, and the dimming of the light about every ten steps.

Notice the many factors involved in this fantasy which facilitate the deepening process. First, there is relationship between hypnotist and subject ("you and I" standing and walking down together). Next, there is the "soft plush carpet" which permits the subject a choice of his "favorite color." The motor concept of "stepping down" by analogy suggests "going down" into a deeper hypnotic state. The increasing darkness also implies a progressive reduction of external stimuli. Repetition and monotony add to the deepening effect.

Variations of this approach involve having the subject go down an elevator in a large building or down a mine shaft as the light above fades out. Sometimes an individual shows fear or resistance to "going down" stairs. Perhaps at a tender age he fell down the cellar steps. In such cases the same deepening effect may be secured by having him walk up stairs into an increasing light until he is "floating on a cloud."

Timed-breathing Approach

Observe the normal breathing of the subject and say to him, "With each breath you will relax deeper and deeper." Then repeat, "Deeper relax,"————"Deeper relax"———— "Deeper relax" over and over, timing it with every exhalation. This can be continued for several minutes.

The Metronome

The same timing method can be employed using a metronome. Set its speed at about sixty beats to the minute and then say to the subject, "As you hear this ticking around you will relax deeper and deeper. It is as if the ticking were saying to you, 'deeper—relax. Deeper————relax. Deeper————relax.'" Time your remarks so that "deeper" and "relax" each coincide with a tick. Repeat your "deeper————relax" ten or more times in synchronization with the metronome. Then inform the subject that he will continue to think "deeper———— relax" with each tick that as he does he will sink into a deeper and deeper state. No more need be said. He can be left, preferably relaxing on a couch, listening to the metronome for up to thirty minutes or more at a time.

The ticking of some metronomes may be quite loud and act as a distraction to deep relaxation. In this case place the metronome in a tall drawer, such as are often part of the ordinary business desk, if this is available in the office. With the metronome ticking inside the closed drawer the sound is muffled and seems to come from a distance.

On occasion, I have found that the subject regresses into a normal sleep instead of an hypnotic state after listening to the metronome for a long time. Although suggestions can often be given during normal sleep to turn it into hypnosis, it is preferable to awaken him and begin the induction again.

Floating in a Cloud

Asking the subject to imagine that he is floating in a soft, fluffy cloud, or that he can feel the soft cloud wrapped around him like a fleecy blanket often deepens the state by encouraging a regression to infantile fantasies.

Revolving in the Cloud

An extension of the "Floating in a Cloud" technique can sometimes be used that involves manipulation of the kinesthetic and vestibular sensations. It might go as follows: "You are now floating in this soft cloud miles above the earth. You can see the tiny houses and people way below you, and you feel a great sense of strength and peace. It seems now as if you are revolving around and around in that cloud so that first you see the earth below you. Then you are rotating backwards so that it is now behind you. Now you are turning so that it is above you. Now, it is in front of you. And you continue floating over backwards, round and around. And the earth continues to change as it is below you, behind you, above you, in front of you. Below———Behind———Above———In front. Around and around."

This can be kept up for some time as the individual feels himself rotating around and around as oriented by the place of the earth "far below" him.

Revolving Wheels Fantasy

A technique to which some subjects react by entering a most profound state is as follows:

"You are in the country lying on a grassy slope. You notice in front of you a large old-fashioned wagon wheel. It is so close and so large that it almost fills your field of vision. As you stare at it you are very aware of the huge hub, the thick oaken spokes and the iron rim around the outside edge. If you look closely at this iron rim you will notice that there are points of light in it imbedded as if they were tiny light bulbs. In fact, there are seven such points of light evenly spaced around the rim of the wheel. Look at each one of them: The first. The second. The third. The fourth. The fifth. The sixth. And the seventh. Now focus your eyes on that seventh tiny point of light on the rim of the wheel. As you stare at it the wheel begins slowly to revolve. It is turning very slowly around and around and you are continuing to focus your eyes on that seventh point of light as it goes with the wheel around and around and around. It seems as if there is a voice also coming from the wheel that keeps saying over and over again, 'Deeper, deeper, deeper.' And as the wheel turns and you follow that seventh point of light with your eyes, it goes around and around and around, and the voice keeps saying 'deeper, deeper, deeper.' Around and around and around. Deeper, deeper, deeper.

"Now you begin to notice that the revolution of the wheel is gradually becoming more rapid. It is going around, and around and around, and the voice keeps saying 'deeper, deeper, deeper.' It is getting harder and harder to keep focusing on the seventh light on that spinning wheel which is going around and around and around with the voice saying 'deeper, deeper, deeper.'

"And now the spokes begin to blur because the wheel is spinning so fast around and around and around. And you can hardly keep focusing on the seventh point of light. In fact, it is now going so fast that all seven lights blend into a fiery ring of light around the outside rim of the wagon wheel which is spinning around and around and around. And the voice with it is saying 'deeper, deeper, deeper.'

"And now it seems as if you are slowly retreating back from the wheel, or as if it was moving back and away from you, and you can see a second spinning wheel coming into the field of view. Now there are two spinning wheels with fiery rings of light around their rims going around and around and around. And two voices saying, 'deeper, deeper, deeper.'

"And the wheels are now getting smaller as they move away from you so that a third spinning wheel surrounded by a fiery ring of light comes into your field of view. There are now three spinning wheels going around and around and around and three voices saying, 'deeper, deeper, deeper.'

"And still they move away from you so that a fourth, then a fifth and then a sixth wheel comes into view. Six spinning wheels going around and around and around and a half dozen voices softly saying, 'deeper, deeper, deeper.'

"As they move away from you even more wheels come into view, seven, eight, nine, ten, eleven, twelve spinning fiery rings and a dozen voices very softly saying, 'deeper, deeper, deeper.'

"And now they are moving so far away into space that it seems like a hundred tiny spinning wheels of light are going around and around and around, miles and miles from you and hundreds of tiny voices are softly whispering, 'deeper, deeper, deeper, deeper, deeper.'

"And the tiny rings of light are slowly fading away, and the whispering voices are getting so soft you can hardly hear them as they say, 'deeper, deeper, deeper, deeper.' And finally all the light is gone and all the voices are gone, and there is nothing left but a great soft warm darkness that fills the entire world, and you feel deeply at peace with the whole universe."

As this narration is being given to the patient the voice of the hypnotist gradually changes. At first, while he is describing the wheel as it beings to turn, his voice is strong but slow. As more wheels appear he speeds up his speaking, "around and around and around." And as there are more voices he softens his until at the last he is saying "deeper, deeper, deeper, deeper" very rapidly but very softly. Finally the fantasy ends in a "soft warm darkness" much like the origins of our life in the womb. This often carries the subject into a profound hypnotic regression.

It should be noted that some subjects cannot respond at all to this fantasy. Others report that they were annoyed by the slow development of the fantasy. One should check the subject's reactions to it after he is alerted. Some enter a state so deep that after about the third wheel they are completely amnesic to the later developments.

Miscellaneous Deepening Procedures

Many other fantasies can be used. Simply listening to their favorite music in hallucination will carry some subject into a deep state. Reading beautiful poetry in imagination or looking at great hallucinated paintings can be effective with others. Individuals tend to respond when the modality that is most natural to them, visual, auditory, kinesthetic, or motor is tapped. The hypnotist learns to adapt his descriptions to the needs of each individual subject or patient.

In general, suggestions tend to build upon one another. This is called "homoaction." The subject becomes increasingly involved in the hypnotic fantasy and gradually severs his perceptions from external reality or other internal preoccupations. The imagined becomes "for real," and his existence for the moment is within that strange state of consciousness which we call a hypnotic trance.

Outline of Chapter 7.
Deepening Techniques

1. Hypnotic "depth" as one of degree
2. The therapeutic value of light and medium states.
3. The relationship between depth of hypnosis and ego participation
4. Characteristics of very deep hypnosis
5. Handling the subject who resists coming out of hypnosis
6. Measuring trance depth
7. Deepening techniques
    a. Fractionation
    b. Summer day
    c. Progressive, warm, heavy feeling
    d. Descending stairs
    e. Timed breathing
    f. Use of metronome
    g. Floating in a cloud
        1. Revolving in a cloud
    h. Revolving wheels
    i. Miscellaneous
        1. Music, poetry and painting fantasies
        2. Homoaction (building suggestions one on another)

Chapter 8

The Hypnotherapist and Suggestive Treatment

Every good salesman knows how to use suggestion. Salesmen and therapists have much in common—both are trying to influence human behavior. In fact, suggestion may well be the most frequent form of therapy ever used, if we consider its employment throughout all the ages of history, in every culture, civilized and primitive, and especially in the placebo effects which operate within every type of therapeutic intervention. Even in psychoanalysis the suggestive factor is constantly operating, concurrent with interpretations and insight. People often change their behavior, feelings, attitudes, and symptoms when told to by someone who holds a position of prestige and respect.

When Suggestive Hypnotherapy is Appropriate

In some psychological treatment approaches great efforts are made to eliminate or minimize the effect of suggestion. However, if our main goal is constructive change of our patient, therapeutic suggestion, within or outside the condition of hypnosis, is an appropriate tactic providing it:

1. Eliminates symptoms or improves the patient's condition.

2. Is successful in maintaining the therapeutic gains, and

3. Is accomplished without the precipitation of some other equivalent or equally severe symptomatic substitution.

In many cases it may well be the treatment of choice because of its simplicity and rapidity, even though the same result could have been accomplished by other psychological techniques.

Criticisms of Suggestive Hypnotherapy

There is a tendency, especially in psychoanalytic circles, to belittle the effect of hypnotic suggestion as superficial, accomplishing only temporary results, and perhaps even harmful ones, and to maintain that anxiety or the formation of substitute symptoms can be expected as a consequence. These practitioners usually argue that only a resolution of the basic conflicts underlying a psychogenic disorder will achieve permanent and complete symptomatic relief. This position was stated by both Freud (1935) and his daughter, Anna (A. Freud, 1946).

Yet the power of suggestion to alter physical and psychological functioning is so strongly established that research these days, on the efficacy of new therapeutic procedures, pharmacological or other, requires very sophisticated designs to rule out the suggestive factor as a significant ingredient.

Regarding the direct effect of hypnotic suggestion on physiological functioning there is little controversy, except the disbelief by many medical skeptics that a purely psychological approach can influence such conditions as "real" pain, that is pain organically "caused" by a known lesion; or that physiological processes can be significantly altered by psychological intervention. The literature today showing the effect of psychological variables on physiological functioning is simply too tremendous to argue this point. However, study is needed to determine those organic processes which are most susceptible and those which are resistant to psychological intervention. What is most surprising is the tremendous lack of knowledge among non-psychiatric physicians concerning the significant contribution to the therapeutics of organic medical problems which hypnotic suggestion is prepared to make. The effects of suggestion on behavior are so obvious that there is little room for argument there. The relative value of hypnosis in the treatment of psychiatric conditions becomes a matter of internal discussion between psychiatrists, psychologists and psychoanalysts.

The Personality of the Hypnotherapist

We are concerned here with the technique of administering suggestions once a hypnotic state has been induced, the timings, the wordings, and the settings which are most efficacious. We cannot stress too much that therapeutic hypnosis is an intensive doctor-patient relationship as well as an altered state of consciousness. It is in the potentiating of this relationship that much of the therapeutic leverage inheres. The skilled therapist utilizes the relationship for all the impact possible. He is prepared to exploit the condition to the fullest in the interests of helping his patient. It has been truly said that it is not only what we *do to* our patient but also how we *be with* him. The prestige factor inheres in this relationship and provides much of the motive power by which the patient is induced, persuaded, or commanded to relinquish his sufferings.

We have already noted the comparative ease with which hypnosis is induced in some individuals by hypnotists who have status as compared to the results achieved by other hypnotists who are not so respected. The same condition holds, and perhaps even more so, when suggestive techniques are employed to eliminate or mitigate symptoms. Unless the patient believes that the "doctor"[1] has power he will probably show little symptomatic change to the suggestions administered, even though a significant degree of trance had been attained. Prestige, of course, may depend on many factors. Some practitioners feel that it is acquired by having a lavishly furnished waiting room, or many diplomas on the walls, by a great reputation in their community, or by charging high fees. All these undoubtedly influence the patient's expectations of success, and hence, the probabilities that he will be influenced by the suggestions. It is indeed true that practitioners who neglect matters of appearance in their manners of dress and their professional offices may reduce the strength of their suggestive influence.

---

[1] By "doctor" we refer to all healing arts personnel who might be employing hypnosis therapeutically whether or not they are physicians.

Many years ago I received a call from a woman in a neighboring city stating that she had read my book on *Hypnotherapy of War Neuroses* (Watkins, J., 1949) and that she would be traveling to my community. She requested, in fact insisted on, an immediate appointment. Since I was engaged then only in part-time private practice I was able to see her the next day.

She stormed into my consultation room and proceeded at once to describe a condition which she felt would be relieved by hypnotic suggestion. At the end of our session she whipped out her checkbook and demanded, "How much do I owe you?" Being relatively unsure of the efficacy of my treatment, but somewhat impressed by her obvious means, I mentioned a sum slightly larger than the usual fee but still relatively modest. Whereupon she scratched out the check, handed it to me with utter disdain and said, "Huh. I make more than that in five minutes." I seriously doubt that the suggestions I had given her had any significant effect. Even as overcharging can impair a therapeutic relationship, undercharging can also mar one's professional image.

Although such factors as fees, office furnishing, diplomas, etc., do add to the image of the hypnotic practitioner, even more significant is an ability to resonate with the needs of the patient and empathically administer suggestions with understanding of the patient's motivations. Expensive clothes, high fees, and a prestigious office location cannot take the place of sensitivity and psychological sophistication.

One of the most significant factors tending to increase probability that suggestions will be carried out is the air of confidence displayed by the doctor. The therapist who is hesitant and administers suggestions in a weak or vacillating voice will transmit this uncertainty to the patient. If you don't believe in hypnotic procedures you will probably instill doubt in your patients. The successful practitioner of hypnotherapy not only is convinced of the efficacy of clinical hypnosis, but is also certain that he can succeed in inducing the hypnotic state and that his suggestions (or at least most of them) will be successfully carried through by the patient. That is why in the earlier chapters of this book relating to induction the factor of supervised practice, initially with good subjects, was stressed. You must *know* that you are able to hypnotize. This doesn't mean you do not recognize that with some individuals you will fail, but it does imply that you must not have an "I-don't-think-I-can-do-it" attitude. This belief in a therapist is fatal to his success. He becomes a negative hypnotist on himself and by such a conviction covertly suggests himself into failure. Hypnotic patients are especially sensitive at picking up the covert beliefs and attitudes of their doctors. Therefore, the trouble that beginning workers in the field often have is not one of failing to learn technique, but one involving their own self assurance.

During a period when I was in analysis I had great difficulty in hypnotizing patients referred to me. My analytic "father" did not approve of hypnosis, and in spite of the excellent insights he helped me to work through, and his skill as one of the recognized old masters of the field, he transmitted in subtle ways his disapproval of hypnosis—one which he had received when he was personally trained by Freud. As a result, during those years I found myself unable to treat successfully by hypnotherapy many of the referrals sent to me, even though at that time I had already written one book, a number of papers and had achieved some recognition in the area. Later, my interest in developing the field of hypnoanalysis by integrating analytic insights with my hypnotic experience enabled me to overcome this temporary inhibition and resume effective practice with hypnotherapy. All this is only to emphasize that if you find difficulty in your initial work with hypnotherapy the problem may lie in inadequate successful experience, which can be corrected by working with good subjects under the supervision of an experienced hypnotic therapist, or in "self-work" to discover and resolve such unconscious blocks, which might be acting as a countermotivation.

Not all practitioners find themselves suited to the practice of hypnotherapy. Occasionally I meet former students who tell me that they never felt safe using hypnosis and that they did not now use it. However, they generally indicated that their training in the field increased their understanding of psychosomatic conditions, their respect for the doctor-patient relationship, and their recognition of the important of unconscious processes in determining behavior and symptoms.

Sometimes further study in the area can correct earlier blocks. A psychiatrist who had taken one of my hypnotherapy workshops at her medical school came back to take a more extensive course I was offering at a different university some twelve years later. She reported that she had seldom employed hypnosis after her initial contact with it, but after the later course she began to use hypnotherapy frequently and successfully in her practice.

The belief that hypnotic suggestion can in many cases be both effective and permanent is essential for the practitioner who would employ the technique successfully. Freud stated that he gave up the use of hypnosis because he despaired of securing permanent cures through it. However, there is considerable evidence (Kline, 1958) that the real reason was because he was a poor hypnotist, and because he did not relish the close interpersonal relationship which is required of the good hypnotherapist. In fact, he stated that he put his patients on the couch because he did not like to face and look them in the eye.

Psychoanalytic Objections to Suggestive Hypnosis

The objection to suggestive hypnosis voiced by psychoanalysts include primarily the following:

1. The results are temporary.
2. This is because the ego is bypassed. Hypnotic suggestions and "insights" received through hypnotic suggestion are not egotized and integrated.
3. Hence, the underlying dynamic causes of external symptoms (and of course, here we are talking about psychogenic, not organically caused symptoms) are not resolved. Soon the underlying conflicts initiate a return of the symptoms or equivalent ones (Meldman, 1960).

Even though these objections have been shown over and over again to be invalid, the prestige of the early founder of psychoanalysis is such that modern day analytic writers (Blanck, G. & Blanck, R., 1974) continue to echo the same criticisms, apparently with no awareness of recent studies and literature to the contrary.

Psychodynamic Reasons Why Suggestive Treatment May be Permanently Successful

When dealing with the impact of direct suggestions on physical conditions, we need not be concerned with this controversy, but for the benefit of dynamically-oriented psychiatrists and psychologists it is necessary to point out several analytically-sound rationales why symptom relief by suggestion may well be, and often is, permanent, though not necessarily always so.

1. Many psychogenically caused symptoms continue to plague an individual after the original conflict which initiated them is no longer present. This is because of their maintenance by secondary reinforcements. Consider the case of a man who developed an hysterical limp because of repressed anger at a mother-in-law whom it was necessary to keep in his home. The offending person dies, but the symptom continues because his sympathetic wife has been for many years pampering him because of it. "I know you've had a hard day's work at the office, Darling, and your leg's been giving you trouble. Just you sit down here in the easy chair and let me mix your favorite martini." No wonder the limp continues. But the real psychological conflict which marked its inception is not now present, and the power for its continuation is not very strong. His resentment at the mother-in-law has long ago been dissipated. Accordingly, such a condition may respond quite well to a session or two of suggestive hypnotherapy in which he sees that he need no longer endure the symptom's inconvenience. This realization will strengthen if following its relinquishment the affectionate concern of his wife for his welfare does not diminish. Undoubtedly many hysterically caused symptoms continue long after the psychodynamic justification for their existence is gone, simply because of the secondary reinforcements which they receive. Suggestive hypnosis is for such conditions the treatment of choice.

2. Psychogenic symptoms which still have some dynamic motivation for their maintenance may be temporarily eliminated through hypnotic suggestion. They do not necessarily return, because the change brought about in the individual's life by their cessation initiates a new motivational system which keeps them suppressed. The world now reinforces the person for *not* having the symptom. Consider the case of the obese woman who developed an overeating habit because of her resentment

at being neglected by her husband. Perhaps he became so involved in his job that he spent all his spare time away from home engaging in business activities. As his wife lost her figure he became even less interested in her. Thus she and her husband are caught up in a mutually destructive relationship. The more he stays away from her, the more she eats and gains weight. The fatter she becomes, the less he is attracted to her.

Now enters a practitioner who suggests that she lose weight through suggestive hypnosis. Reluctantly she tries it and soon finds that she can get along with lowered food intake. As she begins to regain an attractive figure her husband develops a new interest in her. "Hey Honey, you're looking swell. Why don't we go out for dinner tonight, and dance a little afterwards?" And then the neighbors flock around. "Mary, you're looking wonderful these days. That new dress is stunning on you." Why should she go back to overeating? She is now receiving that attention whose lack motivated her neurotic eating behavior. If sufficient reinforcements from her world continue, the symptom is gone, and it doesn't return. Through hypnotic suggestion a permanent change in her life has been achieved. No insight was required.

Symptom suppression can be much more than temporary when the entire reinforcement structure is changed as a result. In such cases deep, psychoanalytic therapy, with much working-through aimed at insight, is an unnecessary and wasteful approach.

3. If hypnosis is an intensive interpersonal relationship experience, then the patient will often introject the voice of the therapist. How many times have we internalized the admonitions, suggestions, and praise of a parent or some other significant figure in our life? It is as if the happy individual travels through his existence hearing unconsciously the praises and positive reinforcements of an introjected parent saying, "Good boy," or "Good girl." "See what you can do. You are very capable; I am proud of you," etc.

In intensive relationship therapy, with or without hypnosis, the good therapist is often introjected. If the therapeutic experience was a significant one, the "teachings," interpretations, and suggestions offered by the important healer become permanently internalized within the patient. They continue to be "said" by the therapist introject within the patient long after treatment sessions with the real doctor have terminated. The suggestions are repeated covertly, and the patient's following of them is reinforced and strengthened. Such an inner dynamic structure may account for many of the innumerable cases where hypnotic suggestion has removed a psychogenic symptom, and for all purposes permanently—to the confounding of traditional psychoanalytic theory.

It is not maintained here that the above three conditions operate all of the time. There are many psychologically caused problems which do not respond to simple hypnotic suggestions. There are many others which, as maintained by the psychoanalysts, are temporarily alleviated but not "cured," and a few in which the removal actually precipitates an even more severe problem. But the flat insistence that suggestion can have only temporary results is simply not true. There are too many cases which prove the opposite. The experience of many hypnotherapists is filled with such examples and these have been frequently reported in the literature.[2]

On the other hand, we cannot side with our behavioral colleagues who claim that the symptoms are the illness, that it is never necessary to analyze underlying "dynamic" reasons for their existence. The most reasonable position seems to be that many organically-caused conditions can be constructively influenced by hypnotic suggestion, and that some psychogenic symptoms will respond favorably and permanently to suggestive therapy. Others may require more intensive and "deep" treatment such as will be described in Vol. II of this work, which is devoted to hypnoanalytic techniques. We reject the claims of both those who cry "never" and those who insist "always" in regards to the indications for symptomatic treatment. The real problem for the practitioner is to

[2]See Cheek and LeCron, 1968; Crasilneck & Hall, 1975; Erickson, Hershman and Secter, 1961 and numerous papers in *The American Journal of Clinical Hypnosis* and the *International Journal of Clinical and Experimental Hypnosis.*

discriminate those conditions which can be handled through hypnotic suggestion, either by simple suggestions or through the more sophisticated suggestive approaches to be described, from those which require some analytic therapy involving insight and personality reorganization. Here, too, hypnosis can contribute, but through more complex methods than suggestion.

Perhaps we can think of hypnosis as an intervention in the psychological equilibrium of an individual. Sometimes this can tip the scales in favor of constructive forces and initiate a benevolent cycle of favorable motivations and reinforcements. For many patients this may be sufficient.

Levels of Hypnotic Suggestion

Intervention in the functioning may be approached at different levels. This is somewhat comparable to the situation in organic treatment where a symptom or harmful process is interrupted at different points. Thus, in the treatment of peptic ulcer an internist might recommend a bland diet, freedom from stress, a gastrectomy, or a vagotomy among other possibilities.

Direct Attack on Symptoms

In suggestive hypnotherapy we may attack the symptom directly, aiming for its elimination, or initially only for its partial alleviation. We may attempt to secure an immediate (one session) response, or we may plant suggestions aimed at a more gradual effect. For example, during World War II I treated, with suggestive therapy, a soldier who had developed an hysterical limp. It was important to him that he gradually relinquish this symptom, since to do so rapidly would imply that he had never really been "wounded." A damaged limb is supposed to take time to heal. Accordingly, I told him under hypnosis that his leg would improve gradually, that he would note its improvement each day, and that within a few weeks he would be fully recovered. In about three weeks he relinquished his cane, and by the time of his discharge only the slightest impairment of function could still be noticed. he could return home and "save face." He would not be charged with malingering; he had had a "real" disability.

In this case a pseudo-rationale was employed, but to the patient it was logical and made sense. An attempt to take the symptom away from him immediately might have provoked severe resistance, resentment, perhaps a refusal to come for further treatment, and even a relapse into a greater disability.

At times, the potency of a psychological treatment like hypnosis can be demonstrated by temporarily increasing instead of diminishing the severity of a symptom. A patient suffering from severe tension headaches complained on being referred for hypnotherapy that, "My headache is real; just talking won't do any good." He was hypnotized and the suggestion given that when he emerged from the hypnotic state his headache would be twice as severe and would remain so until he was touched on the shoulder. At that time it would return to its normal level of discomfort. He emerged from trance and accusingly said, "Your treatment has made me worse; my head hurts more than when I came here." I replied, "Of course. I made it that way; see, now I will bring it back to the condition it was in when you came into the office." The shoulder was touched and the patient immediately noted the difference. He was then told, "You see, this treatment is strong enough to influence your symptom. If it is strong enough to make it worse, it can be strong enough to make it better." The patient was convinced of the potency of a "talking" therapy and immediately became more responsive to suggestions aimed at alleviating his distress.

Indirect Effects through Non-specific Suggestions

Sometimes instead of working directly on a symptom one can direct the suggestions toward the general strength and well-being of the patient.

"You are beginning to feel much better. As you do, a sense of confidence starts to go all through you. You realize that your body is mobilizing to correct this condition. Each day you feel more confident that you will succeed in regaining your health." Here the suggestions are aimed simply at inducing the patient to mobilize his own resources; indirectly we may be stimulating his immunological systems and thus helping him to increase antibody development, improve circulation, and stimulate those physiological processes which operate to distinguish between the patient with low morale and the one who fights to overcome his illness or disability.

Ego-Strengthening

Closely related to this in the psychiatric-psychological area is the use of hypnotic suggestion to strengthen the ego. If an individual has a strong ego he is capable either of repressing discordant elements in his personality and maintaining the repression, or he is strong enough to confront them and resolve them through insight therapy. Either way a strengthening of the ego can be beneficial. Accordingly, we might tell him under hypnosis, "You are developing a sense of inner vitality. Each day you realize that you are building a stronger and stronger personality. You notice how much more frequently you are successful in achieving your goals and what a feeling of adequacy you are beginning to develop. You are more and more convinced that you can reach your goals," etc.

The Cumulative Effect of Suggestions

Suggestion can have a cumulative effect. This principle is well known by the advertising business. Advertisements are repeated over and over again as the public is taught through repetition to say to themselves that which the manufacturer wishes them to think. Thus, almost everybody knows today what brand it is "that tastes good like a cigarette should." Or which kind is related to "You've come a long way, Baby." A most effective beer advertisement of a few years back repeated over and over a musical jingle, "What'll you have?" Millions of people learned to respond with, "Pabst Blue Ribbon." Note how the thought of a particular brand was tied to the question which most bartenders ask a new customer. Suggestions which are tied together in this way under hypnosis are especially potent in conditioning the desired responses.

Tying Suggestions Together

One approach which I have found successful in getting individuals to stop smoking uses this "tying-together" technique as follows:

The patient is hypnotized and then told, "Whenever you feel the urge to smoke this will evoke in you a voice that says, "No! I don't have to smoke. I will not smoke." The stronger the urge to smoke, the stronger will be the voice denying it. As soon as you have said that to yourself you will take a couple of deep breaths, and upon completing them you will note that the urge to smoke simply fades away. A deep sense of calm relaxation takes its place. Shortly after you have enjoyed this period of relaxation you will experience a strong feeling of triumph and it will seem as if you are in control of your world."

In the previous set of suggestions each one was tied to the previous one. We started with the urge of the patient to smoke and used it as the stimulus to evoke the "No" response, in fact the strength of the "No" response was made contingent on the strength of the urge. The "No" response was then followed by a specific conscious action which the patient would then perform, namely, taking "a couple of breaths." Completion of this response would then be rewarded by an immediate lowering of tension and the urge to smoke, and then followed by their replacement with a sense of relaxation and well being. Here we use the principles of behavior therapy by providing an immediate positive reinforcement for the action of *not* smoking. This was further reinforced by stimulating a longer-term sense of mastery in the patient.

By tying together these suggestions which were first given under trance, repeated under trance, practiced under trance, and then instructed that they would apply post-hypnotically, we have maximized their impact.

Aligning Suggestions with the Patient's Motivations

The more we can integrate suggestions with already existing motivational systems within the patient the stronger they are. Examples might be as follows:

To a five-year-old, "By picking up his toys, Johnny can prove that he is really grown-up like Dad, who always picks up his tools when he finishes working with them in the shop."

To another child, "Geraldine is very brave, and she shows it when she goes to school all by herself."

"As your breathing becomes calm and your pulse slows down during these difficult situations you demonstrate once again that you are in control of your emotions, that you are a very strong and mature person."

Authoritative vs. Persuasive Manner in Giving Suggestions

While confidence in the hypnotherapist is an essential ingredient in any approach, he may choose to use a very direct, authoritative manner; "When I place my hand on your shoulder the pain in your back will leave immediately; and when I count to five you will become alert and feel no suffering."

On the other hand, the doctor may elect for a more persuasive approach, such as: "When I place my hand on your shoulder, the muscles in your back will begin to relax. You feel a sense of warmth in them as you recognize that the blood circulation there is improving. This is because you are learning to release the tension which is causing the pain."

Suggestions Administered under Hypnosis and Post-hypnotically

Sometimes it is desirable to remove a symptom under hypnosis but defer its relinquishment for a while after the patient has returned to the normal state. This can be done to test whether or not the symptom can be influenced under hypnosis—a great deal, slightly, or not at all—and is especially indicated when the symptom may be psychogenic and serving some dynamic function. It is often surprising to note that when the symptom has been removed under hypnosis, but (by suggestion) reinstated before bringing the patient out of the trance state, he may give it up spontaneously within a comparatively short time. It seems that by demonstrating to him (unconsciously) that he does not need the symptom he, on his own, can arrive at this conclusion on a more conscious level. He then voluntarily eliminates the symptom and does not feel that he was pressured prematurely by the doctor into doing so.

For many conditions, especially organically caused pain, one may choose to keep the symptom removed or alleviated after the patient has emerged from the hypnotic state. Accordingly, if the symptom has been removed under hypnosis he can be told before being removed from the trance that the change will continue after he "awakens." The subsequent length of time during which the symptom is gone, (an hour, a day, a week, a month, etc.) tells us something about the severity of his condition, and in the case of a neurotic disorder the strength of underlying motivations for developing and maintaining the symptom.

Symptom Substitution

A technique that is sometimes used in treating neurotic disorders is to replace the presenting complaint with a less disabling symptom. A concert pianist who has developed an occupational neurosis involving stiffening of the fingers may accept a transfer of this stiffness from the hand to the foot. He can still be administering a "punishment" to himself, if that is the dynamic reason for the condition, but it no longer prevents him from earning his living. Although there are reports of the successful use of this technique (Erickson, 1954) this writer much prefers to use approaches aimed at the resolution of the symptoms rather than their transfer or substitution.

Hypnotic Suggestion as a Tactic within Insight Therapy

Even though a psychotherapist may be aiming at a personality reorganization of his patient by analytical treatment, hypnosis can often be useful in helping the individual through (let us say) a period of sleeplessness. Or suggestion may be used as a tactic within a hypnoanalytic therapy. For example, a blocking of drinking or smoking behavior, which dams a patient's impulses, may temporarily increase his drive for movement and process in the insight treatment. Resistances can be mobilized and thus brought to the fore where, through analysis, they can be resolved. We do not always resolve the symptom, but, by the suggestions, we have activated the conflict which underlies it.

Finally, it should be noted that hypnotic suggestions can be directed against not only symptoms and behaviors, but also toward attitudes, feelings, motivations, prejudices, or even relationships. The possibilities for their use are infinite and limited only by the practitioner's conception of the structure and scope of the disorder with which he is confronted, plus his own ingenuity and skill in applying this potent tool. In the next chapters we will consider specific conditions which can be treated with hypnotic suggestion and case examples which illustrate hypnotherapeutic technique.

Outline of Chapter 8. The Hypnotherapist and Suggestive Treatment

1. Suggestive hypnotherapy is appropriate when it:
   a. Eliminates symptoms or improves the patient's condition
   b. Is successful in maintaining the therapeutic gains
   c. Is accomplished without the precipitation of some other equivalent or equally severe symptomatic substitution.
2. Criticisms of suggestive hypnotherapy come primarily from:
   a. Psychoanalysts who believe the results are only temporary
   b. Organic-minded physicians who don't believe that psychological interventions can truly influence physical conditions
3. The personality of the hypnotherapist
   a. The therapist's prestige and relationship to the patient
   b. The therapist's self-confidence
4. Psychoanalytic objections to suggestive hypnosis
5. Psychodynamic reasons why suggestive treatments may be permanently successful
   a. The need to differentiate between cases which can be treated suggestively and those requiring an analytic, insight therapy
6. Levels of hypnotic suggesion
   a. Direct attack on symptoms
      1. Authoritative
      2. Persuasive
   b. Indirect effects through non-specific suggestions
      1. Partial or temporary elimination only
      2. Gradual alleviation over time
      3. Suggestion directed against underlying attitudes
7. Ego-strengthening
8. The cumulative effect of suggestions
9. Tying suggestions together
10. Aligning suggestions with the patient's motivations
11. Authoritative vs. persuasive manner
12. Suggestions administered under hypnosis and post-hypnotically
13. Symptom substitution
14. Hypnotic suggestion as a tactic within insight therapy

Chapter 9

Hypnosis in Surgery, Anesthesiology, and the Control of Pain

"Ouch! It hurts, doctor." How many times has the physician or dentist heard such a remark? Nobody wants to "hurt," so it is no wonder that one of the most rewarding uses of hypnosis is its ability to influence the perception of pain. In this area it can make a substantial contribution to the disciplines of surgery and anesthesiology, since the control of pain remains one of man's most pressing problems and one which engages much of the time and efforts of the physician. If only the pain problem of a patient could be quickly and easily solved, the effective application of many other procedures to the treatment of his disease or disability would be greatly facilitated. Moreover, hypnosis can contribute to the management of many other aspects of surgical procedures, preoperatively, during the operation itself, and in the post-operative recovery period. Central to all of these, however, is its ability to alleviate or eliminate pain.

The Experience of Pain

Pain is an almost universal experience, one which we seek to avoid. For centuries it was regarded as an inescapable accompaniment to disease or damage to the body, and the acceptance of it as a necessary burden has been part of many religions. Thus, the Bible teaches that because of Eve's transgression in eating the forbidden fruit, women shall bring forth children in pain.

The use of various drugs, including alcoholic beverages,

for the alleviation of pain had been practiced long before Morton discovered ether in 1846. This was about the time that Esdaile was employing hypnosis in India as an anesthetic for both minor and major operations.

Recently, there has been an increased interest in studying the causes of pain, both physiologically (Lim, 1970) and psychologically (Melzack, 1973; Hilgard, E. R. and Hilgard, J. R., 1975).

Many different pharmacological and surgical interventions have been developed for the treatment of pain (Bonica, 1974). Nor have the possible psychological contributions to pain therapy been neglected. Besides hypnosis, various techniques of behavior modification have been successfully applied, such as operant conditioning (Fordyce, 1973, 1974) and cognitive dissonance (Zimbardo, Cohen, Weisenberg, Dworkin & Firestone, 1966).

The more it has been investigated the more complex the phenomenon appears. As an inner experience it can no longer be viewed as a simple reaction to a stress, disease, or tissue damage. Not only are there tremendous differences between individuals in their perception and tolerance of pain, but the discomfort from a specific lesion can vary greatly from time to time depending upon the interplay of various psychological factors. Motivation, attention, distraction, learned habits, perception, interpersonal relationships all play roles which influence both the perception of pain and its suffering.

Melzack (1974) reports numerous studies which have attempted to differentiate the qualitative and component aspects of pain. In a study undertaken by himself and Torgerson (Melzack and Torgerson, 1971), some 102 terms were found necessary to describe the different aspects of pain. They categorized these descriptive terms under three headings: *sensory pain*, which included such adjectives as throbbing, pounding, pinching, cramping, etc., *affective*, such as those depicted as fearful, terrifying, and *evaluative*, these latter being described as annoying, miserable, unbearable, etc.

Sensory Pain and Suffering

Two specific components of pain appear to have been identified by most contributors, namely, *sensory pain* and *suffering*. Sensory pain provides needed information to the individual that something is wrong which requires treatment and often indicates the site of the disturbance. Accordingly, it serves a protective purpose to the organism and should not be eliminated. People have been known to die because of the failure of their bodies to provide the warning of sensory pain.

However, it is the realm of suffering that shows the greatest variability, the least constructive value to humans, and the greatest opportunity for therapeutic intervention. Morphine, for example, does not knock out the sensory pain but considerably influences its suffering. Furthermore, pain itself interferes with healing.

The "Gate Control" Theory of Pain

Many theories have been proposed to account for pain. Currently the *gate control* theory proposed by Melzack and Wall (1965) seems to account for the various aspects of pain better than any other. According to this theory pain stimuli are transmitted to the higher brain centers through two different sets of pathways called respectively the *sensory-discriminative* system and the *motivational-affective* system. The first of these is concerned with the location and severity of the pain. The second transmits those impulses which involve suffering. These two systems appear to be anatomically verified. Briefly it is hypothesized that pain stimuli in both the large and small fibers ascending the spinal cord pass through a *gate control system.* At this point the impulses from both interact and serve to modulate stimuli transmitted to the motivational-affective and sensory-discriminative systems by certain transmission cells. It is thus possible through surgical, chemical and psychological intervention[1] at this point to interfere with stimulation of the sensory-discriminative system while permitting normal passage of the impulses through the motivational-affective system.

It is precisely such an intervention in which we are interested either through chemo- or hypnoanalgesia. To alleviate suffering without impairing functioning or eliminating nature's protective signals becomes our therapeutic goal. Since we are concerned here primarily with hypnotic techniques which can assist that objective we will not proceed further

[1]In this respect hypnoanalgesia appears to fade at about the same rate as chemoanalgesia. A patient whom I once treated was alternated between hypnoanalgesia and pain medication. In each case she would remain pain-free for about three hours.

into the complexities and theories of pain. Ernest and Josephine Hilgard (1975) have published the most thorough treatise on this as related to the use of hypnosis. Practitioners who are concerned primarily with pain control should consult their monumental work.

The decision to use hypnosis in controlling a pain involves a number of considerations prior to applying any of the hypnotic techniques. Since pain can be referred from an originating site to another where it is apparently experienced, application of a specific hypnotic analgesia at the point where it hurts may result simply in its referral to another area.[2] A more generalized approach may be required. This is especially true if the pain is serving a psychodynamic function as, for example, the individual's need to be punished for some transgression, real or imagined. In such cases suggestive hypnosis is not likely to solve the problem, except perhaps temporarily. The patient may require a more intensive and insightful kind of treatment utilizing approaches such as will be described in Vol. II., and practiced by clinicians who are trained in analytic psychotherapy.

Contrary to widespread belief, hypnotic suggestion is more effective in relieving organically caused pains than those stemming from hysterical or other psychogenic sources which involve underlying needs in the patient. Moreover, the individual suffering from a severe organic pain is usually highly motivated to accept any promising treatment and consequently is often more hypnotizable.

We are concerned at this point with procedures for alleviating pain by hypnotic suggestion, not through some hypnoanalytic resolution of unconscious conflicts. If the patient is found to have such neurotic mechanisms as underlying guilt, masochistic needs, etc., these psychological conditions may well require to be treated first before hypnotic suggestion becomes effective. Vol. II will describe techniques useful in this latter objective which can be employed by the psychotherapeutically sophisticated practitioner. One other type of pain in which hypnotic suggestion is probably contraindicated is that of hallucinated pain in the psychotic.

---

[2]In a recent experiment involving the hypnotic suppression of pain a subject's hand was hynotically anesthetized and then thrust into ice water, thus creating what is called "cold-pressor" pain. The subject was unmoved and reporting having no feeling in his hand, but about a minute later developed a violent stomach ache.

"Covert" Pain and the "Hidden Observer" Phenomenon

The Hilgards (1975) have discovered that while direct suffering is related to overt, consciously experienced pain there is also a component of pain which is "covert." This is registered at unconscious levels. Thus, the experience of pain can be hypnotically suppressed in laboratory subjects who have a hand placed in ice water. They report feeling only numbness and will hold the hand in the solution long past the time when they ordinarily would have removed it. However, their reactions to the following query are interesting:

"Although you are hypnotically insensitive to pain, perhaps there is some part of you which is experiencing it. If there is, lift the index finger on your other hand." In many cases the finger lifts, and the individual communicates at hypnotic levels the fact that he is "unconsciously" suffering. Hilgard has termed this phenomenon the "hidden observer" and describes it as a dissociated cognitive structural system. Accordingly, we must reckon with the fact that pain can be both overt and covert. For specific analgesic purposes we are concerned primarily with overt pain, and we adjudge our therapeutic efforts successful if we can alleviate it. However, it would seem that the repression of some part of the pain into covert levels must involve effort and may well have an effect indirectly on other functioning, even as unconscious motivations are well known to play a significant role in the formation of neurotic symptoms.

The suppression of any stimulating source such as covert pain has both its advantages and its potentialities for influencing psychological equilibrium. In this connection it may be wise to inquire about possible disturbing thoughts and dreams through which suppressed or repressed stimuli may manifest themselves. Cheek (1962) suggests that information about the meaning of a pain can be obtained through the use of an unconscious finger signal technique. The patient is asked when and where the pain first became important to him by questions which can be answered "yes," "no," "maybe," or "I don't wish to answer," these replies being transmitted under hypnosis back to the therapist by the lifting of different fingers which have been conditioned to such responses. This technique may also be employed to find out the patient's underlying reaction to various procedures or his predictions of possible outcomes.

Studies have shown (Hilgard, E. R. & Hilgard, J. R., 1975) that the trance state itself seems to have little effect on the perception of pain. It is the suggestion administered in the hypnotic modality which determines that result. Therefore, the induction of hypnosis should be considered as only a preliminary and preparatory procedure to the skillful use of suggestive therapy.

On the other side of the question Barber and his associates (Barber, 1969, 1970; Barber and Calverly, 1969) have shown that hypnotic phenomena can be elicited in subjects who were given "task motivation" suggestions without a prior induction. However, these represent primarily laboratory studies and have not yet been shown to have widespread applicability in anesthesiology and the treatment of pain.

Simulator studies (Orne, 1974) have found that highly hypnotized individuals were able to eliminate pain completely while subjects asked to simulate or fake hypnosis were not able to do so. Hypnotic suggestion also seems to be different from the placebo effect common in the administration of drugs. In fact, the Hilgards (1975) found that highly hypnotizable subjects responded less well to placebos than did unhypnotizable ones, thus lending weight to the trance theories which hold that hypnosis is a unique, altered state of consciousness.

While the reality of hypnotic analgesia seems quite firmly established among informed workers, one controversy on this point was quite interesting. Sutcliffe (1961) demonstrated that the GSR (galvanic skin response), which tends to be elevated when people are experiencing pain, was also raised in hypnotized subjects who were given suggestions of analgesia. An electrical shock stimulation involving a combined buzzer and shock was used. Even though the hypnotized subjects denied that they felt pain, they showed an equal or greater rise in GSR as did control subjects who heard the buzzer but were given no shock. Sutcliffe argued that the analgesic subjects were either misperceiving or misrepresenting their true feelings, since if the hypnotic analgesia truly relieved them from pain they should have shown less elevation of the GSR than the control subjects.

Bowers and van der Meulen (1972), however, evaluated the GSR responses and heart rate in a group of seven dental patients whose caries were treated under hypnoanalgesia and compared them with a control group of seven patients whose caries were treated under chemoanalgesia. Both the heart rate and the GSR increased dramatically for all subjects. There was no difference between those who received the chemoanalgesia and those who had the hypnoanalgesia. The two analgesics were equally effective. Apparently both analgesics affect the perceptual factors of the pain experience, but not the physiological concomitants. There is some evidence that these two different analgesics can influence each other. Thus hypnosis can be used to potentiate chemoanalgesia, and mild doses of analgesic drugs make hypnotic analgesia available for more people.

Hypnoanalgesia has been used successfully with a wide number of conditions. The published case reports in which it has been found to be effective include: cancer (Sacerdote, 1972, Butler, 1955), phantom limb (Cedercreutz & Uusitalo, 1967), tic doloreux (Golan, 1971), migraine (Harding, 1967), intractable pain (Lea, Ware & Monroe, 1960). It must be generally concluded that hypnosis is an effective analgesic in many types of cases and should be an integral part in any program of pain control.

Hypnotic Techniques for the Control of Pain

The various hypnotic procedures used in alleviating pain can be classed under three major headings: direct suggestion, altering the experience of pain, and directing attention away from pain. Let us consider a number of techniques under each.

Direct Suggestion

The first and simplest approach would be merely to inform the hypnotized individual that he will no longer feel the pain. Here the authority of the doctor and his relationship with the patient is pitted against the pressure of the pain stimuli in an effort at suppression. At times this is effective, especially with highly hypnotizable people who have great faith in their doctor. In fact, by placing all his prestige against the pain, the doctor is using a powerful interpersonal relationship tool, but this can also be a double-edged sword. If the suggestibility of the patient is weak or weakens, if the impact of the pain stimuli becomes overwhelming, not only may the pain return in force, but the credibility of the doctor is jeopardized. Sometimes, when commanded to give up their symptoms, the patients give up the doctor instead. This is especially easy to do if the patient resents what appears to be an attempt to dominate him. A rebellious "child-within" is mobilized. He comes back to report (sometimes with ill-concealed pleasure) that, "Doctor, your treatment didn't work." This demanding, authoritative approach (which Ferenczi termed "father" hypnosis) may be indicated when there is a genuine emergency, and temporary pain relief is a vital necessity.

It is amazing how easy it often is to hypnotize and administer therapeutic suggestions successfully to a patient in whose eyes one has considerable status and respect—or sometimes even affection. The same patient may have been relatively unhypnotizable by another practitioner, or at least have achieved only a light trance. Although some patients appear to resist hypnosis, no matter who is the doctor, the situation can often be improved if one will follow an old injunction which is good in almost any type of therapy, "When in doubt work on the relationship."

If, as is so often the case, the pain is one which requires relief every few hours, two approaches are suggested. First, make a cassette tape recording of the entire induction and the suggestions of pain alleviation including the termination of the hypnosis at the end, such as by counting up to five. Whenever the patient feels the need of relief again from the pain he simply plays the tape. Because it has been made by the therapist specifically for him, and the suggestions are timed to fit his speed of response, the effect is to repeat the hypnotic experience with the doctor and to emerge with the same result, one which generally holds about the same length of time as the original.

Since part of the experience of clinical hypnosis is the close interpersonal relationship with the doctor, it is possible that the effects of the unreinforced tape may wear off after a while. These can usually be renewed, either by another face-to-face session with the therapist, or by playing the tape in his presence. This re-establishes the relationship and potentiates the suggestions again.

Self-Hypnosis

The second approach, which can be used when it is not possible for the therapist to come personally and administer another hypno-suggestive treatment, is to teach the patient auto or self-hypnosis. (See the technique of "Self-hypnosis" proposed by H. Watkins and described in Chapter 6.) If an auto-hypnotic procedure is indicated, it would be well for the doctor to use a similar approach during his initial induction of the patient. Thus, the technique of focusing the eyes on the uplifted hand and suggesting that its heaviness will cause it to lower can be adapted equally well to an induction by the doctor and later as an auto-hypnotic technique. This simply teaches the patient to say to himself the same suggestions that the therapist would. One individual indicated that it was more effective to her if she visualized the doctor speaking the suggestions (induction, deepening and therapeutic) to her and imagining herself as listening to them. This seemed to re-establish the close interpersonal relationship she felt with him even when he was not present.

Visualization is a very effective method of presenting suggestions. That which can be pictured in the mind has more power to affect behavior and experience for most people than simply words. After all, words are supposed to be stimulus cues to behavior, but if they do not have genuine meanings they will probably have little effect. For example, a successful approach to the pain of migraine headaches has been described by Harding (1967). He used suggestions of visualization such as: "—migraine headaches are caused by the blood vessels in the head becoming excessively swollen. Now, picture the blood vessels in the head. See them large and swollen. Now picture them growing smaller and smaller, returning to normal, carrying the normal amount of blood to the brain." Images such as these seem to have more effect on autonomic processes than simple commands or instructions.

Since migraine is considered to be caused by an excess of blood in the cranial blood vessels and their distension, relaxation may be facilitated by suggestions of increased warmth in the hands, arms, legs, or other parts of the body. The net effect is to reduce the blood supply in the head. Suggestions such as these are much more effective than merely telling the patient that his head will not hurt.

Some patients are more kinesthetic minded than visually oriented. If they are unable to visualize a vascular bed or a single blood vessel, suggestions which stress feelings of warmth, comfort, tingling, relaxation, etc., may provide a better reaction for them. When one is uncertain as to what sensory modality is most significant to a patient (visual, auditory, kinesthetic, gustatory, olafactory, or touch), suggestions which incorporate vivid impressions from several or all of these can be employed. Thus, an individual being relaxed might be asked to picture a peaceful scene, see the clouds and the blue sky, hear the gentle murmer of a stream, feel the warm air on his skin, and smell the delicious scent of the wildflowers. The more vivid the suggestions and the more significant sensory modalities they employ, the more genuine they become to the patient, and the more he can throw himself into a meaningful, realistic experience.

Changing the Meaning of Pain

Since the impact of hypnotic suggestion is to alter the "suffering" component of pain, not its presence, the pain experience can be modified to make it feel different. We may tell the hypnotized patient that the discomfort in his arm will be sensed as a mild pressure. He will know it is there, but he will not suffer from it. He may be informed that the dull ache in his back will be felt as a slight sensation of warmth. Such suggestions probably disrupt normal physiological pain processes less than attempts to eliminate them. While little experimental evidence has yet been produced to assess the relative effectiveness of different approaches, one might reason that the complete suppression of pain impulses travelling through the nervous system requires a greater counter force than the permission of their expression in more acceptable ways. Furthermore, if there is an underlying dynamic reason why a patient needs to have pain, such as for self-punishment, the fact of its creation and presence might meet this need. For example, the body often turns unacceptable emotions into pain. Thus, the individual who cannot express his rage at a spouse may instead experience some anginal pain. As soon as he can express the anger, truly "get it off his chest," the pain subsides. The suppressed rage on the one hand initiates heart spasms, and on the other hand is displaced into the consequent "suffering." The patient does not experience anger; he feels pain. The displacement of its suffering component into a more benign form significantly reduces the patient's disability. By such procedures we help an individual to "live" with his discomfort even though we may not be able to eliminate it.

In some cases it is possible to teach him to ignore the pain. Thus, a fifty-year-old woman with breast cancer was told, "You need not pay attention to any uncomfortable feelings coming from below your shoulders. You will ignore them because you are so busy and interested in listening to good music, enjoying television, reading books and conversing with friends." In this case we were using distraction as a technique. That which we do not pay attention to need not bother us.

Numbness can be suggested in one area and then permitted (requested) to "travel" to other areas where it is needed but which are less accessible. It is also best "imaged" when the suggestions are tied to memories such as, "You can remember when the dentist injected novocaine into your tooth. Re-experience it now in relation to—", the afflicted area which it is desired to render insensitive. The "numbness" can often be made more effective if it is established as the opposite of the pain. Hence, the patient is told, "When you have numbness you can't have pain there."

Dissociative Techniques

The psychological mechanism of dissociation is an extremely complex process which we do not understand very well as yet. In its extreme forms it is seen in the multiple personality case where one part of the self may not even know of the existence of another part. We prefer to consider these part-person entities as "ego states," and they will be discussed in considerably more detail in Vol. II. Amnesia represents another example of dissociation. The individual does not remember experiences and behaviors which happened to him at another time. Perhaps normal forgetting is a dissociative process; however, when a person is found in a strange city unable to recall his name, home, or family, we recognize it as an abnormality and consider it a "mental illness."

The hysterical paralysis of a part of the body so that it no longer functions within the individual's "body ego" is comparable to the dissociation of a part of his experiential life so it is no longer a part of his "mental ego." The separation of some part of one's physical or psychological functioning so that it is no longer felt as within one's "self"—as "me" is a fascinating study which can be initiated or un-done and more effectively by the use of hypnosis. We will consider its theoretical and technical manifestations later at considerable length. However, for the moment let us accept the fact that dissociation of bodily and mental processes does exist, that it is possible to manipulate this phenomenon by hypnosis, and that, accordingly, we can effectively employ it for the treatment of various conditions, both psychological and physiological.

In a sense we had already begun to use it when we told our patient to "ignore" unpleasant sensations coming from some part of the body. It is only necessary to extend these suggestions further. We might say to him: "Your right arm is no longer a part of you. Your self stops here at your shoulder. *The* arm has no feeling or movement. You cannot move it, because it is no longer connected to you. You feel that there is a space between the end of your shoulder and the beginning of *that* arm. Therefore, there is no connection between *it* and yourself. Since it is no longer within your own being it no longer has the power to send you painful impulses. It is dead and attached like a board to your shoulders. You experience no sensations coming from it."

We have temporarily "dissociated" the arm from the rest of the body. Accordingly, any impulses coming from it will be ignored. The patient does not respond to them; he has no feeling in that arm and experiences no pain there. Notice that during the suggestions which were given (except for the initial reference) the arm was described as an "it," "the" arm, etc.—not "your" arm. We were attempting to make this limb an object, to remove it from subject, from self.

Not only can a part of the body be dissociated, but even the entire body itself. Suggestions of dissociation such as, "You are now standing by the door in your room looking at *that body* over there in the bed which looks like you. *It* may be suffering in pain, but you are not because at the present time you and it are not the same." In Chapter 10 the use of this procedure in childbirth will be described. The dissociative technique is one of most dramatic procedures within the armamentarium of the hypnotherapist, and usually requires a subject who is highly hypnotizable. If it is to be maintained for some time, the suggestions for its initiation generally must be given with the patient quite deeply hypnotized. Dissociation in its pure sense is difficult in the individual who can enter only a very light trance.

Ego-Strengthening as an Approach to Pain Reduction

If one thinks of the human "ego" as a kind of "mental muscle," an organ of the person developed to aid him in adjusting to reality, then his ability to cope with distress is related to its "strength." Individuals who become emotionally devastated at minor frustrations are considered psychologically to have a "weak" ego. Coping with pain is much like adjusting to any other of life's adversities. The strong individual can carry a greater load. If he is physically strong he can lift a greater weight, if psychologically strong, a greater life burden. Accordingly, if we can strengthen a weak ego in a pain-ridden patient, we can teach him better how to ignore the pain, dissociate it, suppress it or endure it.

Hartland (1966) uses suggestive hypnosis specifically aimed at building the patient's ego, a procedure which can be useful in a number of therapeutic goals, including the relief of pain. He suggests repetitively that the individual will feel physically stronger and fitter each day, more alert, more energetic, and will tire less easily. The patient is told that he will become "deeply interested" in whatever he is doing, that his mind will become calmer and that he can think more clearly. It is suggested to him that he will be less easily disturbed, more relaxed and imbued with greater confidence, and that each day he will feel more optimistic.

The number of such positive suggestions could, of course, be extended indefinitely. There is some question as to whether the ego is strengthened most by much repetition of a few suggestions, or by a wide variety. However, there is no doubt that many individuals respond quite favorably to such an approach and develop both an improved outlook on life and increased motivation to cope with their problems. Hartland's approach to using hypnosis is not unlike Normal Vincent Peale's "Power of Positive Thinking" (1952) or Coue's (1923) "Every day in every way I am getting better and better."

Hypnosis in Anesthesiology

When a patient first enters a hospital for an operation he is rapidly bereft of his belongings and his defenses. He is interviewed by impersonal hospital personnel and signs the operative permit. His valuables are checked and dentures removed. This is followed by blood tests, venipunctures, enemas, x-rays, etc. No wonder even the hardiest individual begins to feel a sense of insecurity which can turn into fear, and in some patients, outright terror.

The anesthesiologist who is willing at this time to visit the patient, introduce himself, and give reassurance can have a significant effect on the equanimity with which the patient faces his surgery and his post-surgical course. Mention of the recovery room will alert the patient to the fact that when he wakes up he will be in a different room than the one in which he departed from consciousness, and surrounded by other patients. This prevents his being startled by the new surroundings. The more details concerning the operation which can be shared with him, the more likely he will be to cope with them. We can usually handle much better that which we understand.

Marmer (1959), who was one of the outstanding authorities in this area, reported four major indications for the use of hypnosis in anesthesiology.

1. To overcome anxiety and fear.
2. To help in providing a more pleasant reaction from anesthesia and as an aid in the post-operative recovery period.
3. To raise the pain threshold.
4. To induce anesthesia and analgesia to reduce the amount of chemo-anesthesia needed or to replace it entirely.

Stress itself often makes a patient more hypnotizable. There is less of that attitude of criticality which needs to be suspended for best results. Accordingly, suggestions of relaxation, freedom from fear, and ability to sleep the night before the operation may be much more effective in helping the patient to be at his best the morning of the surgery than a simple prescription of sedative medication. The less the patient needs to be medicated prior to surgery the more likely it is that his post-operative recovery will be rapid. Furthermore, suggestions to the effect that he will remain relaxed in the operating room and will feel comfortable there can do much to remove both initial fear and post-traumatization. Surgical patients have occasionally been so traumatized by their experience that a long-lasting anxiety neurosis or phobia has been initiated, one which requires an extended period of psychotherapy. The more relaxed and comfortable the surgical patient, the less likely that we will have a psychiatric patient later. The principle of mastery over an experience determines whether it terminates in mature growth or leaves a frightened and ego-weakened individual. Both Marmer (1959), and Crasilneck and Hall (1975), who have had much experience with hypno-anesthesia, stress this relationship factor in the reduction of pre-surgical tension.

Few major operations can be performed with hypno-anesthesia alone. Many have been done, but unless the hypnotic treatment is supplemented with chemo-anesthesia, the patient needs to be an excellent subject, capable of a somnambulistic trance, who has had adequate training and conditioning before the surgery begins. Only about ten percent of patients meet these criteria. The greatest value for hypno-anesthesia appears to be its integration with chemical anesthetics so that less medication than usual needs to be administered. When considered from this viewpoint, hypnosis is prepared to make a significant contribution to many surgical cases.

The desirability of using hypnosis is especially indicated where the patient has a phobia of anesthesia, perhaps a carryover from a previous operation. In some cases the patient is allergic to sedation medication and hypnosis is indicated. There are also poor surgical risks in which the chemo-anesthesia alone poses a genuine hazard. In such cases hypnosis may be the anesthesia of choice.

Patients should never be pressured into accepting hypnosis. However, if they prove to be highly hypnotizable they may well consent, providing they are assured that other anesthetic agents are available for immediate use should they feel the need for reinforcement of the hypno-anesthesia. The wise anesthesiologist, even when working with a highly hypnotizable patient, is prepared for any unforeseen eventuality which may require his full repertoire of procedures.

The range of operations which in recent years have been performed with hypno-anesthesia as the sole or principal anesthetic is indeed broad. Kelsey and Barrow (1958) reported using hypnosis successfully to maintain a pedicle graft when it was important for the patient to be "locked" in a fixed and immovable position for a long period of time. Marmer (1959) described specific cases involving laminectomy, thyroidectomy, vein ligation and stripping, rectovaginal repair, urinary bladder cystectomy, cholecystectomy, hernia repair, hemorrhoidectomy, hysterectomy, pneumonectomy, mitral commissurotomy, and cardiac poudrage, to mention but a few. In each of these cases he indicated either that hypno-anesthesia was used alone, or, if in combination with drugs, the amounts and types of chemo-anesthesia employed. He also described the specific surgical techniques and the post-operative courses.

In cases requiring only local anesthesia suggestions can be made specific by touching or stroking the areas indicated. Thus one might say to the patient, "As I touch this area on your hand, it will become numb. It will feel as if covered by a leather glove. There will be no sensation of pain in it. You can ignore this hand while I work on it." Suggestions of this kind can by pyramided, that is, the patient can be told that, "Each time I touch the hand the feeling of numbness will increase."

A useful variation is to suggest that a piece of ice is being held on the area which is to be anesthetized. The feeling of coldness is built up through repeated and vivid picturizations. It then is experienced by the patient as an hallucination.

During the period of hypnotic induction, including the suggestions of anesthesia or analgesia undertaken by the anesthesiologist prior to the actual operation, the effectiveness of the hypno-anesthesia can be checked by clamps. Tests of this type should be given prior to the actual surgery, assuming that there has been adequate time for orientation and conditioning of the patient beforehand.

In the treatment of burn patients two problems often arise for which hypnosis may provide a solution. Debridement of dead tissue and the changing of dressings can be very painful, and it is not normally possible to spray the afflicted area with a chemical analgesic, since it is under the old dressing. Although sedation medication may be of help a general anesthesia would not be indicated. In such cases the patient can be taught to develop a glove anesthesia on one hand, and then instructed to transfer this anesthesia to the afflicted area by pressing his anesthetized hand lightly over the area covered by the dressing. The anesthesia is transferred, and the dressing can be removed with minimal or no pain.

Another common problem in the management of burn cases is that of anorexia. Here hypnosis is used to stimulate feelings of hunger and appetite. Images of delectable foods pictured to the hypnotized patient, combined with suggestions of desire to eat, can often work wonders with such cases. Of course, the same kind of suggestions can be used in treating anorexia stemming from other reasons.

Erickson (1967a) describes an approach for the management of pain in which the patient is instructed under hypnosis to "compress" his pain experience into a very short and intense period. Thus, by suffering intensely for a minute or two he can then be pain-free for many hours. This approach appears to be promising, but no objective data as yet have been reported as to its efficacy in comparison with other techniques of altering pain.

J. Watkins (1978) describes a cancer case which initially was resistant to hypnosis. He was successful the next day in inducing trance and relieving the pain after analysis of two of his own dreams which were experienced on the night following the failure. These dreams pointed to his personal investment in being successful with this case as a demonstration of the potency of hypnosis in order to impress skeptical medical colleagues. Resolution of his "ugliness" enabled him to establish a more resonant relationship with his patient the next day, one which she sensed as committed to her welfare for its own sake rather than an attempt at a "therapeutic trophy." This case illustrates the importance of a sound doctor-patient relationship as a prerequisite to success in hypnotherapy.

One of the greatest drawbacks for the use of hypnosis in surgery is the amount of time sometimes required to induce a deep enough level of trance. Esdaile often spent many hours with each patient before operating. Today, the amount of surgery being done, and the many demands upon the time of the anesthesiologist and surgeon, often preclude the expenditures of many hours in conditioning a patient, which may extend over a number of days.

The patient frequently arrives in the hospital the evening before the surgery is scheduled. There is time at best for a brief visit from his doctors, and so much needs to be accomplished in such a little time. Furthermore, if the doctors involved must charge relative to the amount of time they spend with each case, the cost to the patient who will be given hypnoanesthesia can be prohibitive. Since so many good chemo-anesthesias are now available, and the technical aspects of using them well known to anesthesiologists, the more time-consuming psychological approaches to pain control, such as hypnosis, tend to be ignored.

Nevertheless, hypnosis can make a substantial contribution to surgery and anesthesiology in many cases, and in some there are special indications which prove it to be the anesthesia of choice, such as a danger of cardiac or respiratory decompensation. Knowledge of its uses and limitations should be part of the training of every surgeon and anesthesiologist, and personnel skilled in its application should be available when needed. After all, while it is not always the most convenient and effective anesthesia, it is definitely the safest.

Hypnosis in Surgery

Surgery is an intervention into the physical body which can alter its functioning in extremely complex ways. Less attention has been focused on the fact that it is also a psychologically traumatic experience. Normal mental and emotional functioning may be highly disturbed as a result of surgery, or before it in anticipation of the feared event. If we view the human individual as a physiological-psychological-social system of equilibrium which functions as a whole, then tissue insult can precipitate a drastic reorganization of psychological functioning.

That patients often get depressed as a result of surgery is a well-observed fact. That the process can also operate in reverse is not nearly as well accepted and understood by physicians. Put succinctly, we are more cognizant that tissue insult can cause psychological disturbance than we are that psychological disturbance can initiate tissue damage. Recently, the role of emotional factors in the maintenance (and even initiation) of malignant processes has been rather clearly demonstrated through controlled research studies (See Achterberg, Simonton and Simonton, 1976). Consequently, the effects on behavior and sensation of such procedures as lobotomies and neural blocks can be equally matched by the consequence of tension, stress, and emotional conflicts on bodily functions (Selye, 1956).

From this wholistic viewpoint the physical technique of performing a surgical operation, plus the post-operative management, represent only a part (albeit the most significant part) of the total impact on an individual. The wise surgeon and anesthesiologist will give much attention to the psychological factors within their patient which can heavily influence the outcome of the procedure. If understood and mobilized, the patient's chances of a successful recovery are greatly enhanced. If ignored and badly handled, his postoperative course may be a rocky one. In some cases these psychological factors will determine the difference between recovery and death.

It should be emphasized here that we are concerned with the total psychological situation of the patient, emotionally, perceptually and cognitively; as he approaches the operation, during it, and in his post-operative reaction to it. Hypnosis is only one of many psychological interventions which may be of value. However, it is a specific technique which can be employed for specific purposes before, during, and subsequent to surgery, to facilitate management. Since it has many well known effects on behavior and functioning in the hands of the practitioner trained to use it, hypnosis becomes an extremely potent therapeutic procedure to supplement and facilitate the surgical intervention. It is common for the physician who has been trained to think primarily in physiological terms to underestimate the value of this more intangible tool.

Every surgeon has been confronted by the anxious, tense, fear-ridden patient who may either relapse into an attitude of fatalistic resignation, become paralyzed with terror, or at times even refuse to accept sound, medical advice. He avoids a needed operation—sometimes at the cost of his life.

Pre-operative apprehension is often a significant complication to post-surgical adjustment. Contrary to popular belief, the individual who manifests complete calm is not always the one who shows the best recovery. Many people achieve this apparent placidity by an excess of control and become post-surgically prone to the development of phobias and obsessions. Thus Janis (1958) found that there was an optimal level of anxiety. Both those individuals who exceeded it and those who were below it showed a less satisfactory post-operative adjustment. However, patients who had been informed about the experiences to be anticipated related to their operation were less likely to become angry or emotionally upset during the period of convalescence.

As an adjunct to providing such information and reassurance, Field (1974) has developed a tape which uses hypnotic relaxation accompanied by instruction given to the patient at hypnotic levels. He found that patients who had listened to the tape during the pre-operative period were less tense on the day of the operation and demonstrated a more rapid recovery.

There is much evident to verify the fact that patients who approach their operations fear-ridden and with negative attitudes are poorer surgical risks than those who can relax, understand the nature of the surgery, and are prepared for maximum cooperation. This initial fear can be significantly reduced if the surgeon and anesthesiologist will give adequate reassurance to the patient prior to the operation.

However, if hypnosis is to be used to assist in an operation on a patient who is undergoing psychotherapy, especially an intensive or analytic therapy, it would be wise to consult the psychotherapist who has been treating him. In some cases hypnosis may be contraindicated for psychiatric reasons.

Consider the initial contact of the patient on arriving at the hospital. he is often questioned in a non-emphatic way about his residence, religion, ability to pay, etc., by an admission interviewer. He begins to feel that he is simply an object, a "thing." He may be faced with the most fearful event of his life, yet no one is considering his emotional needs. At this stage his phobias about the operation and his questions may well be brushed off by the contacting person, who more often is a representative of the business office than a member of the professional staff. He finds himself in a strange, impersonal environment, surrounded by efficient people who nevertheless have little time for his emotional needs. Friends and relatives may leave or be escorted out, and he is free to conjure up the worst in his mind.

It is at this stage where a contact with his surgeon, however brief, can be of tremendous support. The doctor who is not in too big a hurry to dismiss the patient's fears, but is willing to allow these to be expressed, will find that the anxiety level will lower, and the patient's preoccupation with them can be directed into constructive questions about the conduct of the coming operation. Our coping mechanisms can handle a known danger more effectively than an unknown one. Accordingly, the good surgeon will at this time, or at least before the operation, rehearse with the patient what will be done. This could involve a step-by-step explanation of each stage of the procedure.

The patient is probably in a highly suggestible mood then.

He will react with greater calm if the surgeon describes the procedures in a quiet but firm manner. This simultaneously informs the patient of what to expect and transmits to him the message from his doctor that, "I know what I am doing. The operation will be conducted competently."

Wording can be very important. Thus "discomfort" is not as alarming a term as "pain" or "hurt." "Separate" may not stimulate as much anxiety as "cut." While the surgeon is rehearsing the operation or thoughtfully explaining it in advance to the patient, he is also desensitizing him. The suggestions which the surgeon implants in the patient at this time may have a powerful effect.

This "rehearsal" of the operation can also be accomplished under hypnosis. The patient is hypnotized by one of the methods described in the previous chapters, and the various steps in the procedure gone over with him. Suggestions in nontechnical language can be given at this time, aimed not only at relaxation and the reduction of tension, but even more positively at stimulating constructive attitudes, hope, and the will to recover. A wording of such suggestions might go as follows:

"Now that you are deeply relaxed you find that you do not have to feel fearful. You recognize that your operation will be skillfully conducted and that you can make a rapid recovery. You understand what is to be done, and you do not need to worry about it. The entire staff which will perform the operation is competent and prepared to handle every stage of the procedure. You know you are in good hands. You look forward to the correction of your medical problem and the improvement in your life which will result. You are very strong. You can handle this situation well. You can let your surgeon, your anesthesiologist, and the entire surgical team perform their roles efficiently while you remain quiet and relaxed under the anesthesia. It is good to know that capable people are taking care of your welfare and that you have no cause for alarm."

Such suggestions can be administered by the surgeon, the anesthesiologist, or by a consulting psychologist or psychiatrist skilled in hypnotic techniques who can assume responsibility for emotional pre-conditioning of the patient. However, it is quite important that the patient meet his surgeon and his anesthesiologist face-to-face. He needs to know just who the significant people are in whose hands he is placing himself, his body, and perhaps his life.

Reactions and questions voiced by the patient should be

listened to carefully. The patient who states, "I am afraid that I may die," is not being merely "neurotic." His concern is genuine, and in fact there is evidence that individuals who enter the operating room harboring such an attitude may indeed be poorer surgical risks. While it is not wise to argue with the patient, efforts should be made to change this belief. It can operate like a self-suggestion. People who believe that they are going to die are indeed more likely to die. Incidentally, some practitioners (Cheek and LeCron, 1968) ask the patient under hypnosis what is the best time for his surgery. This is a question directed at his unconscious processes. His reply may have substantial validity.

Individuals who have had their anxiety lowered by an explanation of the procedures to be done, reassurance, rehearsal, and positive suggestions aimed at improving attitudes (either in or out of hypnosis) will often require much less pre-operative medication, thus enhancing the chances of recovery. There are times during surgery when it would be desirable to secure a response from the patient following some procedure. Under chemo-anesthesia this may not be possible; however, it is almost always possible when hypno-anesthesia is the method being used.

Cheek and LeCron (1968) have extended their "ideo-motor" method of communicating with patients to elicit replies from covert processes during surgery. Under hypnosis they suggest that when a question is asked, "the unconscious" will answer by lifting a finger on one hand to indicate its reply. Thus, a lifting of the forefinger might signify "yes," the middle finger "no," the little finger for "I am not certain," and the thumb for "I do not choose to answer." They have found that it is possible to communicate in this way with a patient when he can no longer verbalize. For example, it has been used to secure responses from dying patients even after they appear to have slipped beyond the realm of communicating. Cheek has reported that through such a technique he has been able to elicit reactions from individuals regressed to pre-verbal levels in the earliest periods of their infancy. He has also used this technique in asking the patient to predict his cure date.

If the patient is hypnotized prior to surgery, suggestions can be given to him such as, "During the operation you will remain very quiet. It will not be necessary for you to move." This assists in providing the surgeon with a quiet field in which to work. Such suggestions also permit the patient to endure long and uncomfortable procedures in cases where a general anesthesia is contraindicated.

It has been assumed that under a general anesthesia, in which deep muscle relaxation is secured, the patient is also unable to hear and react to words spoken in his presence. However, researchers have found that patients who were subsequently hypnotized were often able to report much of what was said and done during their operation (Cheek, 1964; Levinson, 1965; Pearson, 1961). Negative or unflattering remarks made by members of the surgical team were received and recorded at covert levels and had a decided impact on recovery. Even though a recent study (Trustman, Dubousky and Titley, 1977) throws some doubt on this finding, doctors and nurses would be well advised to guard their tongues while operating. A remark such as, "I don't think this old crock will make it," may be devastating and have an effect similar to what one might occur if the patient were hypnotized and then told, "We don't respect you very much and we expect you to die." In the high surgical risk case such a remark could make the difference between recovery and death during the postoperative period.

If patients under anesthesia can react to negative suggestions, they can also be constructively influenced if the surgeon, anesthesiologist, or other professional takes advantage of this period to make remarks emphasizing successful completion of the various stages of the operation and instilling suggestions aimed at enhancing post-operative recovery. Wolfe and Millet (1960) have demonstrated the value of this procedure. Suggestions might go as follows:

"There, that's been taken care of. It should not bother you any more. When you wake up you will not feel excessive discomfort. You will be able to sleep soundly, pass water, breathe well, and cough if necessary. You need not feel nauseous."

Of course, the entire surgical team should be aware of the importance such suggestions may have when the patient is apparently completely anesthetized, and be sympathetic to the possibilities of constructive psychological intervention at this time. Otherwise, these remarks will be received with derision by those doctors or nurses who are ignorant of the findings regarding their significance.

There should be no hesitation in suggesting such aspects of cooperation and recovery as are desired. Among the most useful suggestions which can be given a patient to improve the course of his post-operative recovery are: freedom from retching, ability to cough without pain, increased fluid intake and appetite for food, the need for lesser amounts of narcotics and sedation, and control of vomiting and hiccoughing. These can be implanted prior to surgery under hypnosis, but they can also be given or reinforced while the patient is still on the operating table.

One use of hypnosis which may be effective in some cases is to restrict bleeding. This possible ability of the modality may well stretch the credibility of some practitioners. Yet hypnosis has been shown to be effective at times in constricting the vascular bed and has been so used both in surgery and in dentistry (Cheek and LeCron, 1968; Stolzenberg, 1955; Cooke and Van Vogt, 1956).

Helen Watkins (1976b) reports a case in which a middle-aged woman whom she had been psychotherapeutically treating for alcoholism decided to secure a facelift, hoping to erase the lines which marked the years of neglect to her health, body, and appearance. Since hypnosis had been an integral part of the psychotherapy, the patient asked her physician if it could be used to assist her through the operation. Upon discussing this situation with the surgeon, the psychotherapist asked him in what ways she might help the patient to undergo the operation. He mentioned first of all the reduction of tension and pain and then remarked, "Of course, I wish her bleeding could be restricted."

The therapist made no promises but when next the patient was hypnotized, after suggestions were administered regarding quiet, peace of mind, and freedom from pain, she was also requested not to bleed. The operation, performed under local anesthesia, was quite successful, and the patient emerged with a greatly improved face and morale. The surgeon noted that there was a small amount of bleeding, but that it was minimal. The patient reported to her therapist later, however, that during the operation she had a very strong impulse to bleed, almost as if some inner compulsion was saying to her, "Bleed, bleed." She would then answer back with another part of herself, "I won't bleed. Helen doesn't want me to bleed." This inner stuggle continued throughout the entire operation, but her apparent relaxation and quiet transmitted none of this to the surgeon. Later, the physician told the therapist the patient's medical record noted that two years previously she had

had a hysterectomy for excessive bleeding, but that the pathology report had shown no evidence of tumor. The therapist and the patient during the course of the analytically-oriented therapy disclosed many evidences and psychodynamic reasons for a self-punitive, masochistic tendency which seemed related to her need to bleed. Bleeding, like many other physical functions, may in some patients have a strong psychogenic component and can therefore be psychologically influenced by hypnotic suggestion.

This particular case illustrates a number of significant points regarding the use of clinical hypnosis. It should be noticed that the intensive relationship with her psychotherapist, developed over many sessions, provided the motive to the patient to inhibit bleeding. The unconscious need to bleed stemming from masochistic impulses was pitted against the therapist's hypnotic suggestion not to bleed. Had the patient (who was obviously a bleeder) sought relief on a long-term basis from this symptom by hypnotic suggestion we would anticipate that the inhibiting suggestion would have soon broken down. Hypnotic suggestions aimed at suppressing symptoms which have a strong underlying psychogenic motivation usually succeed only temporarily. The suggestive approach, therefore, would probably be inadequate in a psychotherapeutic treatment of this condition. A deeper, more complex, and dynamically oriented psychotherapy would be required to eliminate it. However, the suggestion to suppress the bleeding symptom was successful in temporarily inhibiting this response during the period of the operation, thus demonstrating how suggestive hypnosis can be successfully utilized for time-limited effects during surgical operations.

One finding which was first noted in the 1840's by Esdaile (1957) was the greatly lowered incidence of surgical shock in patients who were operated on while under hypnosis. This suggests that such shock may be as much a psychological reaction to the trauma as physiological. At least, it is a phenomenon which deserves to be much more carefully researched.

Many minor procedures in which a general anesthesia is not indicated can often be expeditiously performed under a hypnotic state, even a light hypnotic state, for example, cauterization, curettment, or the debridement of wounds.

Cooper and Erickson (1959) have shown that the sense of time is capable of manipulation hypnotically. Thus, through suggestion, an operation which requires many hours can be made to appear experientially to the patient as if it lasted only a very short time. Likewise, long dreary hours in the recovery room can be "shortened" by the hypnotic suggestion that the patient will experience each hour as if it had lasted only a few minutes.

Hypnosis will probably never again be used as extensively and exclusively in surgery as by Esdaile, since many other methods of anesthesiology and pain control are now available which are applicable to a broader number of patients. Surgeons, because of their training, have been most comfortable with objective, tangible physiological procedures. However, as they become increasingly cognizant of the significant impact psychological factors can have on their success, and as more of them become trained in hypnotic procedures, it seems probable that the modality of hypnosis will become increasingly utilized as an integral part of their specialties.

Outline of Chapter 9. Hypnosis in Surgery, Anesthesiology and the Control of Pain

1. The experience of pain
2. Sensory pain and "suffering"
   a. Hypnosis in the relief of "suffering"
3. The "gate control" theory of pain
   a. The "sensory-discriminative" system
   b. The "motivational-affective" system
   c. The ability of hypnosis to affect the "motivational-affective" system
4. "Covert" pain and the "hidden observer" phenomenon
5. Hypnotic techniques for the control of pain
   a. Direct suggestion
      1. Use of tape recordings
   b. Self-hypnosis
   c. Changing the meaning of pain
   d. Dissociative techniques
   e. Ego-strengthening
6. Hypnosis in anesthesiology
   a. To overcome anxiety and fear
   b. Providing aid in the post-operative period

    c. To reduce or eliminate need for chemo-anesthesia
    d. Specifically indicated when there is a danger of cardiac or respiratory decompensation

7. Hypnosis in surgery
    a. Preparation of patient for surgery
    b. Wording of reassuring instructions and suggestions
    c. Ideo-motor method of communicating with anesthetized patient during surgery.
    d. Determination of psychodynamic meaning to patient of symptoms, anesthesia, and of the operation
    e. Possible reduction of danger of "surgical shock"
    f. Employment of time distortion

Chapter 10

Hypnosis in Obstetrics and Gynecology

OBSTETRICS
Hypnosis in the Relief of Childbirth Pain

Pain during childbirth seems to be an affliction of women from the more civilized races. Both animals and primitive women bear their children relatively painlessly, at least in comparison with unmedicated deliveries of today. Hypnosis has been used in some form for over a hundred years to relieve labor pains. Throughout the middle of the 1800's there were various reports (especially in Germany and Austria) of deliveries carried out under "mesmeric trance."

A tradition extending from the medieval period to the Victorian age held that pain was a proper accompaniment of childbirth. This view probably stemmed from a strict religious interpretation of the Book of Genesis in which the Lord is supposed to have punished Eve by decreeing that, "In sorrow shalt thou bring forth children." In 1853 Queen Victoria delivered Prince Leopold while under the influence of a chemical anesthetic, thus lending an official sanction to the newer concept that such suffering was unnecessary.

The Grantly Dick-Read and Lamaze Methods

In 1933 Grantly Dick-Read (1968) introduced a technique of delivery which aimed at reducing pain by teaching the expectant mother to relax. He termed it "natural childbirth." Read held that it was tension which produced the pain, and that this tension was a consequence of the fear with which a woman approached labor and delivery. To reduce this fear, he would teach his expectant mothers the facts about childbirth, since we are less prone to fear that which we understand. He followed this with exercises in breathing, relaxation, and the use of suggestion. At first, he insisted that his suggestions were in no way related to hypnosis. However, later he admitted that the combination of relaxation followed by suggestions was very similar to the procedure practiced by hypnotists.

Currently a very popular approach toward "natural" childbirth is the "Lamaze" method (1958). This was brought from Russia by a French physician of that name. His teaching includes the facts of pregnancy and delivery, plus respiratory exercises, neuromuscular control, and conditioning methods of eliminating fear. It is theorized that an individual develops a recurrent and self-reinforcing cycle of fear—tension—pain, which in turn creates new and greater fear, etc. By breaking this cycle through knowledge and relaxation, the delivery approximates that which is more natural and like that of other species of mammals. All of these same elements enter into the tactics employed by the skilled hypnotherapist of today who is employed in the field of obstetrics, be he the obstetrician, an anesthesiologist, or another skilled professional trained in the field of clinical hypnosis, such as a psychologist or psychiatrist (Samuelly, 1972).

Theoretical Conceptions Concerning the Ability of Hypnosis to Relieve Childbirth Pain

Just why women under hypnosis seem to experience a less painful delivery has been a matter of speculation by a number of workers in the field. Meares (1961), who believes that hypnosis is a form of atavistic regression, holds that the hypnotized individual regresses or returns to a type of experiential existence which characterized humans during the stages of his evolutionary development from an anthropoid animal into primitive man. This then re-establishes abilities of pain isolation and control which were characteristic of humans then, abilities which have been lost by civilized man. Meares also holds that the conscious experience of mother love becomes possible when chemo-anesthesias are not used and that this enables the mother to achieve a more total and realistic anesthesia. The conscious experience of delivery results in a closer mother-child bond than when it is blurred by a chemical anesthetic.

It will be recalled that Rank (1952) held that birth was traumatic to the child and the original source of neurotic anxiety since it involved separation from the mother. Whether or not this is correct, certainly the addition of chemo-anesthesia, which drugs the child prior to separation, could not but add to the hazard the infant faces in coming into this world. There are reports published by therapists indicating that a birth which was traumatic to the mother may be equally traumatic to the child, and may have strong unforseen effects upon its later emotional development.

Nevertheless, the birth experience is an extremely significant one to the mother. If it is accomplished without undue pain, attitudes toward the child may be more positive than if the baby's delivery was accompanied by much suffering. It is the beginning of the mother-child relationship. It should be started under the most favorable circumstances possible for the future well-being and emotional health of both.

Since hypnosis is not suited to all individuals, the judgment as to whether or not to use it as an anesthesia and analgesia in the case of a gravid patient should be made early and should consider many different factors. A last-minute decision to employ hypnosis (perhaps as the woman in labor is being wheeled into the delivery room) may well result in failure and traumatization. Although some individuals are highly hypnotizable and can quickly enter a deep trance this fact should be known beforehand, since most people require a period of conditioning if they are to achieve a pain-free state. Both advantages and disadvantages of hypno-anesthesia should be considered, whether it is to be the sole anesthetic or more likely is to be employed in conjunction with chemical anesthetics and analgesics.

Advantages of Hypnosis in the Practice of Obstetrics

Kroger (1977), one of the most experienced authorities in this field, lists the following advantages for hypnosis in the practice of obstetrics:

1. Fear, tension, and pain may be reduced or eradicated before and during labor.

2. The amount of chemo-analgesia and anesthesia can be reduced and in some cases entirely eliminated.

3. By controlling the painful uterine contractions the

mother can decide herself whether or not she wishes to experience the sensations of childbirth.

4. There is often decreased shock and consequently a more rapid recovery.

5. Since the patient can cooperate better, there is a lowered incidence of operative delivery. By relaxation and anesthesia of the perineum, delivery, episiotomy, and suturing are facilitated.

6. Since there is little or no chemo-anesthesia needed, many undesirable post-operative effects are avoided.

7. Hypnosis shortens the first stage of labor by two to three hours.

8. Hypnosis raises resistance to fatigue.

9. Hypnosis is especially useful in cases of premature delivery, debilitated patients, and in those who have ingested food shortly before delivery.

10. The hypnotic relationship is such that rapport can be easily transferred to a nurse, other doctor, or husband if necessary.

11. No special training beyond those normally employed in the Read and Lamaze methods is generally required, since they are all modifications of hypnosis.

12. Hypno-anesthesia, unlike chemo-anesthetics, cannot harm either mother or child. In this respect, the noted specialist in obstetrics and gynecology, J. B. DeLee (1939), stated that, "The only anesthetic that is without danger is hypnotism."

13. Most mothers find childbirth under hypnosis an extremely gratifying experience.

14. In some cases of emergency, such as abruptio placentae, the use of hypnosis can be life-saving.

Kroger presents a number of contraindications and limitations, including the small percentage of patients who can attain a sufficiently deep hypnotic state, the occasional occurrence of a hypnotized woman breaking "trance" upon hearing the screaming of other patients, the added time required to achieve a deep enough trance state, and the need for a trained hypnotherapist who is continually available during labor. He also notes the common attitude of suspicion and misconception in both professionals and laity which often prevents patients from cooperating in hypnotic procedures. He feels that hypnosis is contraindicated in the case of psychotic individuals, or others who are borderline,[1] unless a skilled psychotherapist is available who is trained to handle such patients.

Some doctors fear that hypnosis will foster too strong a dependency. Of course, patients are always dependent on their physicians, but such dependency is usually only temporary, and hypnosis need not bring this about any more than a non-hypnotic doctor-patient relationship does.

Who Does the Hypnosis during Obstetrical Delivery

The best individual to administer the hypnosis during an obstetrical delivery is the obstetrician himself. He is the doctor who has had the most contact with his patient. He is the one whom she trusts to see her safely through this experience. He is the one who can be counted on to be present at the time of delivery, and the one who knows what medical complications might occur in her case. He bears the final responsibility from her first consultation with him, presumably early in pregnancy, through labor and delivery. His relationship with the gravid woman has been a long one, established over a number of months. Accordingly, one might anticipate that, since clinical hypnosis is an intensive interpersonal relationship experience as well as an altered state of consciousness, he would be the one to whom she would most likely make a positive hypnotic response. Furthermore, he (or she) is generally endowed with the characteristics of a nurturing parent figure in a natural transference reaction established by the patient at this time. The obstetrician's influence should be most potent during the induction of hypnosis and the administration of the therapeutic suggestions.

This presupposes, however, that the obstetrician has been

[1]In the past it was commonly taught that borderline psychosis was a contraindication for the use of hypnosis because there was great danger that one could precipitate a full-blown psychosis. This belief is less prevalent now. Many hypnotherapists work with borderline or incipient schizophrenics and no major psychotic reaction is precipitated. However, this should be done only by experienced therapists who have established a very close interpersonal relationship with their patient.

trained in hypnotic procedures—a situation which should be strongly encouraged. Since many doctors have had little or no training in hypnosis or find that the practice of clinical hypnosis is not to their interest, then once the decision to use it has been made, it is necessary to find or select a well-trained professional in this area to carry out the procedures. Recognizing that hypnosis is a time-consuming technique, many OB doctors find themselves simply too busy, and handling too many patients to use this approach, even though they know its value.

An anesthesiologist, trained in hypnosis, makes a second-best choice. While this doctor probably does not have the long and continuing relationship with the patient, he is skilled in all the other procedures of anesthesia, and can best handle an emergency such as the last minute failure of the hypno-anes-thesia to be effective. However, he, too, may not have the time to employ hypnosis, and may not be conveniently available at the time of labor and delivery. The labor, of course, may require many hours, and the professional who will act as the hypnotist should be able to spend considerable time with the patient throughtout this period, as well as being present at the time of delivery.

Should the obstetrician be untrained in hypnotic techniques, and an anesthesiologist so trained also be unavailable, then a psychologist, psychiatrist, or other psychotherapist, who is skilled in these procedures, is the most suitable practitioner. These applied behavioral scientists are accustomed to communicating over long periods of time with patients, and, if they are competent, have developed many interpersonal relationship skills which can make them invaluable in dealing with the frightened or disturbed gravid woman. If the patient has been in psychotherapy, and her therapist is skilled in hypnotherapy (especially if this technique has been used in her psychological treatment), such an individual should be ideal to work with the obstetrician.

Some obstetricians maintain a continuous colleague relationship with this professional and arrange for this person to be involved in the early education and conditioning of their patients throughout the period of pregnancy. He/she then becomes most naturally a part of the "obstetrical team," and no new element or person is introduced to the patient at the last moment with whom she has to cope. Such an arrangement promotes a general feeling of security. If the doctor has not been personally acquainted with such a professional, and does not have full knowledge of the training, experience, and skill that the hypnotist has to offer, then a few suggestions can be offered here which should help any physician to select a well-trained specialist in this field.

Most legitimate, ethical, and well-trained workers in the field of hypnosis belong to one or both of the two major hypnosis societies, the Society for Clinical and Experimental Hypnosis, and the American Society of Clinical Hypnosis. Many qualified psychologists are associated with Division 30 (Hypnosis) of the American Psychological Association. A few highly experienced practitioners are also diplomates of one of the sub-boards of the American Board of Clinical Hypnosis. These are the American Board of Medical Hypnosis, the American Board of Psychological Hypnosis, and the American Board of Hypnosis in Dentistry. Affiliation with any of the above organizations does not guarantee a successful hypnotic experience for your patient. However, it does assure that the individual has had qualifying courses in the field and is recognized by the respective membership committees or Boards as being trained to use hypnosis.

Members of these groups are all qualified people in their recognized professions: medicine, psychology, dentistry, etc. They are not simply "hypnotists." They have full training, usually doctoral, in their major fields and have learned hypnotic techniques in addition. Accordingly, they have worked with many other "patients" and are bound by the same principles of ethics and responsibility which inhere in the practice of medicine. While there are occasionally other individuals who have had specialized training in hypnosis, the obstetrician or other physician who seeks their services should exercise extreme caution in using them, since there are currently a number of "hypnotists" attempting to offer their services to physicians who have neither the medical nor psychological background to be entrusted with this delicate and sophisticated psychological procedure. To hypnotize can be easily learned; to apply hypnosis skillfully and with appropriate precautions during clinical practice is an entirely different matter. Even a simpleton can cut open a belly with a scalpel; this does not make him a surgeon. Psychological sophistication does not come from a course in how to induce a trance, and the practice of clinical hypnosis or hypnotherapy is a job for a clinician, not a technician.

Training in Hypnosis During Pregnancy

If hypnosis is to be used during labor and delivery, training in the procedure should be started early, preferably by at least the third or fourth month of pregnancy. Training may be individually or in groups. Each approach has certain values and limitations. More attention can be given a patient when seen by herself. Moreover, the techniques of induction and deepening can be adapted to her individual needs. The doctor-patient relationship may be closer at this time. By observing her unique responses to the induction procedure, the doctor is better prepared to take maximum advantage of these during the period of labor and delivery.

However, these advantages can frequently be offset by certain plusses which inhere in a group training situation. In the group an esprit-de-corps rapidly develops which involves both social motivation and competition. In order to win approval from the doctor, patients may vie with each other in trying to reach deeper levels of hypnotic response. The amount of time which is spent for induction practice can be considerably increased without tremendous cost if patients are conditioned in groups.

As each woman new to the group observes more experienced subjects demonstrate hypnosis, her own suggestibility is increased. Two-hour meetings, held about twice a month, are recommended. The value of the procedure in the eyes of the trainees is further increased as those who "graduate" return with their babies to relate their experiences to the group. Group motivation and support are powerful facilitators of the conditioning process.

Whether done individually or in groups, the training steps are the same. They involve first answering questions about hypnosis and desensitizing the patient. Emphasis is placed on it as a "natural" procedure. Anxieties are resolved which might have occurred as a result of viewing horror films, listening to old-wives' tales, and countering the resistance which often is engendered by friends, family members, and too frequently even by doctors and nurses who are committed to tangible chemo-anesthesias with which they have had experience.

The period of questioning and desensitizing is followed by relaxation exercises accompanied by simple inductions such as eye-fixation or arm drop (See Chapter 5). The aim is to help the patient to raise her pain threshold and to teach her to be able to establish a glove anesthesia.

Suggestions to induce a glove anesthesia following an induction might be administered as follows: "Concentrate on your left hand. As I (or you) stroke the back of that hand all of the hand including each finger will become more and more numb. The hand begins to feel like it was made of wood. Sensation is being withdrawn from it, so that when it is pinched you can feel no pain. It feels like it is made of wood and covered with a leather glove. Your arm above the wrist is normally sensitive to all touch, but not the hand. It is almost as if it was no longer a part of you."

Such suggestions should be repeated many times, especially during the early training sessions. Anesthesia can be tested by pin pricks applied both to the hand and to the other hand or the arm above to demonstrate to the subject the reality of the loss of sensation. Such a demonstration is important and should be performed several times before the patient enters labor so that she will have developed a solid conviction of her ability to shut out pain. Inability to establish an anesthesia after several sessions suggests that hypnosis cannot be relied upon to be of much help during the time of labor and delivery. Really good hypnotic subjects will, after training, demonstrate the ability to remain in hypnosis while opening the eyes. This can be another useful test of hypnotic "depth."

Obstetricians who use hypnosis seem to favor the more gentle method, involving relaxation, over an authoritative approach. This is especially true where the woman has many aggressive needs, may have a strong masculinity component, or shows considerable resentment against being dominated by men. During the period of their relationship the gravida will usually let her doctor know how she feels about her husband, the kind of relationship they have, and whether or not she feels controlled by him, and if so, whether she accepts it or resents it. If she seems to have strong strivings for independence from masculine control, an authoritative manner in the doctor may well stimulate resistance to hypnosis.

Hypnosis in the Management of Pregnancy

A number of problems which occur during pregnancy may be substantially lessened once the patient has been conditioned to make hypnotic responses. These include nausea and vomiting, difficulty in voiding or problems with urinary and bowel control, insomnia, and excessive salivation. Skillfully planted suggestions can alter these processes in constructive ways which may obviate the necessity of frequent drug prescriptions. Other problems which will often respond favorably to hypnotic suggestion are backache, fatigue, cramps, and regulation of appetite where the gravid patient loses appetite and consumes an inadequate food intake for herself and the unborn child, or overeats and makes an excessive weight gain.[2]

Nausea and vomiting are special situations which deserve psychodynamic consideration. If it appears that they represent a symbolic rejection of the child, hence an unconscious desire to expel it via the mouth, then hypnotic suggestion alone may not only be inadequate, but since it is directed at an underlying motivation, might precipitate other difficulties, possibly hemorrhage or abortion. Direct evidence is lacking on this point. Furthermore, the entire problem of symptom substitution is still controversial. However, psychological prudence dictates that when a symptom seems to be related to some unconscious need, attempts to remove it suggestively be conservative, undertaken with precaution, and with the recognition that the patient may require a more dynamic and insightful therapy. Urinary and bowel control might be attacked more directly, perhaps combining hypnotic suggestion with behavior therapy techniques. Excessive fatigue can often be alleviated by short periods of hypnotic relaxation during which suggestions aimed at instilling a feeling of rest are administered. ("You will wake up feeling as if you have had a good night's sleep.")

One of the most serious problems facing the obstetrician is, of course, persistent vaginal bleeding, with the continuous danger of spontaneous abortion. A number of case reports have been published which describe the effective use of hypnotic suggestion to reduce bleeding time in various conditions (Edel, 1959; Stolzenberg, 1955). Crasilneck and Fogelman (1957) reported a controlled study on the effect hypnosis had on such factors as clotting and bleeding time between the waking control state and hypnosis. Their results were negative. However, it must be constantly reiterated that hypnosis with volunteer experimental subjects is not the same as hypnosis

[2]Suggestions for handling eating problems are presented in Chapter 12.

in the clinical situation with patients who have a close relationship with their doctor.[3]

During the period of pregnancy, not only does the woman's body shape change, but frequently also there are significant alterations in self concept, in her attitude toward the unborn child, and in her relationship with the child's father. In some cases these should receive some kind of psychological treatment which might include support, ventilation, and suggestion, with or without hypnosis. Since this is a time of stress for the patient, a psychological approach to the entire problem of pregnancy, labor, and delivery should be given significant weight. The obstetrical case cannot be considered as having been well handled if as a result of neglect of these factors the mother is traumatized, a pattern of rejecting her child is established, or long-lasting emotional maladjustments are set off, even though the delivery was accomplished without physical harm to either mother or child. In a program of psychological conditioning for expectant mothers hypnosis can play an important role for many of them.

In cases of possible abortion Cheek recommends use of his finger response technique (see Cheek & LeCron, 1968 pp. 131-133) as a way of communicating with unconscious attitudes within the patient. Underlying motives may be uncovered which will throw valuable light on such questions as whether the expectant mother wants the child or not. Decisions as to the best types of psychological treatment to be initiated can be more wisely made, and at times even questions of whether or not the child should be put up for adoption might rest on such communications.

A high percentage of the hemorrhages which occur during the first trimester do so while the patient is asleep. These may be accompanied by frightening dreams related to labor. Such emotional disturbances should receive early psychotherapeutic treatment, either hypnotic or otherwise. Kroger (1963) suggests that prolonged sleep under hypnosis is one of the best methods to ward off a threatened spontaneous abortion.

---

[3]Further studies related to the control of bleeding and techniques used in suppressing it are given in Chapter 14.

Modification of Attitudes About Labor and Delivery

Many women begin their pregnancy burdened by doubts and fears which have been implanted in them by their mothers and neighbors who may have regaled them as children with the horrors of childbirth. These are the patients who so often develop complications which require special psychological attention. If certain individuals can be hypnotized and given suggestions which may have a long-lasting effect, one should consider how these same people may have received unconstructive and harmful suggestions earlier in their lives, suggestions about the pains of childbirth, which now are creating great anxiety in them. Kroger and other practitioners hold that these women were in a sense hypnotized and given anti-therapeutic suggestions as children. In these cases the use of hypnosis is indicated to counter-condition them to the harmful suggestions which they already have received. Attitudes of fear can be offset by continuous suggestions of confidence, relaxations, and peace of mind as pregnancy progresses. These suggestions tying together childbirth and pain have often been repeated to the patient over many years. No wonder they are built-in and difficult to eradicate. Furthermore, even when not voiced, these fears afflict many women who have been taught that it is not appropriate to express fear. Today, since so many anesthetics are available, expression of fear tends to be suppressed. The wise doctor will not attempt to stifle with hasty reassurance the genuine fears his patient has of her coming ordeal. Through ventilation and acceptance, the strength of such anxieties tends to decline. Reassurance and counter-suggestion should come *after* the patient has had full opportunity to voice her misgivings and to reveal her true attitudes about childbirth.

Some practitioners have advocated that suggestions should be given the pregnant women that her child will be a "joy" to her so as to build up her expectations. For most women this technique is probably constructive. To a few, especially those who are angry at being pregnant, such a procedure may backfire. The child does not meet her expectations. She feels cheated and may take it out by a rejection of the infant.

During the period of pregnancy much can be done to counter harmful beliefs and attitudes which have been suggested into patients when they were children. Suggestive hypnosis should be employed to modify such attitudes, and this may be of equal value to training in the producing of anesthesia. As the attitudes improve, so also is the pain threshold raised. Likewise, as the gravid woman learns to produce anesthesia, such as in her hand, her confidence improves and her attitudes of fear should lessen. The psychological approach is a wholistic one, involving her entire being. It is not an isolated set of piecemeal tactics which try to deal singly with each single symptom. A wholistic approach results in a general strengthening of the ego, thus making her better able to cope with pain or any of the other frustrations and discomforts associated with pregnancy, labor, and delivery.

Equally important with modification of unconstructive attitudes within the patient is the learning of favorable attitudes about clinical hypnosis and its benefits by the nursing staff. Unsympathetic nurses can, by their remarks, nullify weeks of careful conditioning in the patient. Attitudes of skepticism, comments to the effect that they don't believe in it, etc., will have a profound impact when made by other health personnel and undermine the relationship of the obstetrician with his patient. Accordingly, if hypnosis is to be used, the nursing staff who will be caring for the patient should have instruction in the modality, including its principles, possibilities, and limitations, and the necessity that they give approval and support to the patient with whom it is to be employed. Their reinforcement will help greatly in bringing the patient to delivery with a strong conviction of its effectiveness.

Nurses who become aware of the suggestive import of their words will show this in many ways when hypnosis is not being utilized. For example, instead of asking, "How are your pains?" they may say, "Are you feeling contractions?" There is an entire language which is associated with pain that can be avoided by the sensitive healing arts person, doctor—nurse, technician, or other. Doctors can suggest doubt and dismay merely by a remark like, "If this doesn't work we'll try———."

Preparation for Labor

At the beginning of labor or just prior to its anticipated onset, a most important session will be held by the patient with her doctor. This is designed to get her psychologically ready for the birth experience. It aims to focus and review all that she has learned prior to this time about constructive attiudes, freedom from fear, and her ability to induce anesthesia. As Kroger and Freed (1951) put it, good obstetric practice should be concerned "with preparation of the woman's mind and less with the administration of noxious drugs...."

If the patient has previously been conditioned to establish an anesthesia, care should be taken that it not be so continuous and automatic that she does not get the warning of the first uterine contractions which warn that it is time to contact her physician and perhaps go to the hospital. If necessary, hypnosis can be induced in the already conditioned patient over the phone, and suggestions of pain relief given.

This is the time for a new dose of reassurance. The patient should never feel that she has made an irrevocable commitment to the sole use of hypnoanesthesia. She can be told that, "If it is necessary, we will supplement with a small amount of chemo-anesthesia," or, "We may need only a little anesthetic," and she should be encouraged to ask for some if she feels she needs it. The situation should never become structured as a test of her courage.

At this time the entire hypnotic procedure should be rehearsed, including a considerable time spent in deepening. If the patient indicates fear that she will not be able to follow her hypnosis training should the doctor not be present, ask her to carry through the procedure and step out of the room while she is doing so. Especially significant will be her ability at this time to self-induce a glove anesthesia. Request that she do so and test with pin prick or clamp.

Management of Labor

Screaming patients in the same or nearby room may so distract the hypnotically conditioned patient as to weaken her conviction about her ability to achieve and maintain a hypno-anesthesia. Wolfe (1961) recommends that the patient is warned in advance somewhat as follows: "You may hear patients in labor in the next room who do not know how to take advantage of hypnosis and are therefore making a great deal of noise. Do not let the noise or conversation of these people, or the use of the word pain, interfere in any way with what you know and have proven you can do."

It is sometimes valuable to make suggestions aimed at eliminating painful memories associated with delivery. In this case, it is recommended that a more permissive wording be used such as, "It is not necessary that you remember—" rather than "You will not remember."

Erickson, Hershman and Secter (1961) have suggested a "feedback" technique to maximize confidence and cooperation in the patient when she is in labor. In this procedure the patient is asked, both in and out of hypnosis, just what she would like to feel during the birth experience. Perhaps she prefers to be awake and alert at the moment the baby appears. Perhaps she wishes to feel the uterine contractions but does not want to endure severe suffering. Maybe she wants to hear the baby's first cry and then go to sleep. The experience of giving birth will be one of the most significant ones in her life. She should feel herself a participant in planning and directing it, not a helpless victim of forces, pains, and numbings over which she has no control. This moment can be one of triumph for her; or it can be a severe trauma with life-long crippling effects.

If she has given birth before, and her previous experience, either under hypno-anesthesia or chemo-anesthesia, was a particularly satisfying one, then suggestions to her that she will remember the exact feelings she had before and fuse them with her present ones may help to secure a replay of the previous favorable labor and delivery.

In making suggestions related to the uterine contractions and approaching delivery, instead of trying to completely suppress all feelings of pain, the doctor might suggest instead that the patient does not need to experience any more difficulty than she is willing to accept.

If a glove anesthesia is to be used and then transferred to the abdomen during labor and to the perineum during delivery, then it should be carefully checked beforehand. It is usually first induced in the hand which is tested with a pin prick. Then the patient is instructed to transfer this anesthetic feeling, by stroking the hand, to some other area of her body. At this time some site is selected which is not experiencing any pain. This secondary area is then tested for anesthesia by a pin prick or clamp. If no signs of flinching occur, and the patient reports feeling no pain, she should be ready to accomplish the same effect during the labor and delivery. Some obstetricians prefer to suggest a numbing sensation over the entire lower half of the body, rather than induce glove anesthesia and simply transfer it to the desired areas. Although a fairly deep degree of hypnotic involvement is necessary to secure a complete anesthesia or analgesia, even a light trance may be helpful in that it lowers the amount of chemo-anesthesia needed to secure the desired result. A post-hypnotic suggestion can be given that this numbness will reappear immediately following a signal to be given by the doctor.

In view of the findings of the Hilgards (1975) on overt versus covert pain it is probably wise to suggest that the patient will "feel" no pain rather than she will "have" none. Their studies have shown that pain has two components, sensory pain, which indicates the location and intensity of the pain stimulus, and suffering, a reaction which follows the first. It is this second reaction which we wish to suppress hypnotically.

A sophisticated and advanced method which can be effectively employed with the patient who can achieve deep hypnotic levels is that of general dissociation. It can be induced as follows: "You are having the feeling of floating out of your body. The body remains here on the delivery table and you are walking over to that side of the room and sitting in the chair, where you can watch that woman lying on the table over there. She looks just like you. She is your size and has the same hair as you do. Her face resembles that which you see when you look in a mirror. She is going to have a baby. The doctors and nurses are there, and you are most interested in observing what happens. She does not appear to have much discomfort, and as you watch her she seems to be looking forward eagerly to her experience of giving birth. You will observe every part of her delivery from the chair in which you are seated across the room."

There is a possible psychological objection to this procedure which may or may not have significance. No research data seems to be available on this matter at present. If the woman over there gives birth to the baby, will the observer across the room feel it is her baby? Or will she feel an estrangement toward the infant which affects her relationship with it? If this were true, it might also be true that anytime a baby is delivered under such heavy sedation that the mother is not aware of the birth, she would have a similar reaction. This possible problem deserves experimental study.

There are a number of advantages which accrue to the use of hypnosis during the period of labor. Through suggestions of rest and relaxation fatigue can be lowered. Furthermore, unlike some chemo-anesthetics, it does not lower uterine activity. Several writers (August, 1961; Kroger, 1963) report that in the primipera the period of labor is shortened on the average by some two hours. Erickson, Hershman and Secter (1961) hold that when chemical anesthesia can be reduced or eliminated there is a reduction of the risks of respiratory and circulatory infection in the mother and baby, such as often results in anoxia. This reduction can be achieved when there is a less prolonged labor. If tension in the patient has been reduced through relaxation, there is less likelihood of the necessity for a breech delivery because of malpresentation of the foetus.

A potential use for hypnosis has been suggested by Rice (1961), who claims that it is effective in inducing labor and that the process can be speeded or slowed by such suggestion.

Once labor has started, the patient's attention can be distracted from pain by asking her to count the average time of each labor contraction by seconds, such as "a hundred and one, a hundred and two, a hundred and three," etc. Another device that may be useful, and which can be related to deepening trance or inducing anesthesia, is to have the patient clasp a wrist tightly and squeeze, especially during the contractions. This mechanism, if it is to be used, should have been established previously as a post-hypnotic suggestion. "Every time you squeeze your wrist you will sink into a deeper hypnosis where you will not suffer discomfort."

Suggestions of relaxation under hypnosis may be effective in preventing a premature onset of labor. If the patient has been conditioned to the doctor's voice, both the induction and the relaxation suggestions can be administered over the phone.

In general, the labor of a patient who has been conditioned to hypnosis, who has learned to enter trance rapidly by a prearranged signal, and who can induce an anesthesia in herself, can be much more easily controlled by the doctor for the reduction of her discomfort and the handling of unforseen contingencies.

Hypnosis During Delivery

If the previously suggested hypnotic procedures have been carried out, then the control which they afford can be extended to facilitate the delivery and reduce or eliminate pain. Cheek and LeCron (1968) suggest the use of ideomotor signal questioning, both during labor and delivery, to ensure maximal understanding by the doctor of the patient's doubts, fears, and hopes. They even recommend this technique to predict the sex of the unborn child. Solid experimental findings are not yet available to determine the validity of this.

The delivery represents the time where the total of all previous hypnosis training is utilized. The patient should be reassured that she is not expected to perform with hypno-anesthesia alone, that if birth occurs naturally she need not suffer, but that other anesthetics are available should they be required. If she is a somnambule, one who goes into hypnosis so deeply that she emerges totally amnesic as to what took place, she should be asked whether or not she wishes to be conscious at the time of the delivery. Some women feel cheated if they are not aware when their baby is born; they wish to participate in the event.

Some obstetricians who use hypnosis do so primarily during the period of labor and during the initial stages of delivery, in which anesthesia has been transferred by the patient to the perineal area from a previously conditioned glove anesthesia on her hand. A local chemo-anesthetic is then used for the episiotomy. Others recommend the combination of a pudendal block with hypno-anesthesia. Most practitioners prefer a combination of hypnosis and chemo-anesthesia and report few deliveries with hypno-anesthesia alone. A few, however, apparently are able to secure sufficient pain control and use it with a large number of their patients. August (1961), for example, lists some one thousand deliveries performed with hypnosis as the sole anesthesia. No figures seem to have been reported differentiating the number of deliveries accomplished with glove-anesthesia versus those in which the dissociation technique was employed. The alteration of what is subject and what object, and how these can be hypnotically manipulated has been described elsewhere (See Vol. II, Chap. 9). Such changes occasionally occur spontaneously. Newbold (1963) reports the experience of a patient whose baby's head was "stuck" in the birth canal. The patient stated that she experienced no pain but felt like another person.

In this respect, some precautions should be made concerning the complete safety of hypno-anesthesia. On the surface the pain has been suppressed or repressed. However, Watkins and Watkins (1979-80), working with unconscious ego states, discovered that although the conscious person overtly felt no pain, the "hidden observers," (which they see as equated with ego states) reported underlying anger and fear. In one case when pain was totally suppressed in the right hand through hypnosis it was transferred to the abdomen and the experimental subject experienced a severe stomach ache, one which ceased as soon as his hypnotically analgesized hand was removed from the ice water solution in which it had been placed. Hypno-anesthesia seems to be quite effective at the conscious level. We do not know whether or not some internal trauma is suffered. But then, neither do we know whether or not this same situation might also hold for chemo-anesthesias. Further research with the hidden observer phenomena may throw more light on this question.

Hypnosis During the Post-partum Period

If the patient has had minimal chemo-anesthesia during delivery, it is possible for her to get off the delivery table and return to her room. This may give her a sense of accomplishment and mastery of the situation which improves morale and speeds recovery. Moreover, she still retains the ability to induce anesthesia in the perineum which should afford less discomfort during this period. Cheek holds that in such cases there is less danger of infection and other complications.

August (1961) advocates the use of suggestion to aid in promoting or suppressing lactation. Cheek and LeCron (1968) agree and hold that this can be achieved within the first 48 hours in those women who wish to nurse. They believe that hypnotic suggestion secures better results than the hormones which are commonly used. Kroger (1963) reports a study published in the USSR which claimed 95 percent success in stimulating milk production in some 77 cases. Specific suggestions to stimulate lactation might include the visual imagery of holding the baby in her arms and feeling its head against her breast. There seems to be evidence that tension itself can inhibit lactation. Accordingly, the use of hypnosis for relaxation is again indicated. Imagery can be further enhanced by inducing the sensation that the milk is flowing.

GYNECOLOGY
Hypnosis in the Relief of Menstrual Difficulties

Amenorrhea has been reported successfully treated by hypnotic suggestion (Cheek and LeCron, 1968; Meares, 1961; Kroger, 1963). The menses are stimulated by suggestion which specify their onset, duration, and frequency. Several techniques can be employed to accomplish this. The actual symptoms which accompany menstruation such as tenseness, pressure in pelvic region, enlargement, and sensations of hotness in the breast can be fed back to the patient. By suggesting the symptoms which are associated with menstruation, the bleeding itself can be stimulated. Another procedure is to have the patient under hypnosis regress to a previous menstruation and rehearse it, reliving her feelings and experiences at that time.

Another frequent problem for which patients consult their physician is *dysmenorrhea*. Many young women are taught by their mothers or others that cramps and pain are to be expected during menstruation. Such communications operate almost like post-hypnotic suggestions. It becomes socially proper to have pains, and since individuals are programmed for it to happen, it does. Hypnotic suggestion can be valuable in breaking the conviction that this discomfort is a necessary accompaniment to normal menstruation. The suffering of dysmenorrhea may also represent a self-punishment need, perhaps for real or fantasied sexual transgressions against the religious or home teaching concerning morality. Cheek and LeCron (1968) and other writers state that this condition is more likely to be caused by psychological factors than organic ones. Consequently, the treatment in many cases (after organicity has been ruled out) should be psychological. Suggestive hypnosis can be tried first. If the condition persists then some deeper, more reconstructive therapy along analytic or psychodynamic lines may be required. Cheek and LeCron also recommend the use of ideomotor finger signals to determine what are the emotional factors which are causing the disturbance and to ask the patient if "it will be all right" if she permits herself to have certain periods of normal menstruation without severe discomfort. She may also be taught how to turn the pain off.

Sexual Frigidity

Frigidity is another problem with which gynecologists and psychotherapists are frequently consulted. Since so many sex manuals have been written which hold that sex without orgasm is incomplete, many women have developed a need to have this experience. Whether or not all women can normally achieve this is controversial, but today it is the socially popular view that without orgasm one's love life is incomplete. Many approaches have been developed and are being widely exploited. Sex education, sex groups, etc., are the order of the day. A most widely publicized approach is that of Masters and Johnson (1970). Volumes have been written on the subject of achieving orgasm. Here, we shall present a few of the approaches involving hypnosis. Most techniques of hypnotherapy can be classed under two major headings: hypnotic suggestion, in which by direct or indirect means a symptom is suppressed or a behavior is elicited; and hypnoanalytic procedures, which involve a reconstructive psychotherapy of the personality, releasing bound emotions and lifting repressions. This second use of hypnosis is based on psychoanalytic conceptions of human personality and considers symptoms to be the overt consequence of psychodynamic conflicts which require resolution. In this section, related to general medical uses of hypnosis, we are concerned primarily with the simple and more sophisticated use of suggestive hypnosis. Many symptoms may be treated first by suggestive hypnosis. If they respond, and no unfavorable sequelae appear, then this is sufficient. Such is the case in most general medical problems, such as anesthesia, pain reduction, etc. However, if symptoms do not respond to hypnotic suggestion, or do so only temporarily, or respond but with the substitution of other equally or more serious symptoms, then the reconstructive therapies such as described in Vol. II may be required.

The treatment of frigidity in the female corresponds to that of impotence in the male. Both involve an inhibition of the full expression of sex and a limitation of the satisfaction received. Although men and women have unique problems, fears, and doubts that differ from each other, we will consider here difficulties of sexual expression in both the male and the female and how hypnosis may be of value in resolving these. The complexities of sexual psychopathology are beyond the scope of the treatise. Accordingly, we will restrict this discussion to a few of the hypnotic approaches which can be of value.

Frigidity is an extremely complex condition, commonly psychological in origin, but one which usually requires more than suggestive hypnosis. Meares (1961) considers that hypnotic suggestion can often do more harm than good and that cases to be treated only with suggestion must be carefully screened. He suggests that the origin may lie in latent homosexuality, parental conditioning, fear of pain, fear of pregnancy, masculine-aggressive personality, or fear of erotic involvement. Other writers note the prevalance of guilt as an inhibiting factor. When the frigidity is due to an unconscious conflict, a more intensive treatment approach will be required.

If one conceptualizes personality in individuals as having a masculine or feminine identification, the woman who identified more with her father and brothers, and repressed her feminine component, may be able to behave aggressively during the sexual act and prior to it. However, her repressed feminine component may exact a kind of frustrated revenge by inhibiting her ability to fully experience the sexual relationship, impairing the feeling of pleasure and stopping the accomplishment of orgasm. Such a psychodynamic situation will probably not respond to suggestive hypnosis and will require a more analytic therapy.

In other cases, a fixation has been developed when the woman as a girl was seduced by some member of the family, perhaps her father or brother. The traumatic experience, heavily loaded with guilt (especially if she had acted seductively toward them), may also have been pleasurable. It had a fixating or impairing effect. Accordingly, she is in the bind that she seeks unconsciously a repetition of that experience; she is emotionally tied to the family member and wants only sex from him. In a sense she remains true to him by being unresponsive to her husband or other men. However, the incest taboo creates such guilt for this unconscious attachment that she resolves the problem only at the cost of being unable to enjoy or participate in sex. Such a dynamic formulation certainly does not apply to all frigid women. However, it is an example of the psychological complexity which may underlie such a condition and which would not be subject to resolution by suggestive approaches alone. A case like this is a job for the sophisticated psychotherapist, not the gynecologist or general practicing physician.

Sometimes, however, a fear of intercourse or of pregnancy is based upon simple misinformation. In this case, reassurance and suggestion by the doctor may be sufficient to relieve the condition. Van Pelt (1963) describes the effective use of such techniques.

The doctor is often viewed as a parental figure in transference. Accordingly, reassurance and permission to enjoy sexual relations coming from this source may be sufficiently powerful to counteract impressions received from over-moralistic, real parents early in life. Parents, in their zeal to protect their unmarried daughters from becoming pregnant, may often try to scare them out of sexual involvement. One girl was shown pictures of female genitals in advanced stages of deterioration from the effects of venereal disease. As a result she was completely protected from becoming pregnant. She developed a life-long pattern of homosexuality.

Erickson and Kubie (1941) carried the principle of "parental" permission to enjoy sex further. They regressed a woman back to the time of her puberty, and the therapist in the role of her mother had a mother-daughter talk in which she was told she could enjoy sex in her marriage. This resolved her frigidity and she began enjoying sexual relations with her husband. Most problems of sexual inhibition involve some form of fear of guilt, and it is these which require treatment. However, in some cases the inability to respond sexually may represent a repressed anger at her mate. It is as if the body is saying, "You anger and frustrate me. I will not respond to you." And in truth many women find themselves unable to respond to their husbands, but highly responsive to an affair with a new individual—thus considerably complicating their problems.

Some women, finding themselves blocked in sexual fulfillment, go about promicuously searching for a satisfactory mate, but the greater their desperation, the more their frustration. The so-called nyphomaniacs can also represent women who have been so mistreated by men early in life that they are imbued with a deep-seated hatred of all men. Seduction is equated in their minds with castration and they go about seeking males to so "castrate" but at the cost of their own sexual fulfillment. Stekel (1943) describes this type of case as the "Messalina" complex.

Sterility

Evidence exists that sterility can be psychogenic in origin. Many cases have been noted where a couple have been unable to have children for years. They quit trying and adopt a child. Shortly afterward the wife becomes pregnant. It is as if some unconscious mechanism, some covert desire not to have a child, has been causing tubal contractions and preventing conception. Once a child has been brought into the home the barrier has been broken and conception takes place.

Several writers have reported the apparently successful treatment of a case of infertility through hypnosis. Raginsky (1963a) discovered under a hypnotic interview that the woman resented the inferior position during intercourse. Hypnotic suggestions were given her that she was free to accept any position she wished and enjoy. He reports that she became pregnant in three weeks. Ambrose and Newbold (1958) report the rather frequent use of hypnotic relaxation in treating sterility. They argue that this condition is caused by "spasms" in the Fallopian tubes, and that hypnotic suggestions of relaxation plus reassurance is the treatment of choice. Other conditions reported successfully treated by hypnotic suggestion include vaginismus, pseudocyesis, pelvic pain and premenstrual tension.

The *menopause* is a time in which many self-doubts and latent conflicts are mobilized. Some women feel guilty at not having borne children, or not as many as they had planned. Others are unconsciously angry at their husbands, who they feel have neglected them, since they are not as young appearing as before. Others develop symptoms related to loneliness, especially if the children have left the home and they had devoted themselves to being almost exclusively mothers, rather than wives and sweethearts to their spouses. This is a time in which depression may develop, but often symptoms that appear may be more related to the suggestions implanted in them by their own mothers and other women to the effect that "all women suffer this way during the menopause."

Hypnosis is certainly not an exclusive treatment for the emotional conflicts which are often precipitated at this time, but psychotherapy combined with hypnosis may be extremely valuable in restoring a sense of dignity and self-pride, in releasing bound up resentments, in giving reassurance and in suggesting worthwhile and meaningful activities for the future. It should be considered by the doctor as a useful adjunct to other forms of treatment at this time.

Outline of Chapter 10. Hypnosis in Obstetrics and Gynecology

Obstetrics

1. Hypnosis in the relief of child-birth pain
   a. Similarity with Lamaze and Grantly Dick-Read methods
   b. Theoretical conceptions concerning the ability of hypnosis to relieve childbirth pain
2. Advantages of hypnosis in the practice of obstetrics
   a. Precautions in cases of border-line psychoses
3. Who does the hypnosis during obstetrical delivery
   a. Obstetricians
   b. Anesthesiologists
   c. Psychiatrists and other physicians
   d. Psychologists
   e. Other health personnel
4. Training in hypnosis during pregnancy
   a. Suggestions for inducing anesthesia
5. Hypnosis in the management of pregnancy
   a. Nausea and vomiting
   b. Urinary and bowel control
   c. Vaginal bleeding
6. Modification of attitudes about labor and delivery
7. Preparation for labor
   a. Orientation of patient
   b. Giving of reassurance
8. Management of labor
   a. Distraction of hypnotically-conditioned patient by nearby screaming patients
   b. Eliminating painful memories associated with delivery
   c. "Feedback" technique to maximize confidence
   d. Initiating and transferring a glove anesthesia
   e. Use of dissociative techniques
   f. Reduction of tension

9. Hypnosis during delivery
   a. Combination of hypno-anesthesia with chemo-anesthesia
10. Hypnosis during the post-partum period
    a. Hypnosis as an aid in promoting or suppressing lactation

Gynecology

1. Hypnosis in the relief of menstrual difficulties
   a. Amenorrhea
   b. Dysmenorrhea
   c. Pelvic pain
2. Sexual frigidity (and impotence)
3. Sterility

Chapter 11

Hypnosis in Internal Medicine and General Practice

The Interaction of Mind and Body

The interaction of mind and body on each other has become a matter of increased interest to health practitioners. Historically, the more tangible and physical manifestations of illness have been the center of focus, as evidenced by the term "physician" applied to the primary health practitioner. Following Freud's discoveries, the role of psychological factors in the creation of symptoms received increased attention, and the term "psychosomatic" or "psychophysiologic" medicine was employed to indicate such conditions. Certain practitioners, such as Alexander (1939), approached the psychology-physiology perspective from a psychoanalytic point of view. Others, including Flanders Dunbar (1938), took a more eclectic approach. But in all these studies psychogenic factors were usually perceived as contributory only to the primary physiological etiology of such disorders as bronchial asthma, peptic ulcers, hypertension, etc. Psychological treatments were then (and still are) considered by most internists and general practicing physicians as secondary and adjunctive to the various pharmacotherapies. However, there has recently been renewed attention to the application of behavior therapy techniques in the problems of general practice, under the heading of "behavioral medicine." Behavior therapists have become interested in applying their procedures to a variety of medical disorders. Some of these combine behavior therapy approaches with hypnosis (Kroger & Fezler, 1976; Dengrove, 1976).

The Effects of Psychogenic Factors on Organic Illness

Raginsky (1963a) noted that half of all medical illnesses are probably functional, hence psychologically caused, and that many emotions are expressed through physiological processes. Furthermore, psychogenic factors are being increasingly recognized as playing a significant role in the etiology of various organic diseases. Fatigue may often be psychological, as intra-psychic conflicts exhaust the patient's energies. While worry and depression can result from a patient's concern about his poor health, the depression, itself, may cause physical symptoms. Sometimes anxiety is channeled into psychosomatic symptoms, and the patient remains unaware of underlying conflicts which are creating the anxiety. Patients of this type are often uncooperative and refuse to listen to their doctors. They do not wish to face the underlying emotional meaning of their symptoms. Such meanings can be primary to their symptoms, contributory, maintaining, or a consequence of them. In fact, they may have a number of unconscious fantasies connected to their illness which can be discovered through hypnotic uncovering. When underlying psychogenic conflicts have played a significant role in creating an illness, the patient who recovers because of the impact of medication may not welcome his return to health, but instead compulsively seeks some other crippling disability. This is why it is important, even in the treatment of ostensibly organic disorders, to understand just what the illness means to the patient. Otherwise, the doctor's efforts to cure him may be like swimming upstream. The motivational current within the patient will be opposing the treatment. The entire individual, not merely his symptoms, must be treated. It is possible that many reported "side effects" of drugs may actually be symptom substitutions in cases which are psychologically resistant to cure.

It should be recognized that even though a disorder is psychogenically caused it may result in physical stresses which in time initiate permanent organic damage. An individual with an hysterically paralyzed hand was relieved of his paralysis by hypnotherapy (Watkins, 1949). However, he had held it for some fourteen months in a tightly-clenched manner resulting in considerable atrophy in his fingers. Much physiotherapy was required to restore their motility, and then it was but partial.

Precautions in the Use of Suggestive Techniques

Some general policies regarding the use of suggestive hypnosis in general medical conditions are in order here. It is wise to attack minor symptoms first and to evaluate the response. Major symptoms are more likely to be rooted in significant psychological conflicts and, therefore, will be more resistant to change. If the minor symptoms respond readily, one can then move to the suggestive amelioration or elimination of the more important ones.

Much has been written about the hazards of symptom suppression through hypnosis, and indeed this factor should be considered. Hypnotic suggestion is an intervention into psychological (and hence physiological) processes which alters disease-health equilibriums. Such interventions may or may not be permanent. The underlying meaning to the patient of his illness and the meaning of the intervention will both determine its efficacy. When the disease process is circular and self-reinforcing, for example, a depression as a reaction to a physical symptom which in turn aggravates the symptom, the hypnotic suggestion may successfully alter the malevolent cycle by providing the patient with coping methods.

The concept that physical treatments such as drugs are appropriate for psychological symptoms like anxiety, depression, and psychotic manifestations is widely understood. And, in fact, at the present time, because of the long period required for successful psychotherapeutic treatment, many psychiatrists are returning to the more somatic approaches to therapy. Psychoanalysis in particular has suffered because of the immense amount of time and effort which a highly-specialized doctor must spend on each case. There is a search for briefer approaches—and hypnosis can be one of these.

That hypnotic suggestion can influence physiological function has been well proven in numerous studies. Since this work is centered primarily on hypnotherapeutic *technique*, we will not try in any comprehensive way to review the tremendous literature available, which has shown that many cardiovascular, cutaneous, gastric, and other physiological functions are subject to influence through hypnosis. For those interested in these areas, the reviews by Barber (1965), Sarbin and Slagle (1979), and by Crasilneck and Hall (1985), are illustrative.

That hypnotherapeutic techniques have been successfully used in altering the factors in psychogenic illness is widely accepted. However, that this modality can influence the course of illnesses considered to be organic is controversial, but attracting increased interest.

As far back as 1958, this writer attended a meeting of the Academy of Psychosomatic Medicine in which a paper was presented by a physician who was using hypnotic suggestion in treating carcinomas, not the pain, but the cancer itself. There was much skepticism among the physicians attending. The doctor presenting made no claims of "cures," but reported that his patients lived much longer than would be expected for the types of cancer which they had. When asked why, he replied, "I increase the resistance of the host." It is in such ways that hypnotic suggestion has proven valuable—by increasing resistance to disease, potentiating drug effects, and perhaps stimulating the immunological system. It has been employed throughout a wide range of physical disorders. We shall not attempt here to report the many studies indicating its validity or limitations, but rather those which have been used successfully in treating these conditions.

Hypnosis As An Aid To Diagnostic Procedures

Many diagnostic procedures which involve penetration of body orifices can be painful. These include such instruments as the gastroscope, bronchoscope, laryngoscope, nasocope, vaginoscope, proctoscope, etc. The relaxed cooperation of the patient is greatly desired during such procedures. If he tightens up he may prevent or inhibit insertion of the instrument and cause damage to the tissues. In extreme cases even a general anesthesia must be considered.

One of the greatest values of hypnosis is to induce a general relaxation, reduction of anxiety, positive attitudes, and willingness to cooperate. Furthermore, since hypnosis permits a focusing of attention (or inattention), the suggestions can be directed toward or away from a specific bodily zone.

One can suggest to the hypnotized patient pleasant reveries which will effectively distract him from attention toward the site of the diagnostic exploration. It is wise for the doctor to inquire about fantasies or sites which are associated with pleasurable and relaxed feelings, then give the hypnotized patient specific suggestions which describe such scenes, so as to encourage him to continue in them during the time the diagnostic procedures are being undertaken. Under a deep hypnosis an amnesia for the entire experience can be suggested, thus removing painful memories.

Diagnostic procedures which do not in themselves bring excessive discomfort may precipitate anxiety because of conflicts over the regions of the body under exploration. Thus, fear of suffocation may cause tension in the patient suffering from a respiratory disorder, so that even the sight of the bronchoscope will initiate a paralyzing fear or a complete lack of cooperation. Violent gagging may follow attempts to do a gastroscopy. In some cases the individual will not relax the glottis sufficiently to permit introduction of the gastroscope. Proctological examination may precipitate anxiety in patients who have conflicts over bowel and anal function. Various hypnotic techniques may be of use here. For those patients capable of a deep level of hypnotic trance, the procedures can be conducted as if they were under a general anesthesia. One can suggest that the patient relax, show no physical response, and be amnesic to the entire procedure upon emerging from hypnosis. It is not necessary to achieve an extremely deep state for hypnosis to be of assistance. General suggestions of calmness, lowering of anxiety, and relaxation of sphincters can aid greatly in completing a satisfactory examination. If necessary, the suggestion of analgesia in the relevant areas may be sufficient to ameliorate pain for those patients who complain of such.

In one case an internist wished to use a string test to assist in locating the site of the gastrointestinal hemorrhage. The patient could not tolerate the string and went into continuous gagging. However, under a light hypnosis she became calm, relaxed her throat muscles, and permitted the string to remain for enough time to locate a duodenal ulcer. For the extremely tense and anxiety-ridden patient, hypnotic relaxation may accomplish as much or more than medicinal sedation without any of the side effects often associated with such drugs. The usual principles applying to hypnotic suggestion (as described in Chapter 8) should be employed.

Poor cooperation of patients in some diagnostic procedures may be due to a deep, unconscious meaning or conflict. For example, insertion of a proctoscope can initiate fantasies of homosexual rape in some patients and precipitate anxieties. In male individuals who have latent homosexual tendencies this sometimes results in a panic reaction. If the patient shows evidence of such a disturbance, no attempt should be made to continue the examination until, through adequate reassurance, relaxation, and suggestion, the problem is no longer acute. The clinician who is intent on the physical examination and who ignores the signs of psychological distress may end up with a psychologically traumatized patient. The internist will not generally, himself, treat the condition of latent homosexuality. This is a job of an experienced psychotherapist; however, his awareness of the possibilities for trauma to such patients can have much to do with averting the creation of a new psychiatric problem.

Hypnosis in the Treatment of Cardiovascular Disorders

Cardiologists have learned not to reveal undue concern to a patient on first listening to a heart murmur. If the patient is alarmed, a fixation may be established on the cardiac region, and a mild or nonexistent heart condition can be elaborated into a cardiac neurosis. Kline (1950) described the case of an individual who reported "heavy pressure around the heart" accompanied by much anxiety. Under hypnosis, Kline regressed his patient back to a previous medical check-up during which the examining physician, after listening with the stethoscope, called in another doctor to do the same thing. This triggered an anxiety reaction. After the patient had recalled and relived the incident under hypnotic regression, the symptom ceased. This technique would appear to be useful in any case of suspected iatrogenic symptom fixation.

Heart beat has been clearly shown to be influenced by psychological factors. It has also been demonstrated that it can be conditioned to operant verbal conditioning. Hypnotic suggestion can be combined with biofeedback procedures to slow down heart beat.

Efforts to *reduce blood pressure* through hypnotic suggestion have not been as successful. However, Deabler, Fidel and Dillenkoffer (1973) were able to decrease both systolic and diastolic pressures through hypnosis. Van Pelt (1950) published electrocardiograms showing that heart beat could be speeded up by direct suggestions, e.g., having the patient imagine an accident during a fantasied car ride. He also induced it to beat more rapidly by indirect suggestions under hypnosis. The entire area needs further investigation, but hypnotic suggestion may be considered as a possible approach when other methods have not been effective. In these cases the patient should be taught relaxation and self-hypnosis (see Chapter 6), and since reconditioning must be continuous, he may need to use such self hypnosis several times a day.

Brady, Luborsky and Kron (1974) used a metronome induction procedure to reduce blood pressure in patients with essential hypertension. Taped instructions gave suggestions of relaxation with the verbalizations synchronized to the metronome ticking at 60 beats to the minute. This technique combined hypnotic induction with behavioral reconditioning. Such an approach can also be integrated with drug treatment.

Relaxation in cardiac patients can be much better secured if hypnotic suggestion is employed to foster fantasies, such as lying on a beach, relaxing on a green, grassy hillside, etc., than if direct verbal suggestions are given like, "You will relax." The picturing of scenes in which relaxation comes indirectly as a consequence of vivid imaginal involvement is much more effective. Kroger and Fezler (1976) have indicated that hypnotic suggestion of warmth paired with relaxation may improve compromised coronary circulation in cases of angina pectoris. They also report success in using hypnotic age regression to ameliorate and relieve *arrhythmias* due to rheumatic fever in childhood.

The effect that hypnotic suggestion can have on a cardiac patient was dramatically illustrated in a reported case by Raginsky (1963b). A patient who had previously suffered cardiac arrest during an operation was induced under hypnosis to relieve his anxiety about that procedure. During this experimental episode, his heart ceased for some four beats as measured on the electrocardiograph. This case illustrates that hypnotic suggestion is not an impotent technique and must be employed with professional skill if unexpected, harmful side effects are to be prevented.

Buerger's and *Raynaud's Diseases* result in restricted flow of blood to the extremities. There are a number of reports of hypnotic treatment of these conditions (Norris and Huston, 1956; Jacobson, Hackett, Surman and Silverberg, 1973; Crasilneck and Hall, 1975). Suggestions were given under hypnosis aimed at increasing flow of blood to the arms, hands, or legs. I have found that having the hypnotized patient visualize putting his hands into a basin of warm water significantly increased skin temperature in the fingers—in one case an average of 4 degrees F. Vivid description by the therapist and clear imagining by the patient are necessary for success with this technique.

Since *overweight* is associated with heart conditions, treatment of obesity in the cardiac patient is frequently indicated. Fortunately, hypnotherapy has been found to be of considerable value in reducing caloric intake. Hypnotic technique for dealing with this problem will be described in Chapter 12.

Hypnosis in the Treatment of Respiratory Disorders

Breathing is a function normally under conscious control. But in certain conditions such as an *asthma* attack,[1] it is closely related to fear and anger. A highly emotional experience may be sufficient to set it off. Afterwards, fear of dying may continue and reinforce the attack. A vicious cycle is thus set up. The disease is considered to be psychosomatic, since either or both the presence of chemical allergens plus emotional conflicts may serve as the triggering mechanism. Allergic reactions may also result from learning or conditioning. For example, some sufferers who have an allergy to roses may produce an asthmatic attack upon being brought into the presence of paper roses.

Since hypnosis is able to produce relaxation and lowered anxiety, its efficacy in the treatment of such conditions has been proven by many clinical reports, both early and recent (Van Pelt, 1949; Marchesi, 1949; Collison, 1975, 1978). Raginsky (1963a) notes that asthmatics are characterized by conflicts related to the suppression of any sort of "intense emotion,

[1]See also Chap. 13. Hypnosis with Children, pg. 306.

threats to dependent relationships and to the security based upon them." He advises strongly that the doctor should not use hypnotic suggestion to attempt to suppress the symptoms, but rather as a modality for getting the patient to ventilate fears, learn to relax, and result of gains in ego strength. Asthmatics have often learned to use their symptoms to control and force significant others to reinforce their dependency needs. Accordingly, direct suggestive assault on the main symptoms often results in a worsening instead of amelioration.

Different practitioners have proposed special suggestions to be given under hypnosis for relieving asthmatic attacks and reconditioning the breathing habits of asthmatic patients. Thus, Jencks (1978) holds that it is quite important for the clinician to time suggestions so that certain ones are given while the patient is inhaling and others during his exhalation. The goal is to reverse the asthmatic patient's tendency to increase the period of inhalation and shorten that of exhalation. She presented a series of respiration exercises and accompanying fantasies as follows:

TABLE 3
Examples of Jencks' Respiration Exercises

Long Breath: for relaxation and a slower breathing rhythm imagine that the inhaled air enters at the fingertips, goes up the arms into the shoulders and chest, and then, during exhalation, down through the trunk into the legs and leisurely out at the toes. Repeat a few times.

Warm Shower: to counteract tension in the shoulder and neck region, imagine water from a warm shower streaming pleasantly over the back of the head, shoulders, and neck. Feel the warmth and relaxation during exhalations.

Imagined Pathways: for easing the breathing or relieving pressures, imagine that the breathed air streams in and out easily at any of the places shown in Figure 1, or at any additional ones where relief is needed. Asthma patients found relief by "breathing through the small of the back;" tension headaches may be relieved by "inhaling or exhaling through the top of the head or the temples;" and "breathing through the holes under the chin" opened up the sinuses.

Opening Flower: to counteract anxiety and feelings of tightness in throat, chest, or abdomen, imagine during exhalations a flower bud opening at the right place, as in a time lapse film. Repeat and feel the opening for several exhalations.

Bellows: to ease the breathing or to increase the vital capacity, breathe as if the flanks were bellows which draw air in and push it out. Imagine that the air streams in and out freely through the flanks.

Golden Thread and Clothes Hanger: for a well aligned posture with an alive yet relaxed feeling, imagine a golden, energizing thread all the way up the spine and through the crown of the head. Imagine being held from above by this thread, so that straightness is achieved effortlessly. Imagine during inhalations that the thread is pulled from above and invigoration streams into the spine from below. Imagine during exhalations that the tissues of the shoulder region are relaxedly draped over the shoulder blades or over a suspended clothes hanger.

Toad: for ego-strengthening, inhale and imagine blowing yourself up to an enormous size, like a toad. Stay this size in your imagination while you relax during exhalations.

A number of workers have also recommended the use of hypnotic "abreactions." In this technique, the effort is made to release bound-up tension and provide other outlets for rage and fear. French and Alexander (1941) describe the asthmatic attack as a "cry for the mother." Abreaction borders between a symptom-manipulation technique and a hypnoanalytic one in which the goal is resolution of psychogenic conflicts. It can be effective in bringing crying relief to the over-controlled patient (see Vol. II, Hypnoanalytic Technique, Chapter 4.

We can but note here again that studies reporting on the efficacy of suggestive hypnotherapy are not valid unless careful attention has been given to the exact wording of the suggestions and the manner in which they are presented. Two hypnotherapists could read off the same suggestive words, but by their manner of rendition, and the way in which they relate to their patients, the results might be quite different.

Most treaters of asthma stress the need for relaxation and the slowing of breathing. Fortunately, hypnosis is a method *par excellence* to induce such a reaction when the patient is highly hypnotizable. It thus becomes a method of choice, even though all too frequently the patient arrives at the office of a hypnotherapist only as a last resort after inhalators and drugs have not proven effective.

Since much of asthma involves a secondary reaction to even a slight breathing difficulty, the patient needs to feel that he can both induce and stop an attack. Brown (1965) stresses the factor of teaching "control" to the patient. Crasilneck and Hall (1975) describe to their young asthmatic patients the television fantasy of horses who are running fast and, hence, breathing heavily. When they slow down and walk normally, their breathing becomes calm, and the wheezing is less. As the breathing of the horses slows, the young patient is taught to slow his own breathing likewise. They then suggest that the patient will have this same experience (e.g., the slowing of rapid breathing) each time he enters a hypnotic trance, and that his breathing will be normal when he is removed from hypnosis.

They reported a case of coughing which accompanied an ulcerative mucosal lesion on the tracheal bifurcation. The coughing continued even after the ulcer had healed. The patient was given suggestions that, "Your throat muscles will be relaxed and at ease. The itchy irritability will decrease. Your breathing will be normal and easy." After five days of suggestive hypnotherapy his cough ceased.

Kroger and Fezler (1976) have reported a number of studies in which behavioral techniques of systematic desensitization combined with hypnosis were effective in reducing wheezing. Highly hypnotizable patients tended to make the best response. They view asthma as a conditioned reflex and perceive the therapeutic task as one of reconditioning. The patient is taught under hypnosis to re-experience a relaxing episode from the past when he senses the onset of an attack.

The use of vivid imagining under hypnosis can be a valuable technique. Thus, the Spiegels (1978) have their patients imagine the tubes in the lungs slowly opening up and follow this with suggestions that they will experience cool, fresh air entering.

Hypnosis in the Treatment of Dermatological Disorders

The skin is an organ most expressive of emotions. Under fear it can blanch. Rage may redden it. Blushing demonstrates embarrassment. Weeping of the skin may act as a substitute for laychrymal crying. Irritations in relationships with others can cause attacks of neurodermatitis. The scratching to relieve itching has been shown to stimulate pain endings. And *psoriasis* has been known to break out in resentful wives to keep the unwanted attentions of husbands at bay. We even use terms such as "irritated," "burned-up," "hot under the collar," "itching for action" to describe emotional feelings. It is no wonder that the skin is reactive to emotional stimuli.

Dermatological diseases are generally multi-caused and

related to bacteria, fungus, allergens, external stimuli, bio-chemical balance in the skin, and emotional stress. This inter-active effect of physical and psychological factors in stimulat-ing a *dermatitis* was clearly demonstrated by Ikemi and Nakagawa (1962). The suggestion to patients that they were passing near noxious laquer trees caused a breaking out of the skin very similar to that observed by actual contact or proximity to such trees. Most practitioners recommend that such disorders should combine the usual medical treatment with some form of psychotherapy: directive, substitutive, or analytic. Accordingly, hypnosis should be considered as only one aspect of the total therapeutic approach.

The skin is the boundary between the organism and its environment, and serves as a protective and defensive organ. Scott (1960) reports that hypnosis has been found effective in a wide variety of skin disorders including pruritis, numular exzema, neurotic excoriation, warts, and especially so in cases of neurodermatitis. He holds that it often achieves per-manent results in disorders which are organically deter-mined. perhaps in no other general medical condition has hypnotherapy been so rewarding as in the treatment of der-matological disorders.

Since the skin is such an expressive organ, the "meaning" of a symptom here becomes especially important if it is to be removed or alleviated. Thus, a middle-aged veteran alter-nated in reporting to the dermatology and psychiatric ward. Psychotic symptoms were relieved by shock therapy, where-upon a severe dermatitis would break out. His skin problem would then receive aggressive pharmacological treatment on the dermatology ward, and as the skin cleared hallucinations would again appear. Such cases require deeper psycho-therapy and are not "cured" by symptomatic treatment, hyp-notic or otherwise.

Although some cases of skin disorders have shown rapid improvement by hypnotic suggestion, it would appear that a general reduction of their severity, step-wise by spaced sug-gestions, is desirable. In some cases it may even be prudent to leave the patient with a residual symptom—a small patch which does not entirely clear up. Strenuous attempts to re-move the last vestige of a psychogenic skin disorder by sug-gestion alone may result in a re-precipitation of the entire condition. Gradual improvement through continuous sugges-tion also has the advantage of permitting the practitioner to detect early adverse reactions.

One of the most difficult problems in dermatological disorders is the sensation of *itching* and the compulsion of the patient to scratch the afflicted area. This is a behavioral consideration and is one of the first aspects in which suggestive hypnosis can make a contribution. A number of different suggestive approaches have been reported by various therapists.

When the scratching is employed by the patient primarily to relieve emotional tension, suggestions of relaxation, maintained post-hypnotically, may be sufficient. Occasionally it is possible to suggest that the scratching will be displaced to other areas of the body, those which are not afflicted, leaving the lesions free to heal without continuous excoriation. As in the treatment of pain (Chapter 9), the patient may be told under hypnosis that "You will be aware of your itching, but it will not bother you," or "You will not have a desire to scratch it."

Itching can also be relieved by changing the nature of the sensation. Thus, a hypnotized patient might be told to imagine that cold compresses were being placed on the afflicted areas and that the feeling of coldness would bring a cessation of the itching feeling. Greenson and Obermayer (1949) have used this technique on warts and added that as the cold surface tingled the warts would fall off.

Crasilneck and Hall (1975) employed a variation of this technique by suggesting the feeling of coldness would occur as the warts were touched with a pencil. Cheek (1974) combined suggestions of cold with those of numbness in the successful treatment of herpes simplex.

Kroger and Fezler (1976) recommend that a glove anesthesia, such as is effective in controlling pain, be used to relieve itching. Sometimes itching has a masturbatory quality, and in cases of pruritis ani or vulvae becomes a way of satisfying erotic needs. Exploration of the patient's sex life may be indicated in such cases.

Other approaches to itching reported by Kroger and Fezler involved displacing the scratching to a doll. They describe a case in which skin-picking at night was turned toward a doll with which the patient was induced to sleep. This represented a displacement of anger from the self to an external object. The patient was also asked to indicate which area he wished to have relieved and to remove any doubt that such would be the case. This gave the patient the option of choice. Kroger and Fezler have also employed finger-twitching as a substitute activity for scratching. After this substitute was well established the twitching was progressively reduced through hypnotic suggestion.

Direct substitutions can be made for scratching as well as for other needs. Painting, sculpture, working with tools, and strenuous exercise may provide both distraction from itching sensations and constructive activity of the hands, so as to inhibit destructive self-excoriation. Inquiry should be made about possible interests which the patient has in such activities. These can then be reinforced with hypnotic suggestion.

Kline (1954) in a classic case involving *psoriasis* suggested that the afflicted areas would change sensation—first becoming warm, then cold, feel light, heavy, feel larger, then smaller, tingle, etc. Surprisingly, the skin soon cleared, although no direct suggestions were given for its improvement. He had used a similar technique with considerable success in the treatment of *neurodermatitis* (1953). One might hypothesize that the therapy lay in "teaching" the patient that he could control skin reactions. If then he was motivated to secure relief he would be able to achieve it. Helping the patient learn how to "control" such autonomic reactions is apparently an important factor in eliminating symptoms. Erickson, Herschman and Sector (1961) employed this technique in the treatment of *hives* in a child. The young patient was taught to turn them on and off, the same way in which biofeedback works. We might suppose, hopever, that patients with a strong masochistic need (and many dermatological patients have exactly this) might not respond favorably. Patients who have strong masochistic or self-destructive impulses should either have these resolved through insight therapy or be provided with substitutive activities which meet such needs in less harmful ways.

Since the skin is the organ most displayed to the world, it is not surprising that it can easily become a means of expressing exhibitionistic impulses. Being noticed (even if not admired) is better than being ignored. Patients with such needs will often express them through gaudy or unusual dress, loud speech, attention-getting behavior, etc. The physician who suspects these motives will do well to inquire into the feelings of inferiority and lack of acceptable recognitions in the patient's life before attempting to remove unsightly skin blemishes through hypnotic suggestion alone. Constructive substitute activities which permit the patient to achieve notice, acceptance, and praise from others may go a long way in making disfiguring skin blemishes unnecessary. If through some form of athletic, economic, artistic, creative, or scholarly achievement the needs for attention can be met, then suggestive therapy, with or without hypnosis, has a much better chance of succeeding.

One method of evaluating the possible effect of hypnotic suggestion is to direct it first only toward certain specific areas of lesion, ignoring others. Thus, Sinclair-Geben and Chalmers (1959) gave 14 patients the suggestion that their warts on one side of the body would disappear. Nine of ten patients judged to be hypnotized showed a complete disappearance of warts from that side in less than three months. The untreated side of the body showed no change. Ths approach permits the practitioner to evaluate the effect which hypnotic suggestion may have in the case of a given patient, without trying to remove all the symptoms at once, in case there is an underlying need for them. Mason (1952) found that aiming suggestions only at one area at a time was very effective in treating a case of congenital ichthyosis erythrodermia.

The "magic-finger" technique can be employed in the treatment of warts. A young girl, about nine years old, was brought in by her mother during a hypnotic workshop for the treatment of warts on the left hand. Her right index finger was anesthetized by stroking it. She was told, "If you will lightly touch the warts on the back of your left hand each day with the magic, numb finger, they will go away." She was taught how to self-induce the numbness by rubbing the finger in the other hand and to release it by squeezing the finger with the other hand. Although this case involved only one treatment without reinforcement, her mother reported that the warts, which had been in existence for many months, disappeared shortly after this session. Warts have been found to be responsive to a wide variety of stimuli, especially when the patient believes in the efficacy of the treatment. (See also Chap. 13, pg. 305).

Cheek (1961) suggested the use of ideo-motor finger signals to inquire of the patient's subconscious mind regarding the meaning of his symptoms and his resistance to their removal. This technique can be employed when the doctor finds a symptom unresponsive to hypno-suggestive treatment for the patient reaches a plateau in improvement.

Ewen (1974), in reporting the treatment of penile warts (condyloma acuminatum), suggested that the affected areas would feel warm, thus producing a dilation of the blood vessels and enhancing the supply of blood. He then told the patient (who was under a light trance) that, "Now your inner mind will lock in on this and maintain this warmth until the warts are healed and your skin becomes normal in every way. You can forget about the warts and turn your conscious thoughts to other things, because your natural healing processes will cure the warts without your having any further concern about them." One notes here that after implanting the suggestion, conscious attention is taken away from it since an "unconscious" motivation is generally more potent than one of which the patient is fully aware. This procedure of hypnotically influencing blood supply to specific areas was also employed by Hartland (1966) to treat rash. He interpreted this to the patient by stating that "more blood will flow through the little blood vessels in the skin—carrying more nourishment to the skin."

Finally, a number of practitioners (Frankel, 1976; Bowers, 1976 and others) have employed guided fantasy and induced hallucinations to influence skin reactions. One of my own cases may be illustrative of this approach.

A nurse in her early thirties requested hypnotherapy for a stubborn *neurodermatitis* which she had suffered for some eight or more years. Although her dermatologist was highly skeptical of the effectiveness of hypnosis, he agreed to respect her wish for this type of treatment. This condition would espcially flare up whenever she had a controversy with the chief nurse, whom she despised.

Although the evidence of a transference conflict related to mother figures was strong, I elected to use first a suggestive approach. She was hypnotized and given the following hallucinatory fantasies: "Imagine yourself taking a warm bath in which has been placed a soothing, healing lotion. You can feel the gentle, soothing relief to your irritated skin." She was asked to visualize and experience this situation for a few minutes and was then told, "Imagine now that you have emerged from the warm bath and that you are taking a brisk, cold shower which has a toning effect on your skin and your entire body. It makes you feel very much alive." She was asked to alternate several times between the "warm, soothing bath" and the "brisk, cold shower." It will be noted that this constitutes a variation of Kline's procedure previously described, but it is implemented by specific images rather than simply the words "warm" and "cold," etc.

After she had bathed and showered several times she was asked to visualize a self-image by a subject-object technique. "Look at yourself in the full-length mirror which is on the door of the bathroom. Notice that the woman there looks exactly like you; she has your hair and your features. However, her skin is pink and clear. There are no lesions. As you look at her, the mirror seems to fade from view and she appears like a replica of yourself standing in front of you. You wish to have clear, pink skin like her, and so you decide to join her—you move over in front of her, turn around, and back into the space she occupies until your body and hers coincide. Your head and hers are the same; your arms and legs are in the same space as hers. You and she are one and the same—now, you look down at your body and you see that the skin is pink, healthy and free of lesions. A sense of great happiness comes over you." Twice a week for some six weeks we used the same visualizations. The dermatitis rapidly cleared.

Two years later I was accosted in the hall by the hospital's personnel physician. "What did you do with Miss X?" he inquired. "I have followed her case for many years. Her skin is now clear and has been so for some time." Rather taken aback, I asked, "What did she tell you that I did?" "Why, she said that you told her to quit scratching." What does one say at this point to a practitioner who had little belief in psychological factors of disease, and none in hypnosis? Do we describe hallucinated baths, subject-object self transpositions, etc.? "Yes," I replied, "I told her to quit scratching." He smiled, apparently satisfied, and proceeded on down the hall.

Hypnosis in the Treatment of Gastrointestinal Disorders

The digestive tract as an organ system is especially sensitive to emotional influence. One does not have to accept the classical Freudian view that "oral" activities represent the first and most elemental stage of personality organization to recognize that the giving of food and drink is a common sign of affection. We take people we like out to dinner. We buy them a drink. We offer a cigarette. We eat when we are disturbed or unhappy. We imbibe alcoholic beverages to quiet our nerves or to relax with our friends. We refer to an individual as having a "sweet" disposition, and to a loved one as a "sweetheart." A person who impresses us unfavorably may be called "sour," and an angry individual is described as "bitter." A manner of personality may be termed "salty," and an individual close to us may be called "honey." Sometimes we can hardly "stomach" dealing with another person who "gripes" us, and it is "shitty" when we are treated badly. A courageous individual may be described as having "guts," while the colloquial term for the anus is used as a sign of derision. No wonder the gastro-intestinal system is imbued with such a rich set of meanings and emotions. It makes sense to expect that tangled interpersonal relationships, struggles between love and hate, problems of fear and rage could be translated into disturbance to the digestive tract or in any of its parts from entrance to exit.

Resistance to oral intake may begin even before the act of swallowing. Secter (1973) describes an interesting imaging technique to alleviate the difficulties some people have in *swallowing pills*. The patient is told to visualize another person who is trying to swallow a pill, but who chokes on it. He is induced to identify with this individual. He is next told under hypnosis to observe that after "our friend" has been given a signal to relax his throat muscles that he is able to do so. The patient is then induced to see himself in the place of the previously imagined individual and prepare himself to relax on signal so as to be able to swallow the pill.

Anorexia nervosa is one disorder which appears to be directly related to psychological problems. Raginsky (1963a) describes the successful treatment of such a case by "nonspecific suggestions for relaxation, comfort and hope." However, a family conflict was also revealed involving dissension between the patient's parents. Agreement of the mother for hypnotherapy, followed by a request from the patient that his mother "feed him," when fulfilled, reversed the process of food avoidance. Although close to death when first seen, he recovered and eventually became a physician. It will be noted here that suggestive hypnosis worked only when the family's emotional problem was treated simultaneously. This indicates that hypnotic suggestion alone may need to be supplemented by at least some relationship or insight therapy.

The *dumping syndrome* has come in for a substantial amount of study. It is characterized by sweating, diarrhea, anorexia, nausea, weakness and food dyscrasias. Although probably organic, it has a strong psychological component. Progressive relaxation combined with hypnotic suggestion has been found to be effective in relieving its most acute symptoms.

Dorcus and Goodwin (1955) reported previous studies which had shown that *duodenal ulcer* patients who developed dumping syndromes following subtotal gastrectomies tended to score high on the Taylor Scale of Manifest Anxiety and on the "Neurotic Triad" scales of the Minnesota Multiphasic Personality Test. In an application of these findings, they administered suggestive hypnotherapy to four such patients. The suggestions were directed towards reducing tension, removal of fear of this condition, enhancing the olfactory qualities of food, and the feeling of comfort with food or liquid intake. All four patients responded favorably.

Bonello, Doberneck and Papermaster (1960) reported symptomatic success in some 56 percent of 36 *gastrectomy* patients. Although these studies utilized primarily hypnotic suggestive techniques, one should consider the possible meaning of the dumping syndrome as involving anger, hate and resentment which has been symbolized in the rejection of food. Accordingly, other approaches which aim at externalizing and releasing such feelings might be found to be effective.

Doberneck, R. C., Griffen, W. O., Papermaster, A. A., Bonello, F., and Wangensteen, O. H. (1960) combined suggestive hypnosis with group therapy in the successful treatment of chronic dumping syndromes.

Lait (1972) reported an interesting case in which he relieved *compulsive vomiting* symptoms in a 31-year-old woman temporarily, first by suggestions of relaxation and relief. When the symptoms returned later, he traced their source through hypnotic regression to an experience when the patient was a child. Her drunken father would beat her and her mother. He often became nauseated after drinking bouts, and would vomit into the bathtub. She hoped he would die, and in fact prayed for his death at those times. Her episodes of nausea as an adult would occur following times in which her husband came home intoxicated. After seeing herself as a six-year-old girl involved in that experience and "forgiving" herself under hypnosis, she apparently lost the nausea permanently. This indicates the likelihood that more complex hypnoanalytic techniques may be required when suggestive therapy achieves only temporary results.

The treatment of *ulcers* has also been frequently tried using hypnosis. Raginsky (1963a) reported that, although hypnotic suggestion did improve patients with peptic ulcers, in some of them other behavioral and somatic symptoms subsequently appeared, suggesting that underlying needs were being bypassed. He affirmed that one should treat gastro-intestinal symptoms through hypnosis with considerable caution and noted cases where successful relief of the bowel symptoms in ulcerative colitis resulted in temporary psychotic episodes.

That gastro-intestinal symptoms are likely to have meanings and, hence, require more than suggestive hypnosis for their permanent resolution is exemplified in another case reported by Crasilneck and Hall (1975). A woman suffering from *globus hystericas* complained about her husband that she could not "stomach the crap he puts out." This was related to being pressured by him into performing fellation. These authors also reported that suggestive hypnosis can be successfully used to keep patients to their prescribed diets.

In general, most clinicians center their therapeutic strategy around the use of hypnosis to inculcate suggestions of calmness, relaxation and thus to reduce excessive gastric motility. Used in this way, it would seem unlikely that any severe sequelae would be induced. However, the therapist must be prepared to utilize more insightful approaches should symptomatic relief be only temporary.

There is a substantial amount of research concerning hypnotic influence on physiological processes. Since we are concerned here primarily with hypnotherapeutic techniques, the reader is referred to Levitt and Brady (1963), Ikemi et al. (1963), Reiter, P. J. (1952), and Sarbin and Slagle (1979).

Cooke and Van Vogt (1956) have published specific suggestions which they employ in treating *constipation*. These involve a "teaching" under hypnosis of the physiology of peristaltic movements followed by suggestions aimed at the relaxation of anal sphincters. They tie together, almost in a behavioral reflex sense, the act of sitting on the toilet to the act of defecation. Their specific suggestions have been republished in *A Syllabus on Hypnosis and a Handbook of Therapeutic Suggestions* (Am. Soc. Clin. Hypnosis, 1973).

Erickson, Herschmann and Sector (1961) report "discussing"

with the constipated patient under hypnosis "the possibility of setting aside a certain time each day" for "emptying the bowel." They also recommend allowing the patient to use the same period "merely to sit and speculate—whether the bowel movement will be a full one or a partial one."

Hypnosis in the Treatment of Neurological Disorders

Ambrose (1963) has found hypnosis valuable in the treatment of petit mal in children. He has his little patients ventilate their grievances, express aggression, and deal with underlying fears and guilts under hypnosis. He believes they can also be taught auto-hypnosis for self suggestion.

Frankel (1976) describes a case of "phobias and temporal lobe epilepsy." These seemed to date from a traumatic episode when the patient was 12 years old. He was alone in a boat rowing away from the shore of a lake when he became very frightened and disoriented. At that time he was diagnosed as heaving petit mal. His fears generalized to all sailing, flying in planes, being caught in traffic jams, and crowded tunnels. Seizure activity increased over the years and were characterized by a blank stare and feelings of depersonalization. The electroencephalogram showed "paroxysmal left temporal discharges." The treatment strategy "was based on having him imagine (under hypnosis) that he was experiencing the situations he had been avoiding. Each situation was dealt with and mastered in a separate session." The hypnotherapy here employed tactics involving abreactions and behavioral systematic desensitization techniques. Frankel noted that, "After a few months he reported no further seizures and an absence of strange feelings related to visual stimuli."

Raginsky (1963a) states that, "A patient suffering from organic epilepsy may be made to have a convulsion while under hypnosis, but that once started it cannot be terminated by hypnosis." This writer confirms that observation. A patient who had a seizure at the dinner table three nights earlier reexperienced the seizure when he was hypnotically regressed to that same meal. The seizure was recorded on the electroencephalograph.

Raginsky also reports a case in which a patient who has been experiencing one to four epileptiform seizures daily was

completely relieved in three, forty-five minutes of hypnotherapy during which the only goal "was to relax the patient
and to set the stage for him to express himself without fear of
reprisal." He remained free of seizures during a 19-year follow-
up.

Kroger (1963) was able to eliminate all further needs for
medication in a 32-year-old woman suffering from grand mal
seizures. She had suffered this condition, involving two or
three seizures a week, for some 25 years. Without detailing his
procedures, he stated that he taught her to become "proficient
in autohypnosis and sensory-imagery techniques." He reported that striking personality changes occurred at the same
time.

Hypnosis in the Practice of Oncology[2]

One of the most intriguing possibilities for hypnotic intervention is the recent attempts to use it in the treatment of
carcinomas. A number of reports have described its successful employment in treating the secondary effects of cancer:
pain, anxiety, depression, feelings of hopelessness, etc. In
this area, the most moving story of "David" by Gail Gardner
(1976) is now a classic in the literature. Gardner, by her sensitive interaction, enabled this 12-year-old boy to master his
fears, to live his remaining months to the fullest, and to die
with dignity. The paper is a "must" for every therapist who
works with dying children (See Chap. 13).

Visualization and imagery techniques under hypnosis
have been reported by Margolis (1982-83), Rosenberg (1982-83),
and others in directly treating the cancer and controlling the
side-effects of cancer therapy. Imagery techniques without
hypnosis had previously been reported by the Simontons
(1975) as having a substantial impact on cancer development
itself. In these, the patient's motivation is stimulated by direct
suggestion, and he is urged under hypnosis to mobilize his
physical resources to fight the cancer. He is also given imagery techniques such as visualizing the cancer in a form of his
own choosing. Thus, he might perceive it as a black mass, or
perhaps symbolically as a castle, which is being attacked. In
a direct or symbolic visual way he is given suggestions to the

---

[2]See also the Oct. 1982-Jan. 1983 issue of the *American Journal of Clinical
Hypnosis* which is entirely devoted to papers on "Hypnosis and Cancer."

effect that this cancer will be attacked by his anti-bodies, that they will "bite away" pieces of the cancer, and that he will imagine these pieces being carried away by his normal eliminative processes.

Meares (1982-83) describes a form of intensive meditation which is characterized by "intense simplicity and stillness of mind." Rather than urging the patient to focus on increasing awareness of such processes as breathing, Meares (as in Zen meditation) helps his patients "not to try," but rather to let themselves effortlessly slip into an altered state of consciousness. He has reported considerable success with certain patients.

A team of therapists at the Newton Center for Clinical Hypnosis in Los Angeles has been researching the use of hypnosis in treating patients with cancer for some eight years (Newton, 1982-83). They use hypnosis especially to relieve incapacitating symptoms such as pain, nausea, insomnia, and loss of appetite, and report substantial success in the treatment of some 105 cases seen for at least ten one-hour treatments over three months as contrasted with 57 cases which were "inadequately treated" by those criteria.

Treatment emphasis was placed on improving the "quality of life" rather than aiming to reverse the disease process—although the latter did occur in a substantial number of their cases. Simple and direct induction techniques were used, aimed at building ego strength and enhancing coping. In some cases intensive hypnoanalytic therapy was employed. Visualization techniques were used but not forced or imposed, and confronting the patient with responsibility for his illness was found to be counter-productive.

Although viewed with considerable skepticism by many oncologists, the data is not yet all in regarding such psychological approaches. Some hypnotherapists have reported remissions of the cancer, others an arrest in its development. While it is to be doubted that psychological interventions will take the place of the usual surgical, pharmalogical, and radiological treatments, the attempt to mobilize and improve natural physiological resistances to neo-plasmic development suggests yet another approach which may be of value. Since the modality of hypnosis has been shown to influence many physiological processes, it would appear that further experimentation in this area is warranted.

Summary

Most illnesses may be "psychosomatic" in the sense that physiologic and psychologic processes mutually interact with each other. This is being emphasized by the recent development of an entire health discipline called "behavioral medicine."

Through its effect on perception, motivation, and covert processes hypnosis can assist in the treatment of many "physical" disorders—if one considers therapy as a mobilization of the patient's natural processes for recovery. A wide variety of conditions have been found susceptible to favorable influence by hypnotic suggestion, and an increasing number of physicians, both general practitioners and specialists, are showing interest in the possibilities for hypnotic techniques in their therapeutic armamentarium. Current research studies in this area are developing improved treatment approaches and determining the relative susceptibility of various disorders to hypnotic intervention.

Outline of Chapter 11.   Hypnosis in Internal Medicine and General Practice

1. The interaction of mind and body
   a. Psychosomatic or psychophysiologic medicine
      (1) Physiological approaches to treatment
      (2) Psychoanalytic approaches to treatment
      (3) Behavioral approaches to treatment
      (4) Eclectic approaches to treatment
2. The effects of psychogenic factors on organic illness
3. Precautions in the use of suggestive techniques
4. Hypnosis as an aid to diagnostic procedure
   a. Hypnosis relaxation in gastroscopy, bronchoscopy, cystoscopy, etc
5. Hypnosis in the treatment of cardiovascular disorders
   a. Essential hypertension
   b. High blood pressure
   c. Cardiac arrest
   d. Buerger's and Raynaud's diseases

6. Hypnosis in the treatment of respiratory disorders
   a. Bronchial asthma
      (1) Techniques with children (See also Chap. 13.)
      (2) Behavioral techniques
      (3) Imaging techniques
      (4) Jencks' "Respiration Exercises"
7. Hypnosis in the treatment of dermatological disorders
   a. The skin as an emotionally expressive organ
   b. The "meaning" of skin symptoms
   c. Dermatological conditions treated by hypnosis
      (1) Dermatitis, Neurodermatitis
      (2) Psoriasis
      (3) Warts
      (4) Pruritis
      (5) Itching—scratching
8. Hypnosis in the treatment of gastro-intestinal disorders
   a. Psychological meanings of oral and gastro-intestinal terms
   b. Gastro-intestinal conditions treated by hypnosis
      (1) Difficulty in swallowing pills
      (2) Anorexia nervosa
      (3) Gastrectomy—Dumping syndrome
      (4) Peptic Ulcer
      (5) Globus hystericus
      (6) Constipation
      (7) Ulcers
      (8) Ulcerative colitis
9. Hypnosis in the treatment of neurological disorders
   a. Epilepsy
10. Hypnosis in the practice of oncology
    a. Pain in cancer patients
    b. Influencing neoplasmic processes

Chapter 12

Hypnosis in the Treatment of Specialized Problems

Hypnotic suggestion may be very helpful in dealing with a wide variety of special problems, such as habits, addictions, and circumscribed compulsions.

Smoking

With the more recent findings that smoking can be dangerous to one's health, many individuals who have been addicted are seeking ways of breaking the habit. This is not easy, since smoking is reinforced in many ways: as a relaxation agent, for the reduction of anxiety, for the inhibition of anger, and for aid in overcoming social shyness, to name but a few. Not only does it meet many different psychological needs for some people, but the smoker soon undergoes physiological changes in adjustment to smoking which result in painful withdrawal symptoms when he attempts to stop. Many individuals have given up smoking only to find that later, sometimes even years afterwards, they find themselves lighting up a cigarette upon slight provocation. The therapist who treats smoking is confronted with a patient whose compulsive habit is strongly reinforced, the cessation of which results in tension, anxiety, and pain, and in which the slightest relapse usually results in a full-scale reinstatement of the symptom.

Many approaches have been devised, generally built around the principle of re-conditioning, and the literature on stopping smoking has become voluminous. Almost every technique described has been able to report results with varying percentages of success, ranging from 20% to 90% in terms of stopping the habit. Follow-up studies, however, have shown a great deal of recidivism as a substantial number of the new abstainers, when finding themselves in smoke-filled company and beset with feelings of tension, are seduced into a resumption of the habit. The research literature reporting studies on the efficacy of various techniques for stopping smoking is quite large and has been better reviewed elsewhere (Bernstein & Glasgow, 1979; Hunt & Bespalec, 1974). Accordingly, we shall describe here only a few of the approaches involving clinical hypnosis which have been found to be successful.

One problem which has so often arisen is that the former smoker, once deprived of the reinforcements of smoking, often begins to overeat and develops an obesity problem. The blocking of one habit has resulted in a displacement of need, and another, equally objectionable, problem has been substituted. This is why treatment of smoking by hypnotic suggestion alone without some attention to underlying motivations often results in only a temporary cessation. The patient is extremely vulnerable to a return of smoking behavior in the face of pain, stress of socializing with smokers, etc.

Spiegel (1970) describes a single-session approach. After the patient is hypnotized, he is asked to close his eyes and concentrate on three basic points:

1. For your body, smoking is a poison. You are composed of a number of components, the most important of which is your body. Smoking is not so much a poison for you as it is for your body.

2. You cannot live without your body. Your body is a precious physical plant through which you experience life.

3. To the extent that you want to live, you owe your body respect and protection. This is your own way of acknowledging the fragile, precious nature of your body and, at the same time, your way of seeing yourself as your body's keeper. You are in truth your body's keeper. When you make this commitment to respect your body, you have within you the power to have smoked your last cigarette.

These three suggestions are repeated and elaborated. The patient is then taught self-hypnosis so that he may practice these by himself. Spiegel reports that, of an initial group of 615 patients, 271 returned a questionnaire aimed at a 6-month follow-up. One hundred twenty-one "hard-core" smokers had stopped for at least six months, and 120 had reduced their smoking.

Dengrove (1970) has adapted Spiegel's approach along behavior modification lines, using both operant reinforcement techniques and systematic desensitization procedures. His method aims at reducing anxiety in the "time between" the cue to take up a cigarette and the actual lighting of that cigarette.

Hall and Crasilneck (1970) report 64% to 82% success in treating smoking over five sessions (an initial evaluation followed by hypnotic sessions on three consecutive days and another session a month later). They used the following suggestions: "It has now been demonstrated to you the complete and total control your mind has over your body and the perceptions you feel. Your mind can block the perception of discomfort, as with the finger, or your mind can control your body, as with your leg. Therefore, your mind will no longer crave for a habit which has affected your life negatively with every drag of cigarette smoke you have taken into your lungs, a habit which has forced your lungs to labor beyond all necessity, stressing and straining these vital organs. But because of the great control of your unconscious mind, the craving for this vicious and lethal habit will grow markedly less until it rapidly reaches a permanent zero level. You simply will not crave nor will you smoke cigarettes again."

Nuland and Field (1970) contrasted certain "old methods" involving technique-centered approaches in which the role of the therapist was as a controller and persuader with a newer "patient-centered, personalized approach with the therapist acting as a catalyst and teacher." They avoided the direct suggestions of "you will stop." In their method the patient's own motives are fed back to him, amplified and vivified, and he is taught self-relaxation or self-hypnosis. They felt that hypnotic depth was a matter of secondary importance. Von Dedenroth (1968) suggested changing brands and not enjoying smoking or having a raw throat.

Rapid smoking as an aversion technique has been utilized

by behavior therapists with considerable success. Barkley, Hastings and Jackson (1977) compared three approaches: rapid smoking, group hypnotic suggestions, and an attention-placebo method in which the subjects were told to quit "cold turkey." The hypnotic suggestions were those employed by Hall and Crasilneck (1970). They reported slightly better success for the rapid smoking (aversion) method in terms of final abstinence rates in 6-week, 12-week and 9-month follow-ups. There was a greater frequency of vomiting among the rapid smokers.

Kroger and Fezler (1976) advocate a "hypnobehavioral" method of aversive conditioning. Under hypnosis, the subject is induced to see himself "smoking past the point of satisfaction, bloating, feeling a distension in his stomach, and becoming nauseated from the taste and his overindulgence in smoking." They advocate restricting smoking to one room and ultimately to one chair. Contingency management, involving the self-giving of positive reinforcements (cola, praise, etc.) by the subject when he successfully resists smoking, is also used by them.

Cheek and LeCron (1968) describe a humorous example of a hypnotic suggestion which misfired. The subject was told under hypnosis that he would find tobacco tasting like castor oil. Apparently, he stopped smoking briefly but then resumed it and, when contacted later, reported that, "I've developed the most remarkable liking for the taste of castor oil." They also reported a case in which, through ideo-motor fingering, they determined that unconsciously the patient (in spite of a bad case of Buerger's disease) did not want to get well. The hypnotic treatment, accordingly, was terminated.

Stein (1964) points out that, although many clinicians believe that one must stop smoking totally to avoid resumption later of one's original rate, there are some who hold that the frequency of smoking can be cut down to the point that it is innocuous. In line with this viewpoint, he describes an approach in which the positive and pleasant *qualities* of smoking are suggestively enhanced, but the *quantity* of cigarettes consumed is greatly reduced by long delays in each stage of the smoking behavior. For example, he tells the patient, "As you hold this clean, fresh, unlit cigarette in your hand, you can notice the clean, pure whiteness of the paper,—Now you can smell the fragrance of the unlit tobacco,—Now you can look forward to striking a match or lighting a flame—and watching the flame—and the pleasure of blowing it out—(this, too, is rehearsed several times, bringing back reminiscences of childhood delights and privileges). Finally, after much forepleasure and delay, the subject gets around to actually lighting the cigarette. He is then encouraged to "take a small puff" and "take a breath of clean fresh room air through your nose,—then blow out everything through your mouth." Finally, before being brought out of hypnosis, the patient is told that he will use this method of smoking from now on.

This approach is conceptually almost the opposite of that advocated by Kroger and Fezler (1976), who believe that no positive reinforcements should be tied to the smoking behavior. Comparative studies between these two approaches would be valuable.

Helen Watkins (1976a) has described an individualized method of treatment which involves five weekly sessions and for which she reports a 78% success in stopping smoking, with 67% still not smoking at the end of six months. She obtains an initial smoking history aimed at the client's reasons for smoking, for stopping, and what feelings he derives from smoking. On the basis of her analysis of the patient's motivations, a series of three suggestions and two visual images are selected from a file of "pre-typed 3 x 5 cards" which seems to fit that particular individual. A "concentration-relaxation" induction technique is used and the patient is presented the selected suggestion and visual image during the second and third sessions. Illustrating the treatment in one case are the following suggestions and visual images.

1. Relaxation Suggestion: You tell me that smoking calms your nerves, that (1) it is relaxing and settles you down, but what's so good about a cigarette that (2) shortens your breath, and gives you a dry, cotton feeling in your mouth? A cigarette may seem relaxing because you pause to reach for a cigarette, remove it from the pack, light it, and take a deep inhalation. It gives you a tension-free relaxing moment. But there are other ways to get the same effect, the same relaxing moment. I'm going to teach you to substitute a way to get the same effect, by taking a deep breath in, letting it out slowly and telling yourself to relax. Do that now. Take a deep breath in, let it out slowly and tell yourself to relax (The numbered inserts apply to this client.)

2. Victory Suggestion: You tell me you want to feel a sense of victory over your smoking habit—a sense of will-power and self-control—a feeling of winning over this vice. You can have the feeling by doing the following: Every time you pick up a pack of cigarettes and put that pack down again, this feeling of victory will come over you. You will feel good and strong. It's like winning one battle after another. Each time you repeat this behavior of saying "no" to a cigarette, either in fantasy or reality, you will be winning one battle after another until the final victory—the victory over your smoking habit. (She has the client experience this scene in fantasy. The good feeling he derives from putting down the pack is the immediate reinforcement which tends to increase future probabilities of him actually putting down the pack without smoking. This is in line with current behavior modification theory.)

3. Anger Suggestion: You tell me that you smoke to put a damper on your anger and frustrated feelings. You can see that smoking is one way to handle anger, but you and I know that smoking is no solution to this problem. Smoking ends up hurting you physically and it cannot discharge or control your feelings. If you are angry at someone, express those feelings in a constructive way. If this is not appropriate, then release that anger energy via exercise, or beating a pillow; or imagine you have a small rubber ball in your hand and knead it as you would dough. Try that now. Just imagine there is a soft rubber ball in your hand and squeeze it. Keep working the ball until your hand is tired.

4. Cost Imagery: Cigarettes cost $1.00 a pack. You tell me that you smoke up to two packs a day. That means you pay at least $2.00 a day for cigarettes. Multiply $2.00 by seven and the result is $14.00 a week. If you multiply $2.00 by the number of days in a year, then the total amount you are paying for cigarettes a year is $730, and what for? For a habit that makes you miserable. Wouldn't you like to use the money for something else— for something that would make you happy instead of miserable? If you stop smoking, you deserve to spend the money you save by buying something that won't go up in smoke. Think now what you would like to buy with the $730 you would save in a year's time, something perhaps

that you have always wanted but felt it was too much of a luxury. In your imagination right now, buy this item and experience using it. Feel the pleasure while I am silent for a minute. (In this imagery, the therapist motivates the client by picturing a desirable long-term goal to which he can commit himself. She suggests to him that after arousal from the relaxation he save the money he doesn't spend for cigarettes in a glass jar and watch the money accumulate daily.)

5. Day-Of-Not-Smoking Imagery: Imagine that the day has come that you no longer smoke. You are walking across the campus to this building. The air is fresh; the sun is shining; and it's a beautiful day. You woke up this morning feeling good about yourself and your world. You like the way you're handling your life. For one thing, the feeling of being a slave to a cigarette no longer haunts you. You are in control, not the ciagarette. You have more energy. Your throat is clear, and you know your lungs are clearing. You feel great, and the more you think about how good you feel, the more energetic your step becomes. Continue walking across the campus now while I am silent for a minute.

Other suggestions are built around the concept of "Excuse-for-a-Break," "Socialization" (showing that cigarettes interfere with socialization and separate the person from others), "Keeping Hands and Mouth Busy," etc. Visual images may involve the aversive experience to tobacco smell on clothes and even a "Hospital Scene" in which the doctor is saying some years later, "I can't do much for you now; I told you years ago you should stop smoking. All I can do now is give you medication for temporary relief."

The patient is next taught self-hypnosis and practices these suggestions and visual images on his own during the last two weeks. An important part of this approach is the therapist's insistence at the end of the second session that the patient is to phone each day for one week and report success or lack of it. No scolding or praise is administered, simply an acceptance of the report, but if the patient fails to call, the therapist calls him on that day. Watkins reports that the greatest difficulty in stopping is for those individuals who use smoking to dampen feelings of anger.

Sanders (1977) has described an intriguing approach. Her

patients were hypnotized as a group and, after first "brain-storming" to produce as many reasons as possible for becoming a non-smoker, were "time-progressed" ("Picture yourself in the future as a non-smoker"). Imagery and hypnotic dreams about being a non-smoker were suggested. This was followed by relaxation practice through self-hypnosis. Sanders reported 84% were non-smokers by the fourth session and 68% remained after ten months.

Nail Biting

Another oral "habit" which some individuals acquire and have difficulty in breaking is nail-biting. Gruenwald (1965), in reviewing the literature in this area, notes that different writers have attributed it to "an ego-integrative search for homeostatic equilibrium through motor channels," "a substitute activity for the release of hostile conflict and libidinal needs," "a discharge of oral-aggressive impulses," "a self-mutilation including both indulgence and punishment," "a depression equivalent in the form of partial, attenuated suicide," "a guilt expiating device with an element of restitution, i.e., nails grow back," "a hysterical conversion symptom and a masturbation equivalent."

Regardless of its etiology, patients seldom seek long, intensive, analytic treatments for it, since it is not usually regarded as seriously incapacitating. However, in the case described by Gruenwald the patient's symptom was tied in with a deep-seated impairment of self-concept and was psychodynamically related to very early childhood conflicts. Gruenwald resolved the nail-biting habit, but the suggestions for its cessation were effective only after much inner conflict had been resolved using complex hypnoanalytic techniques.

Kroger (1963) makes the process complicated so that it becomes a chore by suggesting to the nail-biting child, "Maybe you would like to start biting the nail on the left side of your mouth first—using one bite from each tooth in succession across the mouth, and then doubling back to the side where you started." Other suggestions follow like, "You can increase or decrease biting the nail selected to the degree that you think necessary." The purpose is to make nail-biting routine and boring. One might also hypothesize that by bringing the behavior under more conscious control its motivation by unconscious factors is lessened. However, Kroger, too, felt the need to treat underlying emotional needs and not rely simply on symptom suggestion.

Crasilneck and Hall (1975) suggest to their patients that "When you begin to put your hands toward your mouth, there will simply be an automatic and opposite withdrawal movement." This is countering a compulsion with an opposing compulsion, hypnotically inculcated. They balance this negative suggestion with one aimed at getting the patient to "respect your fingernails—and be proud of them." "One needs to discuss with the child the particular dynamics involved. He is asked to wonder which fingernail he needs to bite most. How much? At what time of the day? How much blood does he need to taste, just a little, or a lot?", etc.

Stuttering (Stammering)

Stuttering is another oral-verbal activity for which many different possible etiologies have been hypothesized (Gregory, 1979) and many different speech therapies employed (Perkins, 1980). Hypnosis is one approach which has shown success in some cases. Meares (1961) reports greatest success when the speech impairment is associated with manifest anxiety. He uses a hypnotic relaxation technique: "You let yourself go; you let yourself go completely. All the nerves of your body are calm and easy and comfortable. The words come easily and smoothly. Calm—easy—confidence is all through you."

Cheek and LeCron (1968) were successful in resolving two cases of stuttering, but only after they were age-regressed to certain traumatic episodes, from which the stuttering apparently started, and induced to relive and master these experiences through abreactions.

It has been noted by many clinicians that individuals do not seem to stutter while under hypnosis, but return to the disability on being brought out of trance. Kroger (1963) considers the symptom to mask a great deal of repressed hostility. He found that making a tape recording of the patient talking under hypnosis and playing it back to him was quite helpful. Kroger's later book with Fezler (1976) reports having the patient read passages in unison with his tape-recorded verbalization made under hypnosis.

Speigel and Speigel (1978) use a speech therapy technique

developed by Brady (1971) combined with hypnosis. They emphasize that people don't stutter if they follow a consistent rhythm, hence, "talking, thinking, and feeling in terms of the beat, always the beat." They employ a metronome set to 65-70 beats per minute and have the patient practice speaking with the metronome. These suggestions are given while under hypnosis.

Raginsky (1963a) reports an interesting case in which a man referred for stuttering showed no speech defect during the initial interview. It turned out that he was "silently" stuttering and controlled it overtly only at great energy and anxiety cost. Raginsky first induced him to stutter overtly through hypnotic suggestions to the effect that he would do so upon emerging from trance. He was then regressed to early traumatic episodes in his life and hypnoanalytically induced to relieve these through emotional abreactions. Subsequently, the stuttering stopped.

Ambrose (1963) held that it was important to use suggestion to induce the patient not to worry about his stuttering. He found that when a child's stuttering was initiated by a faulty relationship with parents, especially the mother, hypnotic suggestion must be combined with counseling with the mother in order to resolve conflicts between them. This suggests that family therapy may be required in addition to hypnotic suggestion for permanent results.

Crasilneck and Hall (1975) note that stuttering may unconsciously represent a desire to speak and a simultaneous desire not to speak for fear of the consequences of speaking. When the onset of the disorder seems related to a specific emotional trauma, a reliving and mastering of that incident often stops the stuttering. Crasilneck and Hall also suggest that it is valuable to have the patient practice speaking in front of a mirror. They reported that if a stutterer is asked to speak in a whisper, either in or out of hypnosis, his speech usually improves.

Erickson, Hershman, and Secter (1961) emphasize ego strengthening and discussion with the patient under a hypnotic trance (even if light) concerning which body movements are necessary for him in speaking. He is also given permission to stammer when he wants to, and told that he need not stammer when he does not want to.

Most of the hypnotherapists who have treated stuttering hold that hypnosis should be considered as a supplemental approach to the usual speech therapies. At times it secures striking results by itself; in other cases it can facilitate the speech therapies.

Hiccoughs

Hiccoughs may be caused by mechanical, inflammatory, vascular, neoplastic, or psychogenic factors. When carbon dioxide inhalation does not succeed in stopping them, resort is sometimes made to chemical blocking of the vagus nerve or even surgical intervention.

Dorcus and Kirkner (1955) reported 18 cases of hiccoughs treated hypnotically. The therapy stressed two points: complete relaxation, and relief of the patient's anxiety concerning his symptoms. Fourteen of the eighteen patients secured permanent relief from their hiccoughs.

Other more recent reports of the successful treatment of hiccoughs by hypnosis are those of Smedley and Barnes (1966), and Theohar and McKegney (1970). Kirkner and West (1950) reported on a severe case involving pernicious hiccoughing in a patient suffering from an adenocarcinoma of the rectosigmoid. Hypnosis was induced once or twice a day, and following suggestion during the initial session, the hiccoughs disappeared for some six days. Subsequenty, remission continued for two to three days after each hypnotherapeutic session.

During the second stage of their treatment, the patient was given a five-minute period of hypnotic sleep before being returned to the waking state. He was then taught how to sleep through auto-hypnosis. They continued this treatment for some five months during which the symptom was successfully controlled. At that point the patient succumbed to his cancer.

Their success following the period of hypnotic interruption of the hiccoughs seemed to be greatly potentiated when the patient was given a period of quiet under "hypnotic sleep." This suggests that Wetterstrand's approach (1902), in which he placed his patients into a continuous hypnotic sleep for several days at a time, might be useful in bringing a more permanent interruption of the neural connections involved in hiccoughs. There seems to be no recent report of this having been tried.

Alcoholism

Alcoholism is an addictive condition in which no therapeutic approach can boast a very high rate of success. Probably Alcoholics Anonymous has had the most effective results for those who stayed with the organization. Psychoanalysis has occasionally been effective, especially when the alcoholism was secondary to long-standing emotional problems of an hysterical or phobic nature. Behavior modification, especially aversive methods, has been effective for short-term relief, but its effect over several years has yet to be evaluated.

Bjorkhem (1956) holds that alcoholics are highly hypnotizable and that hypnotherapy is one of the most effective approaches to treatment. He reports "excellent" results even when the trance state achieved was light. He states that his results were often achieved in a single session. Apparently, he selected only patients highly motivated to stop drinking. An example of the suggestions he employed is as follows:

"Now the desire for alcohol will disappear, and you will really be able to keep your resolves. What is best and strongest in you will now wake. You will never again take any alcohol. Alcohol tastes bad. The desire for alcohol is disappearing for good. You feel perfectly healthy, and you want to be healthy. You can really feel how you are becoming healthier; you feel that you can keep your resolves; what is best and strongest is awaking in you. You can keep your resolves, and the desire for alcohol will disappear, disappear."

In contrast, Crasilneck and Hall (1975) hold that direct symptom removal should never be used with alcoholics. They recommend combining it with counseling, psychotherapy, group therapy, or marital counseling. Their suggestive verbalizations emphasize relaxation, securing restful sleep, ease, and a general strengthening of the ego combined with statements to the effect that the patient will be "secure in the knowledge that you are changing this habit." They recommend reinforcement with self-hypnosis several times a day.

Kroger and Fezler (1976) emphasize the behavioral approach of aversion combined with hypnosis. Under hypnosis, they associate unpleasant tastes and foul smells with drinking liquor, describing these with most picturesque imagery—such as observing another person sitting beside them in an airplane vomiting their drink. This, of course, is a variant, using hypnosis, of the in-vivo method of aversive conditioning often used in alcoholic sanitariums wherein the patient is induced to drink whiskey containing an emetic.

Wolberg (1948, Vol. II) claims that alcoholics can sometimes be diverted into hobbies which so intrigue them that they become completely absorbed. Hypnotic suggestion can be used to stimulate such activities. He, also, recommends aversive conditioning methods under hypnosis, but notes that regular reinforcement of these suggestions will be required for a considerable period thereafter.

The aversive conditioning method often has dramatic initial success. However, criticisms can be directed against it from several viewpoints. If the patient is "forced" to give up his prized drinking rapidly, and without meeting the needs which impelled him to drink in the first place, then he may choose instead to give up the therapist. His basic immature, dependent personality structure has not been altered, and soon it is likely to express its needs, either by a return to alcoholism, or by some other destructive habit such as drug addiction. One patient I treated (and was successful over several years of hypnoanalytic therapy) had previously been treated by a straight aversion approach (without hypnosis). He gave up drinking and developed an addiction to bad check writing. He was sent to me for treatment by the court. These patients especially may exhibit the tendency to revert to their symptoms or equivalent ones when their difficulties have only been hypnotically suppressed, without resolution of underlying problems.

Drug Addiction

The difficulties that inhere in hypnotically treating alcoholism apply even more so to the drug addicts. Success has been limited.

A particularly comprehensive study using group hypnotherapy was reported by Ludwig, Lyle and Miller (1964) at the U. S. Public Health Service Hospital in Lexington, Kentucky. This article contains an excellent description of how to hypnotize a group. These groups consisting of six to ten patients were trained in hypnosis by "the method of high eye-fixation while making continual suggestions for tiredness, relaxation, drowsiness, and sleep." They were then given "educational talks" under hypnosis in which drug addiction was explained to them, inspirational suggestions designed to enhance self-confidence, and encouragement to live up to their potentialities. The evils of taking that first shot of drugs were emphasized. Suggestions were given to increase group cohesiveness.

This *teaching-under-hypnosis* is a method which, perhaps, deserves more attention than it has previously received. The general ineffectiveness of cognitive explanations and reasoning to patients is quite well known by therapists. Usually, such explanations are brushed off, rapidly forgotten, and prove quite ineffective in the face of strong emotional needs and unconscious motivations. However, the inculcating of such material under a hypnotic state may well have more effect than simple conscious, intellectual arguments. Resistances are lower under hypnosis, and the possibility of significantly imprinting new and more constructive attitudes in patients appears better. I have done much "dynamic education" of patients under hypnosis regarding their underlying motivations and conflicts, and have consistently noted that the results were more significant than when the same material was presented to the fully-conscious, alert subject. This area needs further investigation.

Other techniques employed by Ludwig, Lyle, and Miller included suggestions given to have the patients mentally return to a time in their lives when they were leading a happy, drug-free existence. They reported that this technique met with only limited success.

A very potent suggestive approach apparently was that in which the patients were told that they would feel a branding iron, that it "was becoming red hot" and they would soon be branding their brains with words, "I must never take that first shot of drugs." Here we see the concept of planting a very vivid and powerful suggestion under what must have been an emotional experience of the subject. This branding-iron technique seemed to have a great deal of appeal to the patients. The authors hold that a strong, authoritative approach was much more effective than a permissive, analytic one. Perhaps that is because of the kind of dependent personalities typical of drug addicts.

Positive hallucinations were given that the patient would see drugs in a designated chair, but upon reaching for them he would overcome the craving through will power, and relax.

This method was effective with only a few patients, apparently those who could achieve a deep enough trance. "Blackboards of the mind" were described to them and they could erase the words "narcotic drugs," "hate," "incarceration," etc. Most patients reported success in employing this technique.

Some sessions involved hypnodrama (see Vol. II, Chap. 6) in which five members of the group played the role of dope peddlers and tried to induce a patient to return to drugs. Other roles included adjustment problems to home and job-getting which they would encounter after being discharged. This technique seemed highly appropriate as a treatment method, and the authors reported that hypnosis facilitated the role-playing considerably.

Facilities for follow-up were not available after the addicts were discharged. However, about one-third of them believed that they had received a "marked" strengthening in the resolve to resist drugs as a result of the sessions.

LaScola (1973) describes an approach to the treatment of drug abuse in which the hypnotized patient is asked to look at himself in his mind's eye and to notice the way he must appear to other people. He is then told to go over all of the unpleasant things which have happened to him while under the influence of drugs during the time the therapist slowly counts to 20. Then the therapist counts again while the patient reviews the "pleasant" things. He is next asked to weigh the two scores. Following this, the therapist leaves him in the room alone (under hypnosis) for a half hour during which he is to review his life from "the very first thing that happened to you that caused you to later turn to drugs." Other suggestions ask him to focus on his changes and to review his associations, asking if he is proud of them. No data is given as to degree of success from this approach.

Ludwig, Lyle and Miller (1964) studied the ability of hypnotic suggestion to influence drug symptoms and withdrawal symptoms. They succeeded with eleven subjects (patient-prisoners) at the hospital in initiating both typical drug symptoms and withdrawal symptoms, perceptual and behavioral but not physiological. They did this by regressing their subjects to prior times when they had been thrown in jail and had to quit "cold turkey." The subjects reported painful symptoms, but not as severe as when under an actual drug. Of most interest to therapists is that in part of their study in which they removed the behavioral and painful symptoms during an actual administration of drugs and subsequent withdrawal, the physiological symptoms remained, but the psychological components were either eliminated or substantially mitigated. This reminds us of the effects secured by hypnotic anesthesia to organic pain (see Chap. 9).

Bauman (1970), in attempting to wean adolescent drug abusers from actually using the drug, tried substituting revivication of "good" drug trips and pleasurable hallucinations under hypnosis which would be more rewarding, intense, and profitable than the original ones. He reported positive results with users of LSD, amphetamines, and barbiturates, but not those who smoked marijuana.

Crasilneck and Hall (1975) recommend hypnosis to substitute a sense of relaxation and well-being so as to offset the narcoticizing effect of the drug, and to build motivation after the decision to withdraw from the use of drugs has been made.

Weight Reduction

One medical report after another has shown that Americans over-eat, that many people are overweight, and that being overweight makes one increasingly prone to a number of diseases, such as high blood pressure and others. Overweight people tend to die earlier than those of more normal poundage. Furthermore, being slim is a beauty attribute which causes thousands of people, especially women, to struggle with their desires to eat rich foods. We shall make no attempt here to go into the many theories and findings regarding overweightness. Readers who are interested might consult Kline, Coleman, Wick and Sullivan (1976) as a starter.

Hypnosis is one of the many approaches which has been found helpful in reducing weight. Hypnotic techniques used in this way range from simple suggestions aimed at reducing appetite, to behavioral therapy techniques applied under hypnosis, to complex hypnoanalytic and ego-state procedures.

The simplest and most direct methods have involved aversive techniques such as suggesting to the hypnotized patient that he/she will find fattening foods tasteless or foul in taste and smell. This approach works for some subjects. However, it pits the will of the hypnotist against the pleasure of eating, and the patient may simply drop out of the therapy. The chances of this are lessened if the relationship between the therapist and his patient is especially strong, and/or the therapist's prestige in the eyes of the patient is very high. If the treatment is not progressing well, an old injunction to psychotherapists, which is always sound, applies here: "When one is blocked, fails to make progress, or is in doubt as to how to proceed, work on improving the relationship." A close and respected relationship is the best "technique" which the therapist has to offer.

Aversive methods, such as are employed by behavior therapists (Cautella, 1967), may involve "covert" sensitization or desensitization. Images are suggested under hypnosis to reinforce the verbal noxious stimuli to be associated with undesirable foods. The patient is induced to experience nausea when thinking or visualizing tempting, but interdicted foods. Less disagreeable are suggestions that the patient imagine eating favorite high-calorie foods, but the taste or flavors are nonexistent. Thus, Kroger and Fezler (1976) illustrate with the following suggestions: "You might like to think of the most horrible, nauseting, and repugnant smell that you have ever experienced. Perhaps it might be the vile odor of rotten eggs. In the future, whenever you desire to eat something that is not on your diet, you will immediately associate this disagreeable smell with it."

However, not all behavioral re-conditioning need be aversive. Helen Watkins (1979) instructs her groups under hypnosis to visualize two tables of food. On the first are all the rich foods which are high in calories. As they see these foods, they feel a complete lack of interest and a desire to turn away. They then look at the other table, filled with salads, cottage cheese, and other high-protein low-calorie foods, and at once feel very hungry. Their mouth waters, and they visualize how good it would be to eat these. In this approach, the aversive factors are minimized and the positive reinforcement of enjoyable eating is suggested, thus lessening the chance that the patient will avoid the therapist and drop out of treatment.

One suggestion which Kroger and Fezler make seems to stimulate a strong motivation to lose weight. The female patient is asked to buy one of the most beautiful dresses that she has ever wanted, but one or two sizes too small. She is to hang it in the closet and think about it frequently. In buying the dress, the patient has made a certain commitment.

Other suggestions of value might be to have the patient

visualize the undesirable foods and to feel a yearning to eat them, but upon turning away he/she immediately receives a "pleasure buzz," that is a sudden and immediate feeling of relief from tension, a pleasant sensation, and a sense of renewed personal strength. These approaches are all in line with principles of behavior motivation as part of what Kroger and Fezler term "hypnobehavioral therapy."

Mann (1959) believed that an authoritative approach with suggestions for rapidly and dramatically suppressing the appetite, and developing anorexia and perversion of taste, was of no permanent value. He instructed his patients under hypnosis to relax and prepare to enjoy eating. He taught them the good foods and suggested that they would have immense enjoyment in smelling and tasting them. They were to eat slowly, chewing and mouthing each morsel and enjoying each bite. After a few bites they would feel full with a sensation of satisfaction. Some therapists use the term "like after a Thanksgiving dinner" to reinstate a feeling of achieved pleasant state of oral gratification. It would seem that this approach has most of the benefits of conditioning procedures without the hazards of the aversion methods. One might hypothesize there would be less likelihood of substitute symptoms being established (smoking, drugs, etc.) since the pleasure needs of the individual are being met, not thwarted.

Mann also conditioned his patients to go into a trance upon counting up to 20 and emerge from hypnosis by counting back from 20 to one. He thus taught them a form of self hypnosis so that they, themselves, would have control of their therapeutic situation. This tends to lower resistance and make many patients cooperative participants in the hypnotherapeutic experience who otherwise might perceive it as a battle of wills.

Cheek and LeCron (1968) asked their patients a number of questions such as: "Do you overeat when you feel rejected?" and "Are you punishing yourself by being overweight?", etc. The patient's unconscious processes answer through ideomotor finger lifting. On the basis of the replies, a therapeutic program and set of suggestions were specifically designed for that patient. Thus, we may discover that food is a reward for "being good"; it may stand for a gift of love; refusal of it may represent anger; and becoming fat may serve as an unconscious revenge against an unattentive spouse. The ideomotor signaling method is one way of ascertaining the possible dynamics in overeating and the underlying conflicts which are maintaining the maladaptive behavior. It may well be that symptomatic approaches to weight reduction will be ineffective until deeper motivations are met and unconscious conflicts resolved. Such treatment gets into the realm of hypnoanalysis.

One young woman was kept fat by a malevolent ego-state (underlying "covert" multiple personality) in the mistaken belief that it was protecting her from men (see Watkins, H. H., 1978). Some 80 pounds of weight were lost once the underlying entity became accepted, reoriented, and turned into an internal co-therapist.

The Spiegels (1978) treated weight reduction in a way like that which they described as effective to stop smoking, namely, by three suggestions to the effect that "Overeating is a poison to my body," "I need my body to live," and "Therefore, I must treat my body with respect." Here again they employed an approach which they termed "restructuring"; that is, interpreting the patient's symptom from a different perspective so as to extricate him from his previously futile battles between self and body. They also did a great deal of "teaching-under-hypnosis" to build cognitive understanding and underlying constructive attitudes. Such sessions may involve rather long, involved explanations and exhortations concerning the harmfulness of overeating and the desirability of maintaining a proper diet.

All the methods of treating obesity, including those involving hypnosis, suffer from the frequent result that, although initially much weight is lost, it tends to be regained later, when therapy has stopped and the patient is faced again with his usual and customary stress of living. Maintenance of weight loss is a problem which has not yet been solved.

Insomnia

A number of theories of insomnia have been proposed. Perhaps the most significant suggest either excessive physiological arousal or excessive cognitive activity. Bauer and McCanne (1980) describe an interesting approach which was successful with two chronic insomniacs. Under hypnosis, the patient is instructed to hallucinate a blackboard and draw a circle on it with the number 100 written within. He is then to place an eraser in the center of the circle and with rotary movements counter-clockwise slowly erase the number, after which he writes the words "Deep Sleep" at the side of the circle. He next writes the number 99 in the circle and repeats the sequence writing "Deep Sleep" again over the first words, making sure that there are no double lines. This process is continued repetitively. The authors reported excellent results.

If insomnia represents excessive cognitive activity, it would appear here that the therapist has interrupted the flow of new intellectual stimulation by a repetitive task, which requires concentration but soon becomes boring and permits sleep to intervene.

Meares (1961) discusses kinds of insomnia based on different etiologies. Hence, he notes that the sleeplessness which is so often a "premonitory symptom" of psychosis should be distinguished from insomnia stemming from normal anxiety, worry, disturbing thoughts, or from anxiety dreams due to repressed material. His treatment approach stresses calmness, relaxation, and teaching the patient autohypnosis.

Erickson, Hershman and Sector (1961) describe a case which was successfully treated after the patient revealed under hypnosis that his insomnia began following a fire which occurred at his home when he was a child and a discussion of parental divorce was under way. This suggests that a reliving and abreaction may be required when the symptom stems from some single traumatic experience.

Cheek and LeCron (1968) note that insomnia in children often is caused by fear, sometimes fear of death. The old prayer "If I should die before I wake, I pray the Lord my soul to take," which was given to children during the days when many died of childhood illnesses, may be very traumatic since it suggests one might die while asleep. If such is the case, this idea requires correcting with reassurance before the symptom of sleeplessness abates. As in their treatment of smoking, Cheek and LeCron use ideomotor signaling in response to questions aimed at eliciting the conditions and causes of insomnia.

While insomnia, itself, is seldom a serious illness, the all-too-human tendency to overcome it by excessive use of drugs can cause addiction and result in more serious consequences. Spiegel and Speigel (1978) teach their patients under hypnosis to relax and suggest to them that they will see in their "mind's eye" a huge movie or television screen onto which they are to project their "thoughts, ideas, feelings, memories and plans." The patient is told that, "instead of trying to fight your thoughts, turn them off—by learning "to direct your thoughts, feelings and fantasies out there on your screen while you are floating here."

Jacobs (1973) uses the television technique with children who suffer from sleeplessness. He suggests that they can watch "Popeye—or Mighty Mouse" for a while each night before falling to sleep. This will make them feel so good that they will just naturally drift off with happy pleasant thoughts. He also makes tape recordings of the suggestions and instructs the mother to play them to the child. Jacobs suggests correcting the prayer "If I should die before I wake" into one which ends with: "I thank thee Lord for thy loving care; it's good to know you are always there."

Study Habits

College students often come to their counseling center complaining of inability to concentrate. This is usually a result of poor study habits. Correction of such faulty habits is assigned to the counseling psychologist who may employ a variety of directive, non-directive, or behavioral procedures aimed at teaching the student how to establish regular hours for study, and how to banish distracting thoughts during those periods. Sometimes the problem is test anxiety, which often requires treatment as one would a phobic disorder. In all of these problems, hypnosis has proved to be helpful.

Erickson (1965) handled a case of "examination panic" by suggesting to the student that he was to pass this examination, but only with "the lowest possible passing grade." Erickson recognized that these problems can stem from self-defeating needs. By such a suggestion, he provided for their satisfaction while still keeping the student above the passing level. He also suggested that each question would "seem to make a little sense," and "a little information will trickle into your conscious mind. When the time is up, you will have answered all the questions."

Verbalizations useful in helping concentration, improving study habits, stimulating memory, etc. can be found in the *Syllabus on Hypnosis and Handbook of Therapeutic Suggestions* (ASCH, 1973, pp. 106-112).

Donk, Knudson et al. (1968) published an experimental study in which they were able significantly to increase reading speed without loss of comprehension, through specific suggestions. These suggestions specified that the subject would remain calm and relaxed when reading, his throat and tongue muscles would remain relaxed, his visual field would increase, he would ignore individual words and would instead have a mental image of the concepts about which he read. The group of subjects increased their reading speed an average of 38.5%.

In an unpublished study, this author suggested to a 19-year-old college sophomore that she was now 29 years of age, had a doctoral degree from a famous university, and could read with enormous speed and comprehension, whereupon she increased her speed 50% and her comprehension 10% on an ophthalmograph reading machine, during which her eye movements were photographed. Although one would not normally distort self perception to this extent in treating study problems, it was established that hypnotic suggestion could very significantly influence reading behavior, at least for a short time. This experiment lends weight to the idea of improving concentration, study, and reading by a hypnotic enhancement of the subject's self-concept.

Hypnosis in Sports

There is recent interest in the possible use of hypnosis to improve athletic performance. Research data in this area is still very scanty. Early reports that physical endurance could be increased through hypnotic suggestion have not been validated experimentally, although there seems to be evidence that it can influence motivation.

Garver (1977) reported improving the performance of gymnasts and professional golfers by having them covertly rehearse in visual imagery their feelings ranging from a level of "complete relaxation," through "waking up," to "increasing alertness," reaching "optimal performance," then back down to "emotional disturbance," and "disorganization." He held that hypnotic suggestion should be strong enough to enable the individual to reach "optimal performance," but that when the person became more "psyched-up" performance suffered. His subjects were taught a scale ranging from 0 (complete relaxation of sleep) to 5 (optimal performance) and back to 10 (disorganization). Under a hypnotically visualized imagery they prepared for competition so as to regulate their motivation to the optimal level at the right time.

Gardner and Olness (1981) described the case of an 11-year-old, anxiety ridden over a coming ice-skating competition. When regressed to earlier ages (8, 9, and 10) she recalled an unpleasant incident. After being induced to "send" it off via pony express her anxiety subsided and she competed well.

Heise (1961), in a popular book, described methods for improving one's golf game under self-hypnosis. His approach was a visual rehearsal of good techniques for holding the club, making one's swing, etc. No supporting research as to its validity was presented.

Richard Morris, a friend and former student of the author (1982), described hypnotic techniques he has used in improving the skill of wrestlers and in combatting batting slumps as a consultant to the New York Mets baseball team. Of interest was his report that he often found destructive "ego states" which emerged temporarily to impair players' performances at these times. He used a hypnoanalytic ego-state approach (See Vol. II, Chap. 10) to resolve the conflicts which seemed to initiate the slumps.

Although relatively undeveloped at this time, it would seem that an increase in research and practice in this area will be forthcoming. If hypnosis can influence behavior then perhaps it can be used to improve physical performance.

Summary

In most of the hypnotic suggestive techniques applied to special problems, full use is made of principles of learning and behavior modification. Suggestions are couched at the levels of understanding of the individual, and the leverage afforded by a good therapist-patient relationship is exploited to the fullest extent. Hypnotherapists today do not approach their treatment expecting or promising miracles, but the increased potency of suggestions administered following induction of an hypnotic state is constantly verified in dealing with such conditions. The tendency of psychoanalytically trained practitioners to write off hypnotic suggestion as ineffective and temporary has not been borne out. Since conservative and simpler treatment methods should usually be tried first in all types of medical conditions before more radical therapy is undertaken, hypnotic suggestion has proven its worth. Some patients may require the deeper and more complex techniques of hypnoanalysis (described in Vol. II), but an effort to find out what effect suggestion under hypnosis has first is usually well worth a try. Often more intensive treatment is not required.

Outline of Chapter 12.   Hypnosis in the Treatment of Specialized Problems

1. Smoking
   a. Spiegel's single-session approach
   b. Dengrove's behavior-modificaton approach
   c. Hall and Crasilneck's suggestive approach
   d. Kroger and Fezler's "Hypnobehavioral" method
   e. Stein's emphasis on pleasure in smoking at the expense of quantity
   f. H. Watkins' five-session approach
   g. Sanders' mutual group hypnosis

2. Nail Biting
   a. Kroger's complicated chore approach
   b. Crasilneck and Hall's oppositional approach

3. Stuttering/Stammering
   a. Spiegel and Spiegel's metronome technique
   b. Raginsky's hypnoanalytic treatment of "silent" stuttering
   c. Erickson, Hershman and Secter's emphasis on ego-strengthening

4. Hiccoughs
   a. Relaxation
   b. Wetterstrand's "hypnotic sleep"

5. Alcoholism
   a. Bjorkhem's direct suggestion approach
   b. Kroger and Fezler's behavioral aversion method

6. Drug Addiction
   a. Group "teaching-under-hypnosis" method
   b. The "branding-iron" technique
   c. Hypnodrama
   d. LaScola's "looking-at-one's-self" method
   e. The use of regression

7. Weight Reduction
   a. Aversive techniques combined with hypnosis
   b. Covert sensitization or desensitization
   c. H. Watkins' visualization of "health" foods and "fattening" ones
   d. Mann's enjoyment-of-eating-approach: quality vs. quantity
   e. Cheek and LeCron's ideo-motor finger signaling technique
   f. Spiegel and Spiegel's respect-your-body approach

8. Insomnia
   a. Bauer and McCanne's hallucinated blackboard technique
   b. Meares' relaxation and calmness approach
   c. Cheek and LeCron's ideomotor finger signaling
   d. The television technique (Spiegel and Spiegel; Jacobs)

9. Study Habits
   a. Teaching how to banish distracting thoughts
   b. Erickson's approach to examination panic
   c. Increasing reading speed (Donk et al.)

10. Hypnosis in Sports
    a. Improving golf performance (Garver, Heise)
    b. Improving skating performance (Gardner & Olness)
    c. Morris's ego-state approach to wrestling and baseball performance.

Chapter 13

Hypnosis with Children

Hypnotic Response in Children

The problems of childhood often call for unique treatment approaches. On one hand, the more sophisticated and verbal psychotherapies may be of little use when dealing with the immature cognitive processes and emotions of the developing child. On the other hand, since hypnotizability seems to reach a peak at about the age of eleven, and since hypnosis itself represents a kind of regression, the use of hypnosis for the treatment of many problems in children is especially indicated. The literature, however, on hypnotherapy with children is quite meager compared with the spate of books and articles on hypnotherapy with adults. The most comprehensive text in this area is that by Gardner and Olness (1981).

Children, in general, are more easily hypnotized than adults. They tend to think more concretely and are more suggestible. Failures in treating them often stem from the fact that the therapist does not reason like the child. The therapist who works with children, whether or not he uses hypnosis, must be able to gear his thinking and feeling modalities to the level of his little patients if he is to be successful. Many people, by the time they have reached adulthood, have so forgotten or repressed their own child states that they can no longer relate to little people in their frame of reference. Such therapists should not be treating children.

Hypnosis is best induced by some form of fantasy or play. Thus, the child may be told to look carefully at her doll. "Dolly is getting very tired. Do you see how her eyes want to close? If you closed your eyes like she wants to do, I'll bet you could still see her as she is relaxing. She feels so good, so nice and warm, and you can go to sleep right beside her," etc.

The use of television imagery is often very effective. The child is asked to imagine he is watching his favorite television show. The doctor draws an imaginary television screen in space with his finger and then asks the little patient to watch until he sees "Scoobie Doo," "Spider Man," "Wonder Woman," or whoever represents a screen character which he/she particularly enjoys. The child can be told then to watch the whole play, that it is funny, and that he is to tell the doctor about it when the doctor tells him to open his eyes. During that time the doctor may fix his teeth, change a dressing, or give an injection.

Children like to play magic. They can be told that if the doctor strokes their finger, it will become magic. It is all numb and has no feeling. They can then transfer this numbness to any part of their body: their arm, their gums, their face, etc. Children enjoy greatly the feeling of power which they have and thus rapidly develop the ability to achieve this type of anesthesia.

Success in the adult world is dependent on rational thinking, on reacting to realistic, external cues rather than internal fantasies. Yet it is precisely this ability to fantasize, which is characteristic of the more hypnotizable adults (see Hilgard, J., 1979), that is found in children. Hilgard found that individuals reared in punitive homes tended to be more hypnotizable. This may result from a conditioning to make unquestioned response to authority, but it may also inhere in the probability that children who are treated very strictly, with considerable punishment, develop their inner fantasy resources as an escape from an external situation which they cannot master. At any rate, as the child becomes older, his level of hypnotic susceptibility becomes more stable (Cooper and London, 1971), and begins to decline with the advent of adolescence.

As children grow and mature, different approaches to hypnotic induction should be utilized. Thus, Gardner and Olness (1981) recommend for very young tots (during the first 2 years), stroking, patting, rocking, music or a whirring sound, visual objects, or holding a doll or stuffed animal. Between the ages of 2 and 4 the telling of stories, describing their favorite activity, speaking to the child through a doll or teddy bear, and watching induction on videotape may be quite effective. From 4 to 6 story telling, television fantasies, and describing their favorite place is useful. Eye-fixation, involving staring at a coin, is effective at these ages and also in the middle childhood range of 7 to 11. More traditional approaches can be employed in adolescence.

One of the most important motivations in children is their drive for mastery and independence. Considering that the world of children is filled with big people to whom one must defer, giants who tell one what to do and how to behave, it is no wonder that opportunities to show independence and to master events in one's world should be attractive.

It is interesting to note that many of these same needs appear when child "ego states" are activated spontaneously (or through a hypnotic regression) in adults. When a child ego state, which was fearful of "monsters," became spontaneously executive in a multiple personality case (Watkins & Johnson, 1982) Helen Watkins taught it to control its fear by shouting "Monster, go away." The hallucinated "monsters" would then disappear, and the child ego state was reassured by being able to master the situation. It would seem that many child therapy techniques can be used with adults when they are in hypnotically regressed states.

Practicing social situations under hypnotic visualization, like going to school by one's self, dealing with a bully, or approaching the other sex in a teenager can do much to build ego strength and minimize traumatization. This is not unlike the dealing with repressed material in hypnoanalysis prior to fully egotizing it in the conscious state.

Many general medical conditions, such as asthma, dermatitis, gastrointestinal disorders, etc., can occur in children as well as in adults. The hypnotherapeutic techniques described in Chapter 11 were primarily for adults. However, by considering the differences in children's modes of communication, many of these can be adapted for use with younger patients. The hypnotherapist who would treat children will need to modify the suggestions in line with children's shorter attention span, their need for independence from adult control and for self-mnastery of situations, their proclivity for nonverbal communication, their concrete manner of thinking, and their imaginative and visualization abilities. The creative child therapist will consider all these factors in applying hypno-suggestive therapy to younger patients. While deep hypnoanalysis is seldom indicated, some knowledge of personality dynamics is of great value, else one may well be swimmng upstream in attempting to stop a symptom which has been generated in response to an unconscious need or a subtle parent-child conflict.

Parent-Child Problems

A source of difficulty in working hypnotically with children lies in the attitudes of parents. The lay public secures so many of its concepts about hypnosis from movies and television that parents often refuse to permit the use of hypnosis on their children, believing either that it is ineffective, or that it is a diabolical instrument of control. Unless parents understand its possibilities and are willing to cooperative it becomes almost impossible to use the modality with their children. The lack of information plus prejudice displayed by many parents is frequently supported by misinformation and prejudices voiced by physicians and other healing arts personnel who deprecate the procedure to both the child and the parents. Such attitudes must be constructively dealt with if hypnosis is to be successfully applied in the treatment of childhood problems.

Parents are usually more cooperative if some time is spent educating them into the possibilities and limitations of hypnosis. On the one hand it can reassure their fears, and on the other, mitigate unrealistic expectations. They also become more cooperative if they, themselves, have experienced hypnosis.

Behavior symptoms, such as enuresis, soiling, etc., are often signs of a child-parent conflict for control. Unconsciously, the child, through such actions, is securing positive gratification in frustrating the parent, and at the same time is receiving much more attention, even though unfavorable. Unfavorable attention is better than being ignored.

Understanding and cooperative parents can become valuable auxillary therapists in assisting their child to develop hypnotic mastery of his symptoms. However, the emphasis should be on "assisting," not controlling. Over-anxious parents sometimes pressure the child to practice self-hypnotic exercises. The child resists, and therapeutic efforts are blocked. Authoritative hypnotherapists can easily be identified with authoritative parents in the minds of children and be reacted to similarly.

Childhood Conditions Which Have Been Treated by Hypnosis

The number of childhood conditions which have been reported as successfully treated in the literature is legion. They include enuresis (Erickson, Hershman & Secter, 1961), thumb sucking (Crasilneck & Hall, 1975), stuttering (Meares, 1961), asthma (La Scola, 1968; Ambrose, 1963), anxiety (Ambrose & Newbold, 1958), tics (Kroger & Fezler, 1976), nailbiting (Crasilneck & Hall, 1975), burns (Bernstein, 1965), childhood cancer (Olness, 1981), adolescent drug abuse (Baumann, 1970), bed wetting (Cheek & LeCron, 1968), school phobia (Crasilneck & Hall, 1975), delinquency (Mellor, 1970), sleep disorders (Gardner, 1978), psychogenic epilepsy (Gardner, 1973). This list is typical of the many reports, but it is by no means exhaustive of the types of problems and medical conditions in children which have been hypnotically treated.

Children's Hypnotic Susceptibility Scales

Hypnotic susceptibility in children has not had as intensive study as that in adults. However, the clinician or researcher in the area of child hypnosis may wish to use one of the currently available susceptibility scales, such as the Children's Hypnotic Susceptibility Scale by London (1963) or the Stanford Hypnotic Clinical Scale for Children by Morgan and J. F. Hilgard (1978/1979). The items and their wordings are much more suitable for children than those in the adult scales (see Chapter 4).

Induction Techniques for Children

Children do not respond to hypnosis in exactly the same way as do adults. Accordingly, techniques must be modified when dealing with young people. For example, the child is so easily hypnotized and so close to hypnosis all the time that he may be in an hypnotic state and yet appear to be acting quite normally at a superficial glance. Children, like hypnotized adults, can become focused and highly concentrated in concrete situations. They are often entirely absorbed to the exclusion of hearing communications addressed to them or other distractions. This narrowing of the field of attention is also typical of the hypnotized adult.

Children are more prone to transient fears than are adults. They are subjected to a heavy diet of TV and movie violence. If they do not show such fears overtly, attempts to hypnotize them may result in failure simply because the hypnotist has not recognized that they are fearful and distrusting of him. Accordingly, time spent in the early contacts with children establishing rapport and building confidence is necessary for the child therapist.

The ability to relate to children calls for a unique set of traits. They resent being talked down to. In fact, children are probably more sensitive than adults in spotting phony overtures. One needs to be genuine and authentic, and at the same time able to think and feel like a child. One lets one's own child ego state emerge and resonate with the little patient. If the therapist is able to do this he or she will be successful in working with children. As important as the therapeutic relationship is with adults, it is even more significant when working with little people. Erickson (see Haley, 1967, p. 4) gives a verbatim example of communicating with a hurt child which demonstrates clearly the importance of anticipating the child's needs and couching one's suggestions in terms which are meaningful to the small patient.

Since the child's life is so imbedded within the context of the total environmental situation in which he exists, it is essential to evaluate the home environment and to infer the nature of the relationship patterns which exist within it if one is to plan a therapeutic program successfully. Children cannot be treated independently of the circumstances and reinforcements which surround them. This is probably true of most individuals; it is even more so with children.

Children have a shorter attention span than do adults. Accordingly, reinforcements, to be effective, must be administered immediately following successfully achieved target behaviors, and more frequently. Inductions will need to be accomplished faster. Eye-fixation objects which are moving may be more effective than motionless points.

Children's thinking is more concrete than that of adults. They tend to fixate upon some aspect of a situation to the exclusion of its general meaning. They may ask why a dead person does not open his eyes. There is a great love of fantasy. What the world does not immediately supply in the form of desired stimulation, most children can create in their own play. This means that fantasy becomes a valuable way of reaching them. "Let's pretend." But the hypnotist who attempts to foist on the child his own fantasy and not that secured from the little patient's associations often finds that he is not communicating.

Stories created by the children themselves may be more effective than ones made up by the therapist. George B., age 9, had suffered a severe burn on the upper back region. Each time the dressing required changing he would scream loudly and had to be restrained physically. The experience was becoming a real trauma. He was referred to this therapist with the hope that hypnosis might mitigate his severe pain to the point where he would become more cooperative. Together we made up a story about a boy playing in a field, a scene which was very pleasant to him. He was told that whenever he had to have his dressing changed he would go back to that field and spend the entire time playing in the field, and that while he was so playing he would not experience any discomfort. His doctor reported that from that time on George ceased to scream, that he lay quietly during the changing of the dressings, and that he did not complain further of pain.

This is an example of the "guided fantasy" induction technique which has been advocated by Gardner (1973, 1974). She suggests avoidance of traditional eye-fixation techniques and long verbalizations, such as are used with adults. However, she does use a variation in which the child stares at a coin. It may be that by holding the coin the child asserts greater independence in the fixation than in the more common method (Chapter 5), in which the hypnotist holds the object or directs the attention. She also uses imaginary television pictures to secure visualization. By combining this with positive reinforcements for inhibiting fluttering in a case of epilepsy she was able in one child to reduce epileptic spells from an initial 113 within a 15-minute period to only 6 after five hypnotherapy sessions.

The arm-drop method of induction (described in Chapter 5) is well adapted for use with children since it allows them to assume control and to practice it when the therapist is not present. When the little patient gives himself or herself therapeutic suggestions they can be emphasized by instructing the child to squeeze one hand into a tight fist or to interlace the fingers of both hands and squeeze them together.

A most useful technique for symptom control, especially in *pain* cases, is to suggest visualization of a "switch mechanism." Every child learns early that by moving switches lights can be made to go on or off. After a hypnotic condition has been induced the child is asked to imagine that a switch is located in his brain which can "turn off the bad feelings" that come from the point of his injury. "They will go off just like the light does when you turn the switch." If the child suffers from a severe or an organically based pain it may be wise at first to suggest a numbness in some other area of the body and have him practice turning it on and off, checking by pricking with a sharp instrument. When the child has achieved control over this area, the "switching mechanism" is then moved to the main problem. It may also be helpful to have him visualize a colored light as being connected to the switch, so that as he turns it on and off the colored light (which is to be identified with his symptom) turns on and off.

When a hypnotherapy session has been especially successful in rendering at least a temporary improvement in a symptom or condition it is a good idea to tape record it. This will involve the induction, deepening and therapeutic suggestions, followed by a clear arousal. Many children enjoy taking such tapes with them and playing them repeatedly for practice.

Hypnotherapeutic Techniques for Specific Problems of Childhood

Tasini and Hackett (1977) have successfully treated multiple *warts* in children. They employed such suggestions as telling their little hypnotized patients that, "The warts will feel dry. They will then turn brown and fall off."

I have found that a procedure involving the "magic finger" technique can be successfully employed in treating children's warts. Children love to have power. Accordingly, many respond to the suggestion that they will develop a magic finger simply by concentrating on it and stroking it, that it will become stiff and numb. This "magic finger" can then be used to stroke warts lightly, in which case, "they will dry up and go away." The mechanism by which this is accomplished is not known but probably involves some alteration in the circulation and immunological system functioning at the site of the suggested attention. (For more details of this technique, see Chapter 11, p. 262.)

Collison (1975) reported excellent results in treating *asthmatic children* with hypnotic relaxation and ego strengthening. The suggestions were aimed at calmness and easy breathing. Children can be taught self-hypnotic techniques to accomplish this when suffering asthmatic attacks. Ambrose (1963) describes an imaginative dissociative technique which achieved very good results with six child asthma cases. Ambrose has also employed a general technique by instructing the child to visualize that unwanted pain, fear, or other symptom is being held in a clenched hand. When the hand is opened the symptom is released and then goes away.

LaScolla (1968) recommends that only suggestive techniques be employed with asthmatic children, but he believes that the hypnoanalytic approaches can be used effectively with adults. He describes (pp. 203-207) an effective dialogue which can be used with an asthmatic child. After hypnotic induction the young patient is told: "Most people think that you wheeze and can't breathe because you can't get the air into the lungs. But you and I know differently. We know it's just the opposite. When you're having an attack, you can't get the air out of the lungs to let fresh air in." The child is then told, "All a person has to do to be able to breathe comfortably is just let all of these muscles relax." This suggestion is repeated. LaScala also uses reasoning suggestions designed to appeal to the child's need to feel superior to adults, such as: "If you were holding a hot potato, what would you do to get rid of it? Would you tighten all of your hand muscles? Of course not. That would be stupid. You'd just relax the muscles and let the potato roll out." This is extended into the concept that it is "dumb" to tighten "the little muscles around the air sacs of the lung and hold the old air in so that there is no room for fresh air." What is stressed here is that suggestions must be adapted to the age of the patient if they are to be effective. The therapist needs to be able to think like a child if he is to use hypnotic suggestions which will appeal to his little patient and be carried out. Fantasies employed should be those which will interest children of the age of the patient.

A unique approach was reported by Gardner and Olness (1981). A child treated by them associated good and bad air with colors green and orange. They suggested to him that he

"Take a nice, deep breath. Watch that orange air go all the way down to the very bottom of your lungs until all you see is orange. Then breathe out and watch all the orange air come up so that your lungs are all green again, from top to bottom." (See Chapter 11 for other techniques in treating asthma.)

Oral-regression needs are sometimes maintained by *thumbsucking.* In addition to being an immature form of behavior it can have serious consequences in alignment of the teeth. Accordingly, the treatment of this condition is important both to pediatricians and children's dentists.

Too often parents and practitioners meet this problem by threats and shaming. These usually have exactly the opposite effect, causing greater regression in the child and more frequent thumb sucking when adults are not present.

Erickson, Hershman, and Sector (1961) described an interesting approach in which a thumbsucking boy was asked, "What would really happen if you stood there in the corner and didn't suck your thumb while the clock moves from here clear down to there?" Then, "What would happen if you waited while the hand moved from here to there and you just stood in the corner without sucking your thumb?" These suggestions were adminstered, progressively increasing the time and changing the place from one corner to another, to some other part of his room, his house, etc., until he demonstrated that he did not need to suck his thumb any time in any place. He was given much praise and other positive reinforcement for each successful experience. (More on "thumbsucking" pp. 334-335.)

In another case of a three-year-old the question was raised with her as to which part of the finger could she feel best, this part, or that part. Next she was asked whether she enjoyed it most on the back of the tongue, the middle of tongue or the tip, etc. As the symptom came under increasing conscious control its function as an expression of unconscious needs became less. It was "spoiled" for such purpose and was relinquished.

Marcus (1963) calls attention to the point that thumbsucking usually is a kind of equivalent of self-love to a child. Direct authoritative attacks on it will be unsuccessful, but if other tokens of affection are given to the child by parents or therapist such behavior can be more easily relinquished and outgrown. Suggestions under hypnosis should be planted to implement feelings of self worth and being loved. It is particularly important to counteract feelings of guilt or shame.

Cheek and LeCron (1968) suggested an ingenious approach

which would appeal to small children. After inducing hypnosis the little patient was told, "I understand that your parents feel you should stop sucking your thumb. I don't see anything wrong with thumb-sucking, do you? There's nothing wrong with it if you play fair. Now I can tell you haven't thought of it this way, because I can see that you've given all of the attention to one thumb. Is that so?" It is suggested then to the child that "to be 'fair' you will suck each of the other fingers just as long as you did the thumb." The therapist then instructs the little individual that when he counts to ten he/she is to suck each finger in turn and to change fingers with each count. They report that after being a "good sport" and "playing fair" the novelty soon wears off. The whole procedure becomes boring, and the child ceases thumbsucking. If it is resumed the parent is to gently remind the child of the promise to the doctor about "playing fair" with all the fingers.

Enuresis is often a reaction to stress, fear and feelings of inferiority. It constitutes a regression to a more baby-like stage of development. It also can represent a hostility action aimed at parents who are unloving or too critical. If this results in much conflict and haranguing within the home it can easily develop into a power struggle. The parent says, "You will stop wetting the bed; you are causing me much trouble." The child resents the criticism and continues to "cause trouble." This vicious cycle must be broken. The basic problem is centered around a parent-child conflict.

A number of practitioners have pointed out that it is important to improve the child's self confidence and to reduce worrying about failures. Parental cooperation is essential. Suggestions given under hypnosis to the child that he will sleep soundly, but awaken each time there is a tension caused by the need to urinate, can be reinforced if parents will comment upon the amount of a bed which is *dry* each morning, rather than the amount which is wet. Thus, the child is given credit because this morning two-thirds of the bed was dry, the next day three-fourths, the next almost all of it, etc. The malevolent cycle is reversed into a constructive and positively reinforcing one.

Crasilneck and Hall (1975) used suggestions as follows: "When you experience a sensation of pressure in your bladder, your sleep will be immediately interrupted, and you will go to the bathroom in 'light sleep' and urinate." If the child is small the suggestion should be phrased in terminology appropriate to his age such as using words like "wee-wee," "pee-pee," etc., rather than "urinate." Let the child tell you what words he/she uses.

It may be desirable to suggest to a hypnotized child that he will feel just the way he does before he has to urinate and that he will at that moment awaken from hypnosis. This serves as a practice for a similar experience during actual sleep.

Erickson (1958) describes an approach with a child who obviously was using bedwetting as a way of expressing anger at his parents. As soon as the child was brought to his office he immediately sided with him by saying, "You're mad—and you think there isn't a thing you can do about it, but there is. You don't like to see a 'crazy' doctor.—Your parents brought you here, made you come. Well, you can make them get out of the office. Let's tell them to go on out." The parents, on being "told," retreated. The boy was left to regard the new doctor positively. Erickson then continued in a very slow and deliberate voice, "Look at those puppies right there. I like the brown one best, but I suppose you like the black-and-white one." He was using an hallucination method of trance induction. The child, taken by surprise, went immediately into a deep hypnosis. Suggestions were given to the effect that "after you've had a dry bed for a month, they will get you a puppy just about like little Spotty there." After a month the bed was dry. When the father said there was a present for him, the boy said, "It better be black-and-white." This was an example of *Erickson's indirect approach*, in which both the trance induction and therapeutic suggestions are initiated at a moment when defenses are down and resistance low or non-existent.

Baumann (1974), one of the most experienced of the specialists who work hypnotically with children, has also reported substantial success in dealing with urinary incontinency. He "teaches" his little patients under hypnosis how to become "boss" of their bladders and how to distinguish between dreams of urination and reality, so that the child will wake up and go to the bathroom rather than dream of going and wet his bed.

Children often develop many *fears*, such as of animals, strangers, going to school, hypodermic needles, going to sleep (especially when they experience nightmares), the dark, and being left alone. While fear can be adaptive, like protecting them from following strangers, avoiding strange dogs or cats, and not wandering off by themselves, a true "phobia" or deep-seated and unreasonable fear requires treatment. Behavioral techniques, such as desensitization, especially when conducted in a state of hypnotic relaxation, can be most helpful. Under hypnosis the child is asked to visualize the feared situation and approach it to the point where anxiety begins to be strong. At this point he is free to retreat for a way, but not to leave it entirely. Sometimes the child can be reassured if the visualization involves taking the hand of the therapist and walking "together" into the dark closet or other feared situation. The child can also be told that, "You can touch my arm or squeeze my hand if you want to when it gets scary." Rehearsal under hypnotic visualization generally has an ameliorating effect on the fear. We are not nearly as afraid of a situation which we have practiced. The "mantle of hypnosis" permits us to approach, retreat or otherwise control a situation in which previously we were helpless.

The use of hypnotic suggeston to induce relaxation and control of children's fears, such as *school phobias*, has been successfully demonstrated by Lawlor (1976). She concluded that such fears could be more effectively treated through hypnoanalysis than by the traditional psychotherapeutic procedures. Illowsky and Fredman (1976) utilized taped suggestions with a group of hyper-active children and reported a significant improvement in 45 out of 48. This was reflected by much better functioning in school.

Laguaite (1976) found that suggestion combined with television fantasies under hypnosis brought significant improvement to 16 out of 18 children suffering from *voice problems* resulting from vocal nodules. In most cases their TV fantasies, spontaneously stimulated under hypnosis, involved images of fights with siblings, which may indicate something about the possibly rage-suppressed origin of such conditions. As a result of the therapy, not only did speech improve significantly, but in some cases the nodules cleared up. See Chapter 12 for other techniques in treating voice problems like stuttering. The limits of psychological-physiological interactions in the treating of many, presumably organic, conditions have not yet been fully explored.

Hypnosis in Terminal Illness

The dying child is confronted with a multiplicity of problems. There is not only the pain of his cancer or other condition with which he must cope. In addition, there is anxiety, worry, questions about death, depression, dealing with parents and well-meaning friends, who may refuse to accept the child's concerns and try to deny the fact of approaching death. The child often knows he is going to die, and must endure a real burden of keeping this knowledge from others and pretending that all is well. Since hypnosis has had some of its best success in dealing with pain, in stimulating morale, building ego strength, and modifying attitudes, it appears to be an extremely useful tool in dealing with a child's terminal illness.

Crasilneck and Hall (1975) described cases of two children (ages 4 and 8) who responded well to suggestive hypnotherapy. Olness (1981) taught self-hypnosis to some 21 patients and secured symptomatic improvement in a majority of them. The hypnotherapist should use hypnotic suggestions, not only to relieve the pain and improve cooperation, but also try the visual imagery suggestions proposed by the Simontons (1975). Under trance the child is asked to visualize his cancer in some pictorial form. Perhaps he describes a monster, or a band of "bad men." He is then asked to describe what the "good cells" in his body are like, those that are fighting for his life. Maybe he calls them the "white knights" or the "sheriff's posse." The child is then induced to picture the battle between them in which the "bad guys" are killed by the "good guys." Skeptical as many physicians may be about this imaginary procedure clinical experience with both children and adults has indicated that the patient's resistance is better mobilized. Even if the child eventually dies he is often more encouraged and comfortable—and frequently lives longer than would normally be expected.

Gardner (1976) demonstrated a wide use of hypnotic techniques in teaching an 11-year-old child, David, who was suffering from leukemia, how to control his nausea, vomiting, and pain. Through a combination of relaxation, guided visualization techniques, and motivational suggestions under hypnosis, David was able to surmount his fears and to function with enhanced living up to a few hours before his death (see also Chapter 11, pp. 269-270).

Dental Hypnosis with Children

There are many applications of hypnosis in the practice of

pediatric dentistry, such as anxiety reduction, pain control, reduction of salivation, relief of gagging, maintenance of comfort during operations, reduction in the amount of anesthesia, and treatment of bruxism. Discussion of these will be deferred until Chapter 14—Dental Hypnosis. The techniques described there can be generally used with children but must be verbally adapted to understanding and modes of communication appropriate for younger patients.

We must conclude this brief discussion of the uses of hypnosis in the treatment of children with the note that the opportunities in this area have barely been touched upon. In view of the fact that hypnosis is a regressive phenomenon, and that most children are hypnotizable, the potentialities for the employment of this modality in therapeutic programs for a wide variety of disorders and behavior problems deserve much greater attention than heretofore they have received.

Outline of Chapter 13.   Hypnosis with Children

1. Hypnotic responses in children
   a. The peak of hypnotizability at age 11
   b. Children are more easily hypnotized
   c. Hypnosis is best induced by fantasy or play
      (1) Children's creativity
   d. Television imagery is effective
   e. Children like to play magic
   f. Children think more concretely
      (1) Less dependent on rational thinking
      (2) Therapist must gear approach to child's manner of thinking
   g. Different induction techniques for different age levels
2. Parent-child problems
   a. Resistance by parents to use of hypnosis
      (1) Misunderstandings
      (2) Educating parents
   b. Unrealistic expectations of parents
   c. Over-control by parents
   d. Needs of child for independence
      (1) Mastery needs
3. Childhood conditions which have been treated by hypnosis

4. Children's hypnotic susceptibility scales
   a. London's Children's Hypnotic Susceptibility Scale
   b. Morgan and Hilgard's Stanford Hypnotic Clinical Scale for Children
5. Induction techniques for children
   a. Guided-fantasy techniques
   b. Eye-fixation
      (1) Coin method
      (2) Shorter attention span in children
      (3) Moving objects
   c. Self-hypnosis
      (1) "Switch mechanism" in pain control
      (2) Arm drop
   d. Tape recording of sessions
6. Hypnotherapeutic techniques for specific problems of childhood
   a. Warts
      (1) "Magic finger"
   b. Asthma
      (1) Relaxation and ego-strengthening
      (2) Ambrose's imaginative dissociative technique
      (3) LaScala's "reasoning" approach
      (4) Gardner and Olness' "color" technique
   c. Thumbsucking
      (1) Erickson, Hershman and Secter's technique of bringing the symptom under conscious control
      (2) Cheek and LeCron's "play fair" technique
   d. Enuresis
      (1) Erickson's "hallucination" approach
      (2) Bauman's teaching approach
   e. Phobias (fears)
      (1) Behavior techniques
   f. Voice problems
   g. Terminal illness
   h. Dental problems

Chapter 14

Dental Hypnosis (Hypnodontia)

History of Dental Hypnosis

Dentistry is a branch of medicine which is so associated with pain that many of its patients come to treatment burdened with anxieties, tensions, and fears. Some individuals needing dental treatment avoid such care with the resulting loss of their teeth. Even when this loss requires the fitting of prosthetic devices there is often considerable discomfort and difficulty in adjusting to new dentures. Since the first use of ether in 1846 by Morton, a dentist, practitioners have developed and utilized a number of different chemo-anesthesias. However, hypnosis has proven to be a valuable adjunct to both dental therapeutics and surgery which has not yet realized its full potential.

Since World War II a small, but active, number of workers have applied hypnotic techniques in their dental practices. As mentioned in Chapter 1, organizations of dentists using hypnosis (especially in the State of Minnesota) pre-date formation of the larger societies involving physicians and psychologists. Since this book has been written by a psychologist, its treatment of dental hypnosis does not reflect his own personal practice in this area. However, we will report uses and techniques as described by major workers in this field such as: Ament (1971), Bernick (1972), Bodecker (1956), Burgess (1952), Crowder (1965), Hartland (1966), Jacoby (1967), Kornfeld (1958), Kuhner (1959), Marcus (1963), Moss (1952), Secter (1960, 1961, 1964, 1965), Shaw (1958), Staples (1958), Stolzenberg (1955, 1959, 1961), Thompson (1963), Wald & Kline (1955).

Psychological Importance
of the Oral Cavity

In psychoanalytic theory the oral cavity is assigned the most significant role in the development of a child's personality. It is the primary "love organ" of the body during infancy. Through the mouth the neonate receives the life-sustaining food provided by the mother, and in this process establishes the first relationship with another individual. The meaning of love and the fear of its loss are reflected in the frequency and way by which the mother feeds the child. Many psychoanalytic studies trace the later development of dependent and aggressive behaviors to the imprinting which the individual received during this early, oral stage of his growth. Fixations at this level or later regressions to it often occur when the child is unable to cope with more mature demands.

A few reflections on our language direct us to the emotional significance of many terms related to the mouth and eating. The word "sweet" applies equally to a taste and to personality attributes. "Putting teeth" into a project, a "biting" remark, "swallowing" one's pride, translate oral terms into descriptions of behavior. Furthermore, one loves one's "honey." A relationship can go "sour," and one may have to learn a "bitter" lesson. An old-timer may have a "salty" personality. We take a person we like to dinner. We kiss each other with the lips, and we can "spit out" angry words during an argument. It is obvious that the mouth cavity is established very early in life as an organ of the greatest emotional significance. It is, therefore, not surprising that manipulations of this organ, such as the repair or extraction of teeth, can provoke primitive fear reactions in many people.

In view of this great psychological significance to the oral cavity the dentist must know more than the anatomy and physiology of this part of the body. He should be very aware of the stress which procedures in this region can induce in his patient, and be prepared to cope with the consequences when they are painful, anxiety provoking, and disruptive to his reparative efforts.

Although the technique of inducing hypnosis can be learned with only a minimal sophistication, the practitioner who crudely intervenes in his patient psychologically may cause considerable emotional harm. Accordingly, it is recommended that the use of hypnotic techniques be learned in a general setting of personality dynamics and psychopathology. Such a background, highly indicated for the hypnodontist, is almost equally so for the dentist who does not yet use hypnosis, since he, too, whether or not he recognizes it, is evoking psychological reactions every time he probes into the oral cavity. Some dental schools have understood this importance and are providing psychological courses within their curricula. However, because many of the brief courses in hypnosis offered by the professional societies as workshops have little time in which to teach the broad psychological background desirable, the dentist who would study hypnosis is advised to supplement such workshops with readings like: Coleman, Butcher & Carson (1980); Derlega & Janda (1978), Janis, Mahl, Kagan & Holt (1969). Books of this type can help the dental practitioner who intends to use hypnotic techniques to practice them with a broader psychological understanding. The study of psychopathology and personality dynamics is to psychological treatment what the learning of anatomy and physiology is to surgery (Wald and Kline, 1955).

Dental Problems in which Hypnosis may be of Assistance

In what areas could hypnosis be of help to the dentist? All of the following have been included in publications on dental hypnosis as reported by various hypnodontists:

1. Patient relaxation.

2. Alleviation of fears and anxiety related to dentistry.

3. Dealing with objections patients have to necessary dental work.

4. Patient comfort during dental work.

5. Getting patients accustomed to orthodontic or other prosthetic devices.

6. Treating bruxism.

7. Correcting faulty habits such as nail biting, thumb sucking, etc.

8. Anesthesia and analgesia during painful procedures.

9. Amnesia for painful procedures.

10. Pre-medications.

11. Treatment of gagging and nausea.

12. Taking impressions.

13. Reducing excessive salivation.

14. Reduction of bleeding.

15. Assisting post-operative recovery.

Precautions and Contra-indications in the Use of Hypnosis by Dentists.

Before discussing hypnotic techniques which can be employed in dealing with these problems it would be wise to consider the conditions when a dentist should not employ hypnosis. These can be reviewed under two headings: first, restrictions of hypnosis to the necessities of dental practice, and second, precautions which should be observed in dealing with certain problem patients.

Hypnosis involves an intervention in depth into internal personality processes. As such, it is not a field for amateurs. Accordingly, it is assumed that the dentist who would employ hypnotic techniques has acquired not only the skills of inducing hypnosis, but has also had substantial instruction in normal psychology, psychodynamics of personality, and in emotional disturbances which result in psychopathology and mental illness. He is not expected to be a psychologist or psychiatrist, but he should be acquainted with the major psychopathological syndromes, such as schizophrenia, borderline states, and severe neuroses. The dentist should be able to recognize when anxieties are within the normal range, and when symptoms are sufficiently severe as to warrant referral to a mental health specialist.

While the possibilities of actually harming an individual simply by the induction of hypnosis are slight, in general it is not wise to use such procedures on patients who are borderline to a psychotic break or who demonstrate paranoid ideation. In the first case, a severe anxiety attack may be stimulated in the person who is close to a schizophrenic break with reality (and in the opinion of some workers hypnosis might trigger such a break). Although this is not a strong likelihood it is probably undesirable for the dentist to employ hypnosis with patients who show considerable emotional instability. In the case of paranoid individuals, those who exhibit suspicion, secrecy, ideas of reference, and feelings of persecution, the attempt to induce hypnosis may cause them to feel they are losing control to another person. If their state of mind is the result of repressed homosexual impulses (as Freud believed) then they might regard the induction of hypnosis as an attempt at sexual seduction. In this case they can become angry and litiginous. These cases are rare, but the dentist should be aware of the existence of such situations. If the patient has verbalized suspicions and veiled hints that he thinks other people are "out to get him," the dentist would be wise to discontinue attempts at hypnosis and have his assistant close by when working on that patient. When in doubt, referral to or consultation with a psychiatrist or psychologist skilled in hypnotherapy is indicated.

Occasionally, a patient will react to hypnosis, or to some fantasy activated by hypnosis, with severe anxiety reaction. Again, these are very infrequent but must be dealt with if they occur. It is of the greatest importance that the practitioner not panic under these circumstances. Such reactions are usually transitory, even if severe. Reassurance should be given in a calm and firm voice: "There is nothing to fear. You are in complete control of your mental processes. As I count up to five you will become alert, wide-awake, feeling calm and relaxed. 1-2-3-4-5." Letting the patient discuss the experiences for a few minutes before returning to dental work can be most helpful. When such a rare occurence does happen, it is wise to forego further use of hypnosis without an evaluation first by a qualified mental health professional.

During the hypnotic state patients are most sensitive to cues presented by the practitioner. If the dentist is awed by the hypnotic modality or filled with doubts and anxieties about its use, these should be resolved. Attendance at advanced workshops, supervised experience with more skilled workers in the field, or further reading and study should provide sufficient desensitization so that the novice can overcome his own uncertainties. The cues he then transmits to his patients will be those of calmness, certainty, and competence. The greatest criticism that can be offered with most brief training workshops in the field is that there is usually inadequate time to provide the experience doing hypnosis so as to desensitize the beginner in the field. A high percentage of those who attend such introductory workshops do not leave with sufficient confidence in their newly acquired skills. They do not follow through and begin to employ the hypnotic modality in their practice. Hypnosis, more than most other therapeutic procedures, tends to activate emotional processes within the practitioner as well as in the patient. If the dentist (as well as the physician or psychologist) who has completed a course in clinical hypnosis does not immediately start to apply the skills he has learned, he may become like many former students I know who have stated that they enjoyed the course, learned a great deal about psychological functioning, but never got around to using hypnosis themselves.

Hypnosis is a fascinating modality since it can open up unconscious processes and underlying layers of personality functioning. The hypnodontist should not attempt to use this modality to practice outside his area of competence. Hypnosis can assist in many dental procedures, but the dentist is not a psychotherapist and should not try to treat psychological disturbances per se. He can use the hypnotic modality to relieve anxiety and mitigate pain in normal individuals, not to suggest away neurotic symptoms or to "analyze" emotional conflicts. Hypnosis is a perfectly legitimate modality for the dentist to employ as long as he uses it to further the dental objectives which he has always treated without the use of hypnosis. Marcus (1963) also holds that hypnosis should not be used when it is not needed, as for example, preparation of a devitalized tooth.

Perhaps one of the greatest obstacles to the use of hypnosis in dentistry is the time-cost factor. Many patients are not susceptible to hypnosis, or at best achieve only light trance states after lengthy inductions. In such cases the use of hypnosis is likely to be discouraging to both the practitioner and the patient. This is sometimes offset in that once a patient has been hypnotized the state can be easily re-established for future sessions. However, it is not economically sound to employ hypnosis with resistant patients when the procedures are minor and they can be handled effectively with chemoanesthesias. In the dental office, hypnosis should be used selectively with patients and conditions for which it is especially indicated.

Occasionally, a catastrophic anxiety reaction may be activated which represents the patient's previous reaction to drug anesthesia. In earlier days it was not uncommon for a few dentists to use forceful, smothering procedures on uncooperative child patients. These may have caused traumas which became repressed over the years but were revived by memories activated under hypnosis. It is wise for a dentist to determine in advance the patient's past experiences with anestheisas, and if unfavorable, to anticipate the possibility of an untoward reaction being stimulated under hypnosis.

While hypnotic suggestion can be utilized to improve the patient's cooperation, it is unethical to attempt by hypnosis to force his agreement to surgeries or other procedures which he strongly opposes in the conscious state. The dentist who violates this rule may get temporary acquiesence at the risk of instilling underlying suspicion and distrust of him at unconscious levels. These may later be manifested in the patient's refusal to return to treatment or in resistance at paying his bill. Logical persuasion can be employed under hypnosis in an effort to induce the patient to approve of needed surgery, just as in the conscious state, but this should not involve direct suggestive pressure.

Techniques of Hypnotic Induction and Deepening in the Dental Office

Most of the procedures described in Chapters 5 and 6 can be used by the dentist as well as by the psychologist or physician. However, certain ones appear to be better adapted to the physical conditions surrounding the practice of dentistry. Additional variations peculiar to the dental chair and dental office equipment become possible. The relaxation and eye-fixation approaches described would seem to be well adapted to the dental office. Some dentists (Moss, A., 1952) have championed the direct-stare method. Although this technique can sometimes induce a subject rapidly, it may be associated by the patient with the hypnotizing of innocent victims by villains as portrayed in some of the Hollywood horror films. A few patients may react with fear. Therefore, its use is recommended only with caution. After all, the dentist is trying to reduce fear in his patients, not stimulate it. Eye-blink, hand-levitation, and arm-drop as described in Chapter 5, as well as the rehearsal and fantasy techniques reviewed in Chapter 6, can be effectively employed by the dentist.

When using fantasies, the sound of the drill or of the saliva ejector can be tied into an image of flying in a jet plane, perhaps in travel to a tropical island vacation. The music which many dentists provide as background in their offices can be integrated into the hypnotic procedure: "As you relax deeper and deeper you will find yourself immersed into beautiful music, concentrating on it, swimming in it, as you sink into a more and more pleasurable state in which you ignore any sensation of discomfort." Here we have combined induction and office music with suggestions aimed toward an anesthesia by dissociation.

Although a deep state of hypnosis is desirable for long and painful surgical procedures, not all patients can achieve a deep trance. However, many patients can attain light and medium states sufficient to reduce discomfort significantly for most dental work. Failure of a patient to reach a deep trance is not contraindicative for using hypnosis. In many cases the amount of procaine necessary to have a numbing effect can be greatly reduced when the patient is in a light hypnotic state even though the need for chemo-anesthesia is not entirely eliminated.

Although force should not be applied to achieve a hypnotic result, the dentist who employs a firm and confident tone to his suggestions can expect much better compliance than one who gives them in a hesitant or vacillating manner. A patient (one who waits) is usually regressed to more childlike attitudes. He "waits" to be taken care of, to be treated, to be told by his "doctor parent" what must be done to alleviate his suffering. He must feel that the doctor knows what he is doing. Hypnodontia, like hypnotherapy, is not a technique for the timid practitioner. Hypnosis requires that the dentist be much more verbal than he normally is, and those practitioners who prefer to work in silence will not find the hypnotic modality congenial to their operation. The practice of hypnodontia requires much more interaction with patients.

Use of Hypnosis by Dental Assistants

There has been considerable controversy among hypnotic specialists as to how much latitude should be granted in training dental assistants to use hypnosis. The more conservative position in the hypnosis societies requires that its use be restricted to psychologists, physicians and dentists. However, in the field of dentistry it is already restricted to suggestive procedures directly related to dental practice. Hypnoanalytic probing is contraindicated.

Since hypnotic induction can be time consuming, and the time of the dentist may be more economically employed in direct treatment, it would seem that hypnotic conditioning might be entrusted to a good dental assistant, well-trained in hypnosis, who is under the immediate supervision of a dentist also trained in hypnosis. Her services in hypnotically relaxing the patient and then transferring rapport to the dentist might improve the efficiency of the office practice and encourage the use of hypnosis more frequently. It should be emphasized that, just as the dentist should restrict his work with hypnosis to strictly dental problems, the dental assistant should restrict her procedures to hypnotic induction and deepening. Morever, she should have had instruction in the handling of untoward reactions, and her supervising dentist should be immediately available if any of these occur.

Reassuring Patients and Reducing their Fear

If hypnotic procedures are to be employed, no attempt should be made to disguise that this is hypnosis. Patients are usually aware these days that they are being hypnotized. Many of them will resent an attempt at hypnosis if they think they are being fooled, or that the doctor is attempting to hypnotize them in a concealed manner. Authenticity is the best policy. Either the patient should be told that hypnosis could be of help to him, or the possibilities should be presented to him. I have found it effective to describe the procedure to be used as "a natural, hypnotic relaxation, in which the use of drugs can be eliminated or reduced, a state in which it is possible to reduce discomfort." Orientation of the dental patient in this way usually avoids the anxiety and resistance which some patients may develop if told that, "We will now hypnotize you." Words are very important and those used to describe a procedure may well determine the patient's reaction. For example, "I will now *put* some novocaine in your teeth" is not as frightening as "I'm going to *inject* some novocaine."

Integration of Hypno-Anesthesia
with Chemo-Anesthesias

Induction techniques can be combined with the administration of nitrous oxide. Suggestions of deep relaxation given at the same time as a diluted mixture of nitrous oxide and oxygen may have just as much effect in pain reduction as a greater concentration of nitrous oxide without the suggestions. When this can be done, the patient recovers faster and avoids the side effects which may occur in some cases. It should be recognized that the administration of the gas is itself a form of suggestion. A placebo effect is therefore secured over and above its pharmaceutical properties. This effect should be constructively utilized and maximized: "As you inhale you will feel yourself sinking into a deeper and deeper state of comfortable relaxation, where nothing unpleasant can bother you." Some dentists have found that by combining hypnotic relaxation with nitrous oxide they not only get a potentiated effect with both, but they also increase their own skill and confidence in employing hypnotic suggestions. They can gradually reduce the concentration of the nitrous oxide while simultaneously increasing the potency of the hypnotic verbalizing.

Fantasy techniques of induction and deepening which are effective in the dental office may involve the vivid description of baseball games, picnics in the meadows, hiking in the mountains, relaxing on the sand at the seashore, walking through an art museum and looking at the pictures, attending a musical concert, going fishing, or reliving a pleasant episode in one's life. The skill lies in picturing these situations so vividly that the patient becomes involved in them and completely ignores the procedures which the dentist is using on his teeth. In a real sense his or her "self" has left the dental office and is experiencing the fantasy, not the uncomfortable dental procedure. Some prior inquiry concerning the recreational activities of the patient may enable one to depict an image into which this patient can throw himself most completely. The person who never goes fishing and has no interest in this activity will scarcely respond to attempts at initiating such a fantasy. Find out what your patient enjoys and build the induction and deepening techniques around that.

Dealing with Resistance in Patients

When a patient is resistant and enters only light hypnotic states after much time spent on induction, do not attempt to accomplish a great deal of dental work at early sessions. Employ the principle of fractionation (See Chapter 7). Put him into the light states and take him out, perhaps several times during the first session and follow with several sessions. Time may be required to reach a state deep enough as to permit dental work to be done without anxiety or discomfort, but in the case of a severe dental phobia it may well determine whether the patient gets the needed work done or loses his teeth.

If one employs hypnosis with several patients it is wise to record their reactions to suggestibility tests, induction techniques, and deepening. These should include the kinds of inductions employed and the time involved in reaching a desired state. A note on a patient's idiosyncrasies, such as anxieties at descending a staircase, slowness of hand levitation, or the description of any untoward reactions may greatly shorten the time for successful induction during the next session. Kornfeld (1958) indicates that immediately following an unsuccessful dental procedure the patient is likely to be more resistant to the hypnotist. This is not a good time to suggest using hypnosis. It is better to schedule another appointment and initiate this procedure later. The dentist's sensitivity to the feelings and moods of his patients will determine the difference between a practitioner who is successful in the use of dental hypnosis and one who finds it unsatisfactory and gives it up.

Specific Problems and Techniques in Dental Hypnosis

Patient Relaxation

One of the most common impediments to the dentist's work is the inability of many patients to relax and remain quiet. Fidgeting, moving about, scratching of the nose, and general restlessness can slow up dental procedures considerably. Therefore, relaxation techniques of initiating an hypnotic state not only will induce hypnosis, but will result in the quiet, passive type of involvement which is most desirable to the working dentist. These can involve eye-fixation and closure plus deepening procedures which combine lowering of muscle tone with stimulation of inner fantasies. While ordinarily we do not use the word "sleep" when a state in which hypno-analytic therapy will be conducted is to be induced, for purposes of relaxation on the dental chair, employment of this term may be desirable. Even though we know that hypnosis is not the same as ordinary sleep, the similarity of sleep to a passive trance state as experienced by the patient renders use of the word legitimate in this case.

The first use of hypnosis in dentistry is simply to promote such relaxation in the dental chair. This is closely related to the method of progressive relaxation (see Chap. 5, pp. 113-115). In fact, such relaxation techniques, which involve teaching an individual to relax progressively different muscle groups, are sometimes used as a pre-induction conditioning. The procedure involves first tightening a group of muscles, such as those in the leg, concentrating for a few moments on the feelings in that limb, and then letting go. Other muscle groups are then treated progressively in the same way until the whole body is relaxed. In this way the patient compares the sensations of tension with those of relaxation. The procedure operates similar to bio-feedback technique. By identifying physiological reactions the patient brings them under control. Progressive relaxation suggestions given to the hypnotized patient may be carried out more affirmatively than when administered in the conscious state. By a reduction in muscle tension the mind becomes calmer, and external stimuli tend to be ignored. This is not unlike what happens when we go to sleep. Even if the hypnotic modality did no more than help many patients to maintain a quiet and relaxed attitude in the dental chair it would be making a considerable contribution. To induce such a state the hypnodontist or his trained assistant might voice repetitiously such phrases as: "A beautiful warm feeling is coming over you. Your eyes are relaxing, your face is relaxing, the muscles in your neck are relaxing, you can feel a sense of relaxation moving down through your arm, the trunk of your body, and into your legs. The tension is melting away. Relax. Relax deeply," etc. After an apparent state of quiet and relaxation has been achieved, the patient can be told: "You will enjoy remaining in this relaxed state. You need not pay attention to the procedures I will use in treating your teeth. Perhaps you would like to think of pleasant matters or remember some pleasant experiences. The work I am doing will not distract you from your relaxation and the enjoyment of your thoughts." Many people who are not deeply hypnotizable will respond sufficiently to such suggestions as to reduce their discomfort and to make the dentist's work easier.

Anxieties and Dental Phobias

Some individuals are so frightened of the dentist they become dental cripples. They avoid all contact and often end up losing their teeth. Even if their friends and relatives can induce them to visit the dentist they are so easily traumatized that at the slightest pain their fears are reinforced. They often fail to return for a second visit. Almost every dentist has contacted such individuals who have a mouth full of rotting teeth which have been neglected over many years. They need a great deal of dental work—and they can hardly tolerate even one minor filling. In such cases hypnosis has a great deal to offer. Something must be done to counteract previous unpleasant experiences and raise the pain threshold. Their first visit must also be so handled that they will return for further necessary work. Specifically, they need a reconditioning of attitude and expectancy toward the dental drill.

A procedure which some dentists have found useful is to have the patient squeeze the arms of the chair whenever the drill is being applied. For normal individuals this may be helpful. For the patient suffering from a severe dental phobia, it will probably prove inadequate. With such people, the possibility of being helped through hypnosis can be broached by asking them, "Would you like to have your fear removed?" If this opens a way for the dentist to discuss hypnosis with them, and if they agree to try it, then the first session or two should be devoted only to orientation, suggestibility tests, and induction. It is often advisable to do no more, or at most to undertake the very minor dental procedure. If the patient can begin with a period of confidence and relaxation, dental work can be performed later.

A behavioral technique used by psychologists to eliminate a phobia can be applied here (Wolpe, 1961). It is called systematic desensitization. The patient is first deeply relaxed and given suggestions of comfort. While in that state the feared stimulus is applied, but in such a minor intensity that the fear reaction is not evoked. Gradually, step by step, the stimulus is submitted to the patient in greater and greater degree until he has been reconditioned to tolerate that which he could not stand. In applying this principle to the reconditioning of dental phobias the hypnotic state is induced and intensified, then a very small bit of dental work is done. At the slightest sign of anxiety and fear the dentist stops the procedure and goes back to the hypnotic induction, reinstating and deepening the hypnotic state, giving suggestions aimed at inculcating a sense of pleasure and confidence. Obviously, little will be accomplished in restoring the teeth during the first session, but if the patient can leave without being traumatized, feeling that he has mastered this first session, he will return, his pain threshold higher, and more can be accomplished the second session. Dentists using this procedure have reported that they were able to complete needed work on many patients who previously would never come to see them, or if they did come, would not return after the first session.

A variation of this desensitization method "covert extinction," (See Cautella, 1971) involves rehearsing forthcoming unpleasant situations under hypnosis in imagination. Instead of actually experiencing them progressively while he is hypnotized, the patient is asked to imagine or visualize them under hypnosis. Minor ones are described first, and he practices experiencing them in his "mind's eye" before they are tried *in vivo*. Through such a rehearsal he becomes desensitized and is better able to master the real thing when it is tried. At the conclusion of a successful session, either in covert imagination or in actual hypnosis, the patient is given ego-strengthening suggestions such as: "When you return next time you will feel stronger and more confident. You have not suffered this session, and you know that you can handle the next one. You will have no fear. You can relax calmly in the chair and preoccupy your mind with other thoughts, paying no attention to the work of the dentist," etc.

Patient Comfort

Closely associated with the reduction of fear and anxiety is the maintenance of comfort in normal patients, those who do not exhibit overt fears, but who could be happier and more cooperative if they felt more comfortable during the dental work. Holding one's mouth open for long periods of time can be fatiguing, or keeping the tongue out of the way, particularly when work is being done on the molars. Since the hypnotized patient is more suggestible, suggestions aimed at relieving fatigue in the lips and facial muscles, or in holding the jaws open can be quite helpful: "Your facial muscles are becoming soft and relaxed. They feel good. All the tension is going out of them. It is easy to open your mouth and to hold it open. It just naturally stays open. You do not need to pay any attention to the muscles which hold your jaws apart." This is partly suggestion and partly dissociation since through suggestion the feeling of "selfness" is being directed away from the jaws and the facial muscles. It may be desirable to suggest to the patient that he will regard his session of lying on the dental chair as a period of rest and relaxation, and that he will look forward each time to the opportunity to set aside worries, cares, and tensions. Some individuals under such suggestions not only are able to exclude painful stimuli from the dental procedures, but seem to resent completion of the session and cessation of the pleasurable hypnotic state in which they find themselves. This maintenance of patient comfort is especially desirable during a long and arduous operation.

Anesthesia and Analgesia

The biggest contribution which hypnosis has to make in dental practice is the reduction of pain. The same principles regarding pain control in dental problems apply to those used in the medical field of anesthesiology (See Chapter 9). However, certain considerations unique to the practice of dentistry need to be added. In most cases where some degree of hypnotic trance can be secured it is usually possible to reduce the amount of chemo-anesthesia, such as procaine or nitrous oxide, required to secure a desired condition in the patient. Where the individual is highly susceptible, and is able to enter a profound hypnotic state, chemo-anesthesia may be entirely dispensed with. Direct suggestions may be given the hypnotized patient to the effect that: "You will completely ignore any unpleasant sensations in your mouth. The entire region of your mouth will be completely numb. It will have no feelings of discomfort." Strong, positive suggestions like this, administered while the patient is in a deep trance, are usually effective. In some cases hypnosis can be used to replace chemo-anesthesias when such are medically contraindicated. The dentist, however, should be prepared to administer the chemo-anesthesias, when not so contraindicated, if the patient shows signs of emerging from the hypnotic state. This cannot always be ascertained by behavioral movements. The Hilgards (1975) have shown that pain can be registered at unconscious levels even though not overtly experienced. Accordingly, the patient may show signs of movement or response and still emerge from the hypnotic state reporting that he "felt" no pain. When such movements do appear it is probably best to interrupt the dental work and deepen the hypnotic state before continuing. Some clinicians recommend suggesting amnesia to the patient before bringing him out of hypnosis: "When you are alert you will have no recollection of discomfort during this past hour," etc.

It is important to be sure that all hypno-anesthesia has been removed before the patient leaves the office, that is, of course, except such analgesic suggestions as might be given to alleviate discomfort during a post-surgical period, or to permit the patient to sleep that night.

When it can be used, hypno-anesthesia has certain specific advantages over chemo-anesthesia in the practice of dentistry. For example, it can be localized. A large area need not be made numb when the work is to be done within a more specific region. Areas anesthetized hypnotically do not need to correspond to those innervated by specific nerves. Any area touched by a finger can be rendered insensitive. Hypno-anesthesia can be applied without the necessity of any abstention from premedication or food. It can be initiated and terminated at the suggestion of the dentist and need not be continued for some time once administered. There is no nausea or sickness stemming from the anesthesia during or after an operation. Once hypno-anesthesia has been induced it can be re-induced very rapidly. Furthermore, since suggestions can be given to render it effective post-operatively, the need for post-operative medication may be eliminated, or at least greatly reduced.

The disadvantages of hypno-anesthesia in dentistry stem primarily from the limited population to which it can be applied. Wookey (1938) held that 35% of his patients could be hypnotized deeply enough for painless dental surgery. However, most hypnodontists believe the number to be lower. The matter of time also tends to restrict its use, especially if the clinician is inexperienced in using it.

Suggestions to a hypnotized patient to produce anesthesia might proceed as follows: "I shall press down on this tooth, and you will feel a sense of pressure in the gums. The more I press, the more numb the gums will feel. I shall count backward from ten to zero. By the time I reach zero all feeling will be gone from the tooth. Ten, you are beginning to sense the numbness. Nine, the numbness is increasing. Eight,— seven,—six, the feeling is going away from this tooth. Five,— four, all you can feel is a slight sense of pressure. Three,— two, the tooth is becoming almost totally insensitive. One, zero. It now does not feel any pain. It is completely anesthetic. You will feel no discomfort during the dental work. Relax deeply. You need not be disturbed in any way."

Moss, A (1952) suggests that the dentist should then press the points of an instrument lightly into the gums while stating firmly, "See, you have no pain." He then follows this by contrasting the sensation with a probing of another, non-anesthetized area, stating firmly: "I shall now press this pointed instrument into the opposite side of your mouth. This time you will feel a sharp pain and draw away." It is our feeling that, while this test is very definitive and quite convincing to the patient when a deep anesthesia has been obtained in the anesthetized area, the probing into the non-anesthetized region should not be so severe as to bring the patient out of hypnosis. Perhaps this second part of the test might be verbalized as follows: "I shall now press this pointed instrument into the opposite side of your mouth. This time you will feel a definite pain and draw away. However, it will not disturb your deep hypnotic relaxation. You will continue to remain in the same state." One precaution should be noted. Since the deeply anesthetized patient may make no response to drilling, it is important that the tool not be overheated and that the same consideration for brief rest periods be given as usual.

With training, subjects can be conditioned to produce anesthesia in any part of their body. This is most easily done by having them focus on the hand or a particular finger and suggesting a numbness in that member. Once numb, the anesthetic feeling can be transferred to any part of the body simply by massaging that part with the anesthetized hand or finger. Thus, the index finger can be anesthetized. The patient can then be instructed to make the gums adjacent to a given tooth insensitive by rubbing his anesthetized finger over that area. In many cases this will be sufficient to permit operative work without further anesthesia. In others, where the numbing is incomplete, the effect will at least be such that the patient will feel no discomfort from the needle during injection of a chemo-anesthesia, and less chemo-anesthesia will be needed. Hypno-anesthesia makes the problem of suturing gum tissue much less painful.

Once he has been hypnotized, and suggestions of anesthesia administered, it is advisable not to question a patient about possible feelings of pain. Assume that they are not present and proceed with the dental work unless the patient himself questions or complains. When in doubt, use chemo-anesthesia. However, hypno-anesthesia should be tried first. Some dentists have found hypnosis useful for premedication especially during short operations.

Post-operative Care

Post-operative sequelae, such as pain and bleeding, can often be mitigated by hypnotic suggestion. There are many reports on the effectiveness of hypnosis for the relief of bleeding. Most clinical studies are positive (Newman, 1971, 1974; Stolzenberg, 1955). However, Crasilneck and Fogelman (1957) were unable to secure significant effects on clotting time. Even though the literature is controversial, the frequency of successful reports suggest that hypnosis should definitely be considered for bleeders, both during surgery and post-operatively. The patient should be informed while in hypnotic state that "there will be no bleeding" during the operation. Some practitioners have had the patient visualize his vascular bed and "see" the blood vessels constricting and the flow of blood being restricted. Moss, A. (1952) holds that bloodless tooth extractions can be generally performed on somnambulistic patients, these who can enter a deep trance state, and that they are successful in some 20% of patients.

To aid in post-operative recovery, the patient should be instructed while under hypnosis that healing will be rapid and that he will not suffer pain. There is, today, considerable new interest in the extent to which psychological motivation in general and hypnosis specifically can stimulate healing processes. Such influences are thought to have a mobilizing effect on natural physiological restorative processes.

Gagging and Nausea

Gagging is a natural reflex which is developed to protect the soft palate from harmful contact. In some individuals it becomes so strong as to prevent any dental procedure, even to the point where it will begin when the dentist's hand is simply approaching the oral region. Severe gagging can make the taking of impressions impossible. A number of techniques have been proposed for controlling this response. Strasburg (1960) taught his patients how to control the tongue as a way of inhibiting gagging. He had them notice that whenever they gagged they would thrust their tongue up and forward, almost out of the mouth. By bringing an instrument into proximity of the oral cavity he would initiate the gagging and call their attention to this tongue response. He then told them that if they held their tongue back, low in the mouth, and almost swallowed it, they would be unable to gag.

Secter (1960) tied the gag reflex to control of the abdominal muscles. The patient was instructed to hold his breath and tighten these muscles. His attention was called to the fact that if there was any lessening of this tension then he was "leaking" air, and he must not leak air. The procedure of having the patient tighten the abdominal muscles and hold them tight was similar to that employed in the method of progressive relaxation previously described. Secter used the direct stare combined with an authoritative manner and maintained that the suggestions must be given very firmly with no tendency toward hesitation or doubt by the dentist.

A commonly used procedure is to induce anesthesia in some other part of the body, such as the hand or a finger, and then transfer it to the entire oral cavity. The patient is then told that, "Your mouth is numb all over, therefore, you cannot gag. It becomes impossible to gag." Secter adds the phrase, "Try to gag and take pleasure in failing." The gagging may not be inhibited directly by the numbness. However, a clear demonstration of hypnotic influence to the patient by the induction and transfer of the anesthesia establishes confidence in the potency of hypnosis. Accordingly, the following suggestion of "It is not possible for you to gag," is believed and followed.

Moss, A. (1952) recommends several approaches as successful. He employed the direct stare coupled with firm, authoritative suggestions, such as: "you are deeply relaxed and asleep. Nothing can awaken you until I do so. A numbness will spread all over your mouth. At the count of five the numbness will become so complete that you will be completely unable to gag. You will not gag. Nothing can make you gag," etc.

Secter (1960) found that many individuals would respond to a variation of Coue's method of self suggestion (1923). The patient is instructed to spend a period each day relaxing and saying to himself such suggestions as: "Every day my dentures will fit better in every way. I will soon stop gagging and have no further desire to do so." He reported that within a week or so the adjustment became satisfactory and the patient ceased gagging. This approach can be used when the patient is found resistant to hypnotic induction.

Accustoming Patients to New Dentures

The problem of accustoming a patient to new dentures can be approached in another way. Under hypnosis a memory of the patient's original teeth is suggested. This is done by regressing him back to the period when he still had his teeth. He is instructed to run his tongue over his teeth in fantasy and to recall just exactly how they felt. He is next told that every time he runs his tongue over his new dentures this will reactivate a memory feeling of his original teeth. It will be one of familiarity. In this technique the tactual memory of his original teeth is hypnotically activated. Then the touching of the new dentures by his tongue is made to constitute the stimulus cue which reactivates that familiar memory again. The dentures begin to feel like his original teeth as he fuses present contact stimulation with past memory experience. This same procedure can be used to secure adjustment to any new formation in the mouth, such as a crown, bridge, or orthodontic appliances, which may feel an initial strangeness. Ament (1955)

utilized the principle of time distortion to suggest to the patient that he had been wearing his new dentures already for a
· long time and that within a short period he would experience
them as if a long period of time had passed.

Since gagging may result from deep-seated unconscious
conflicts related to the oral region, hypnoanalytic therapy has
been effective. Sometimes it is essential when none of the
more suggestive or directive approaches succeed in the face
of powerful underlying motivations to the contrary. However,
hypnoanalysis is not a procedure that will ordinarily be used
by the dentist. It should probably be employed only when
these simpler suggestive procedures have failed and when
the symptom is part of a more severe neurosis.

Shaw (1958) presents an entire chapter describing in detail
the hypnotherapeutic treatment of a stubborn case of gagging. In three sessions he reconditioned the patient to inhibit
her gagging, stabilized this positive attitude, and suggested
that she could now return to her regular dentist, free from
gagging. If the dentist is untrained in hypnotic methods, a
psychologist or psychiatrist may be called upon to treat the
gagging and provide suggestions transferring control to the
patient's dentist.

Salivation

Excessive salivation may be inhibited by suggesting to the
hypnotized patient that his mouth will feel as if it is full of dry
crackers. The principle involved here is to suggest a condition
associated with a physiological response and allow that response to emerge indirectly as a consequence.

Correcting Faulty Habits

Thumb sucking in child patients can be inhibited by suggesting to them under hypnosis that the thumb will taste
bitter. Another approach is to displace the response to one in
which they clench the hands. The two can be combined. The
sucking is inhibited by the bitter-suggestion response. The
need to suck is then transferred to the hand movement or
perhaps to some less harmful oral activity such as a greater
enjoyment of food during mealtimes. The same procedures of

inhibition and possible displacement may be successful in reducing tongue thrusting (See also Chap. 12, pp. 307-308).

Secter (1961) reported the successful employment of behavior therapy reinforcement techniques at a time before behaviorists had fully developed such procedures. A child who was given both to tongue thrusting and to nail biting was induced under hypnosis to visualize a very disgusting scene which initiated in her "bad" feelings. This was replaced by a beautiful scene which caused the bad feelings to dissipate and new pleasant sensations to be experienced. The first scene was then tied by suggestion to the stimulus of tongue thrusting. Every time the patient employed tongue thrusting she would experience the bad feelings. But as soon as she ceased the activity the unpleasant sensations would leave, and the pleasureable ones would emerge. This procedure, of course, employs both the principles of punishment and positive reinforcement to extinguish an undesirable response (tongue thrusting) and reinforce a constructive one (the cessation of tongue thrusting). After the linking of the bad feelings with the tongue thrusting and the good feelings with its absence the procedure was repeated with nailbiting and succeeding in eliminating that response also.

Marcus (1963), in dealing with thumb sucking children, called their attention to the fact that while it was all right to suck when one was little, grownups did not suck their thumbs, also that one becomes "prettier" when one does not do so. Little girls might be asked if their dolly sucked her thumb. The important point is that children should not be shamed for such behavior since fear and shame are often one of the basic causes of these responses. Rather, a careful consideration of the motivational needs of the child (such as wanting to be grownup) will enable the practitioner to plan his suggestions and images to maximize the child's natural drive and to harness these in the interest of eliminating faulty habits.

Bruxism

Among the harmful dental habits bruxism, or the grinding of teeth together, frequently during sleep, appears to be one of the most detrimental. Some individuals will completely wear away the enamel and must have their teeth extracted. A number of procedures, some utilizing hypnosis, have been employed in treating this condition.

Stolzenberg (1961) used a behavioral technique. Under hypnosis his patients were told that they would sleep with their teeth slightly apart. If the teeth touched they would immediately awaken. However, as soon as they parted the teeth again they could go right back to sleep. Here a punishment paradigm is being employed. The unpleasure of being forced to awaken is tied to the stimulus of touching the teeth. By taking them apart again the patient is rewarded by being able to resume sleep.

Other approaches revolve around the fact that the teeth-grinding individual is very tense. Teaching him to relax when awake and to transfer this to the sleeping state will often reduce this activity. Psychoanalytically, such an individual is often viewed as having a great deal of repressed anger which he expresses, dream-like, during his sleep. The psychodynamically-oriented therapeutic approach would then require that, through abreactions or other analytic techniques, the repressed rage must be released, the origins of it discovered, and a re-integration of the personality achieved. This may be necessary if the behavioral approaches, like those suggested above, are unsuccessful. However, such a treatment is a very complicated procedure and normally would require referral to an analytically trained psychotherapist.

Hypnosis cannot replace the many chemo-anesthesias, analgesias and other dental techniques which have been developed to their present stage of effectiveness. But it can serve as a valuable adjunct, and in some cases will provide the leverage which makes possible successful treatment of previously impossible cases.

Dentists who become experienced with hypnosis not only have available another modality and additional techniques for the improvement of their practice, but in the course of studying the modality they will learn much about the psychology of human behavior. They are better prepared to deal with the entire patient as he reacts to interventions in the oral cavity.

Outline of Chapter 14. Dental Hypnosis (Hypnodontia)

1. History of Dental Hypnosis
   a. First use of dental hypnoanesthesia by Morton in 1846

b. Development in field following World War II
2. Psychological importance of the oral cavity
   a. Oral words as related to descriptions of personality
   b. Importance for psychological sophistication in dentists
3. Dental problems in which hypnosis may be of assistance. Precautions and contra-indications in the use of hypnosis by dentists
   a. Possible hazards
     (1) Borderline psychoses
     (2) Latent homosexuality
     (3) Paranoid reactions
     (4) Precipitation of severe anxiety
   b. Time-cost factors
4. Techniques of hypnotic induction and deepening in the dental office
   a. Relaxation
   b. Eye-fixation
   c. Direct stare
   d. Eye-blink
   e. Hand levitation
   f. Arm drop
   g. Fantasies
5. Use of hypnosis by dental assistants
6. Reassuring patients and reducing their fear
7. Integration of hypno-anesthesia with chemo-anesthesias
8. Dealing with resistance in patients
9. Specific problems and techniques in dental hypnosis
   a. Patient relaxation
   b. Anxieties and dental phobias
   c. Patient comfort
   d. Anesthesia and analgesia
   e. Post-operative care
   f. Gagging and nausea
   g. Accustoming patients to new dentures
   h. Excessive salivation
   i. Correcting faulty habits
     (1) Tongue thrusting
     (2) Thumb sucking
     (3) Nail Biting
   j. Bruxism

Chapter 15

Precautions, Dangers, and Contra-indications

Hazards from the Use of Hypnosis

It has been said that there is no modality of treatment strong enough to do people some good that cannot also do harm if misused. So is it also with hypnosis. Possible hazards from hypnosis will be discussed under two general headings: 1. Those which might result from inappropriate or improper applications of hypnotic techniques, and 2. The possible utilization of hypnosis for the initiation of anti-social behavior on the part of unethical practitioners, this last being controversial among clinicians and researchers.

Qualifications of Hypnotic Practitioners

Hypnosis as an altered state of consciousness and as an intensified interpersonal experience is not in itself harmful. People are normally subject to many different states of consciousness such as sleep and trance. They are not harmed by such states. And close interpersonal relationships with other individuals are not dangerous unless the other persons are malevolent. But hypnosis is a psychological intrusion in depth into the personality structure of an individual and, like surgical insertion into the body, should not be done except by one who is professionally and ethically prepared to take the necessary responsibility.

In addition, his or her background should include instruction in psychology, psychopathology and psychodynamic processes, as well as courses in clinical hypnosis. It means both practice on subjects and supervised treating of patients. Even then, one cannot guarantee that the hypnotic practitioner will never make mistakes which could be injurious to his patients or clients. Clinical hypnosis is not a field for psychological amateurs, however well-meaning.

Ability of Hypnosis to Lift Repressions and Suppressions

One of the attributes of hypnosis which has been previously described is its ability to penetrate ego defenses and activate material which has been repressed or suppressed. Such material has usually been repressed because the conscious ego did not feel equipped to deal with it. In some cases it represents only negative self concepts which are unpleasant to face and which cause cognitive dissonance with the self-image one wishes to maintain. In other words, the repression is maintained because not to do so would initiate anxiety. There is a great deal of difference between how much anxiety one is able to tolerate and how much he comfortably chooses to undergo. In many cases the anxiety caused by the hypnotic lifting of the repression is unpleasant but not devastating. The bringing to awareness of such material is not harmful and may even be beneficial in helping the individual to master and integrate it.

Possible Activation of Psychosis

However, some people possess very little ego strength, and there is much repressed material which is too frightful for them to handle, perhaps death wishes against a loved one, sadistic impulses or other deviant desires. If the material is released because of the hypnotic lessening of the ego defenses, and the ego is not prepared to cope with it, then the confrontation may be experienced as a trauma and precipitate a catastrophic emotional reaction. In extreme cases, if the individual's defenses were already precarious, there would be the possibility of activating a full-blown psychotic reaction. This possible hazard was once considered more likely than it is today. It used to be taught by some hypnotherapists that one should avoid hypnotizing the borderline or pre-schizophrenic. One might still recommend caution in such cases. However, if the relationship between the patient and therapist is good, there is little likelihood that an irreversible emotional reaction will be precipitated or that psychotic behavior will be initiated which cannot quickly be dealt with. In such cases the patient should be alerted and given a great deal of immediate environmental stimulation, such as directing him to stand up, walk, shutting off psychotic talk, and questioning him about reality experiences that are not emotionally loaded in his life.

I was asked one time by a psychoanalyst to try to help a patient of his to sleep. She had started an analysis but for several days had been unable to sleep. She was very tense and filled with much anxiety. Accordingly, he had placed her in a sanatarium to reduce outside responsibilities and in the hope that she should be better able to rest there.

I found that she had attended the same university at which I had done graduate study and had taken classes with several professors with whom I had been acquainted. After establishing some type of friendly relationship I asked her to lie down on the cot in her room, and, seated across from her, perhaps ten feet away, I began giving her suggestions of relaxation. Her eyes soon closed, and she seemed to be entering a hypnotic state.

Suddenly she said, "You're leaning over me, aren't you, Doctor?" I denied that I was this close to her. In a few moments more she began to scream in high alarm, "There's a big black cloud that is going to engulf me. It's trying to swallow me up."

Immediately, I had her get up off the couch and walk back and forth rapidly across the room. It occurred to me that the "big black cloud" might represent an impending threat of the invasion of repressed, prelogical (primary process) material which threatened to break through repressive barriers and inundate her ego, or in other words a psychotic break. Accordingly, I tried as rapidly as possible to restore "cathexis" to her body through activity and movement. It was desirable to get her up from the passive posture on the couch, to orient her toward responses in the external world, and to shut off the world of inner, and possibly psychotic, fantasy. While she was striding back and forth, I fired at her many questions about her days at the university and experiences with the various professors whom we both knew. Her physician was summoned, and he "snowed her under" with an injection which removed the ego from contact entirely. Primitive material is most likely to emerge during the "twilight zone," that condition of consciousness between the totally alert state and that of profound sleep or coma.

The next day I administered a Rorschach test, and not surprisingly it showed many of the signs of a pre-psychotic condition (such as form-minus responses, confabulations, contaminations, etc.). Not only was it undesirable to have attempted to hypnotize her, but she should also not have been in analysis until ego-strengthening therapies could bring her enough stability and intergration so that she could tolerate the weakening of defenses, either through hypnosis or on the psychoanalytic couch.

Cases like this do occur, and the clinician should be alerted to the possibility of his patient being in a borderline psychotic state. In working over many years with hundreds of patients I have seen only two who demonstrated such a reaction. Most of the time the ego will defend itself, by refusing to respond to hypnosis, or by some other psychodynamic maneuver which will maintain its continued integrity. This remote possibility is, however, a good reason for insisting that the hypnotic practitioner be adequately knowledgeable in psychology, psychopathology, and psychodynamic personality reactions. This is especially true if he proceeds into the more complex and analytic hypnotic techniques rather than limiting himself to suggestive procedures.

It has been proposed by some therapists that a similar situation can exist in regard to latent homosexual reactions. The unconscious erotic needs of the patient might be activated in the hypnotic transference and result either in overt attempts to engage in homosexual acting-out behavior with the therapist, or in some cases precipitate a full-blown paranoid reaction, if homo-erotic impulses are violently denied but only precariously repressed. Since hypnosis has the quality of focussing attention and of energizing unconscious processes, this is possible. Although I have known of such cases in the psychoanalytic situation, I have never seen an example when using hypnosis.

One prominent worker in the field has warned about the

possible precipitation of a psychotic depressive reaction which might result in suicide (Rosen, 1953). He cites several cases as examples. This, too, is a remote possibility. However, most practitioners consider this danger to be very uncommon. When it does occur, it probably represents the ineptness or failure of the therapist. It is not due to the nature of the hypnotic modality.

Psychotic reactions and suicides occur in many psychiatric treatment settings, hospital or outpatient. They can result from an incorrect diagnosis, failure to appreciate the current state of the patient, inadequate attention to the therapeutic relationship—and in pure chance which nobody could have forseen. Hypnosis is no more dangerous than any other type of intensive treatment which must deal with highly disturbed patients. In case of doubt the hypnotic practitioner who is a dentist or a non-psychiatric physician should seek a consultation with an experienced psychiatrist or clinical psychologist, who not only is well-trained in psychopathology, but is also knowledgeable in the field of clinical hypnosis.

Some criticism has been directed at the use of hypnosis with people of schizoid disposition on the assumption that it might teach them to dissociate more. Again, this may be possible in a few cases, but the experience of most practitioners is that this is not likely. Rarely do we see an individual who is continually going into states of hypnosis spontaneously. A problem like this should not be blamed on hypnosis. Its maintenance should be sought in the personal dynamics of the psychological state of the patient.

There are some dangers to hypnosis, however, that seldom occur with the reputable, professionally trained hypnotherapist. These may be initiated by the amateur, would-be therapist, or stage hypnotist who is psychologically naive and who is not prepared to take the professional responsibility which should be required of a person who hypnotizes another, however well-meaning.

Hazards in Stage Hypnosis

Stage hypnotists are interested in providing entertainment. They usually travel about giving demonstrations in one community after another. Since they do not maintain a continuous residence, nor assume responsibility for what happens to their subjects after they have left, phobias, compulsions, and inner conflicts can be precipitated which become manifest after the hypnotist has gone. In most cases of stage demonstration, the natural defenses of volunteers protect them from harm. But since there is no time to make evaluative or diagnostic studies, individuals with borderline adjustment may be hypnotized, caused to perform amusing antics, even humilated before the audiences, and then dismissed. The stage hypnotist may instill various compulsive behaviors and then fail to remove them completely. He has learned how to hypnotize and to entertain, but he is not trained in medicine or psychology, and is not prepared to provide the necessary psychotherapy if he blunders. Furthermore, the public demonstration of unusual hypnotic phenomena can stimulate other lay people to try hypnotizing friends and neighbors.

Many years ago I used to give demonstrations of hypnosis before undergraduate college classes until I discovered that some of the students were copying my induction techniques and experimenting in the fraternities and dormitories, hypnotizing associates and girl friends, often with unethical intent. Hypnosis belongs in the clinical treatment office, the professional graduate classroom, and the scientific research laboratory. It should be practiced only by those sufficiently trained in psychology and psychopathology to assume the necessary responsibility for their subjects or patients. Its use as a parlor game or in stage entertainment should be legally abolished. Such use tends to discredit it as a reputable treatment modality.

Possibilities for Anti-social or Unethical Use

When it comes to the question as to whether anyone can be hypnotized against his will, or whether it can be employed to initiate criminal behavior or take unethical advantage of another, such as sexually seducing them, there is controversy among the knowledgeable experts in the field. Numerous articles have been written strongly advocating the position that such suggestions are impossible (Orne, 1972; Conn, 1972, 1981). This position is the one presented in most textbooks. Many other papers have been published presenting cases and contending the opposite, namely, that anti-social behavior can be hypnotically initiated in some subjects, and that in a few cases people have been hypnotized against their will. A number of symposia have been held at national meetings in which the pros and cons of this controversy have been argued (see April 1972 issue of *The Int. J. of Clin. & Exp. Hypnosis*).

A resolution of this conflict is desirable if intelligent laws are to be enacted governing the practice of hypnosis. If nobody can be made to do anything which is normally wrong to him through hypnosis, if no one can be hypnotized against his will, then the argument that its practice should be restricted to well-trained members of the legitimate health professions, who are bound by professional codes of ethics, has less weight. Amateur hypnotists and stage performers cannot do much harm, and there is no need to regulate them by law.

This writer happens to be one who has consistently maintained that some people can be hypnotized in spite of their active resistance and that anti-social behavior can be initiated in some subjects through hypnotic suggestion which has been skillfully applied (Watkins, J. 1947, 1972, 1985*).

In one case (Watkins, 1951), a highly-hypnotizable young nurse who had served a year earlier as a volunteer subject during a demonstration before the hospital staff was discussing her experience with me, a female psychiatrist, and another nurse. She said, "I could never be hypnotized against my will." Sensing an opportunity for an experiment I informed her that I did not feel she could resist going into hypnosis and placed a dollar bill in front of her which was to be hers if she successfully resisted. She said, "You placed no restriction on how I was to resist." She then closed her eyes, put her fingers in her ears, and engaged in incessant jabbering so that she could neither see nor hear me. I whispered near her ear that she was developing a severe headache, and that it would get ever more excruciating until she went into hypnosis. After a few minutes, she pulled her hands away, shouted, "Here, take it," threw the dollar bill back at me, and slumped into a deep trance. The two observers were quite indignant. When the subject was brought out of hypnosis she stated that the pain was so severe she could not have tolerated it for another minute, "not even if you offered me a check for a million dollars." I published a report on this case but never repeated that particular experiment.

Two other studies (Watkins, 1947) seem especially signifi-

---

*Several well-documented cases were presented in which a number of reputable women were seduced under hypnosis, in one case by a physician and in another by a policeman.

cant. In one, a WAC soldier who had volunteered as a demonstrated subject before a large group of professional personnel at an Army training school was asked to role-play being captured by the enemy and questioned by their intelligence officers. Prior to hypnosis she stated she would only give her name, rank and serial number—the proper military response. After she was hypnotized, the experimenter took the role of her commanding officer and started questioning her. She then began to describe her (real) research work in a special unit of the Army's Edgewood Arsenal. At this point the demonstration was stopped by an intelligence officer from the Edgewood Arsenal who knew about the work of that unit. He stated that she was revealing highly-secret information before this large audience.

In the second case, a young lieutenant was given the distorted perception under hypnosis that he was back in combat and was being attacked by an enemy soldier with a bayonet. Another lieutenant, his best friend, was then instructed to approach him. Suddenly the hypnotized subject reached into his back pocket, pulled out a knife, and dove at his friend. We had to intercept him to prevent a stabbing. It should be noted that no suggestion was given that he kill a friend, only that he was being confronted with an attacking enemy. He then behaved as if the hallucination were real. Had the stabbing not been prevented the lieutenant might well have been held responsible for it—especially if professional witnesses had testified that anti-social behavior cannot be induced under hypnosis. This situation might be comparable to known cases of individuals committing crimes while walking in their sleep.

Rowland (1939) designed a study to see if deeply hypnotized persons could be induced to harm themselves. They were asked to pick up a large rattlesnake which was coiled ready to strike. The snake was behind invisible glass, so that the hands of the subject could not actually reach it. Three out of four subjects complied and would have been bitten except for the invisible glass partition. Critics have argued that the glass was not really "invisible." Rowland also induced subjects to throw sulphuric acid into the face of the experimenter (which was similarly protected by invisible glass). Real acid was used and was so demonstrated by putting zinc in it prior to the test.

Reiter (1958) published a classic case in which he reported on a criminal in Denmark who was apparently induced by a hypnotist to carry out a number of robberies—two of which ended in murders. Orne (1960) has intensively reviewed this case and concluded that "the relationship" between the perpetrator of the crimes and his hypnotist, rather than "hypnosis," was the significant factor. He felt that the crimes could have been suggested and carried out without hypnosis.

This, of course, brings us back to the controversy as to just what is hypnosis. If one believes that hypnosis is as much an intensive interpersonal relationship as it is an altered state of consciousness, or rather an altered state induced within an intensive interpersonal relationship (Watkins, 1954), then there is no conflict in the views. The question remains as to whether the hypnotic induction permitted the relationship to become intensive enough to make possible the suggested anti-social behaviors.

Erickson (1939) attempted to induce subjects to steal under hypnosis, but was not successful. He concluded that individuals have built-in controls that will protect them from carrying out suggestions which are contrary to their moral standards. Young (1952), reviewing the literature up to that time, criticized Erickson's methodology. He noted that the highly-skilled Erickson, who in his therapy used a wide variety of complex, dissociative techniques, failed to use any of them when attempting to get his subjects to carry out anti-social actions. In these studies, Erickson employed simple, direct suggestions only. Young compared the "pro" studies (Brenman, 1942; Wells, 1941) plus the previous experiments by Watkins and Rowland, with several "con" reports by Erickson and by Weitzenhoffer (1949) and Wolberg (1948). He concluded that the key differences lay in the manner in which the attempts to influence the behavior was suggested. When hypnotized subjects were simply instructed to carry out unethical or criminal behavior (actions which they were aware of as being anti-social), they refused. However, when their perception of the situation was hypnotically altered so that they interpreted their actions as protective (as in the case of Watkins' lieutenants), they often carried it through. Young also pointed out that a malevolent hypnotist would be most likely to use just such hallucinatory suggestions to accomplish his aims.

If we regard hypnosis in the light of Hilgard's dissociative theory (1977), then whether or not an individual would carry out such behavior will depend on the extent to which the anti-social suggestions are dissociated from the person's conscience, or "super-ego." This whole area of dissociation will be explored further in Vol. II (See Chap. 9, Dissociative Procedures and Chap. 10, Ego-state Therapy).

One can argue that if it is possible to anesthetize and paralyze an arm by hypnotic suggestion so that it no longer can feel or be moved, then it is also possible temporarily to "anesthetize the conscience" so that it also cannot carry out its protective and integrative functions within the ego. Furthermore, since most people harbor anti-social impulses at the covert level (as has so often been disclosed during psychoanalytic treatment), then the inhibition of super-ego controls hypnotically may well permit more primitive and unethical motivations to become dominant. Every person is a dynamic system of equilibrium with a balance between impulse and control. Hypnosis, being also a regression (Gill and Brenman, 1959; Meares, 1961), can turn the balance toward the impulse and make possible more immature behavior.

Some who hold that hypnosis has no unique position in initiating anti-social behavior point to the studies by Milgram (1963). Milgram demonstrated rather conclusively that normal experimental subjects (unhypnotized) could be induced to undertake actions which they, themselves, perceived as harmful to other subjects—if they were urged to do so by the experimenter. This involved the administering of painful electrical shocks to subjects in another room on the pretense that this was part of a learning study. The shock administrators had reason to believe that the shocks were of dangerous intensity, and the "victim" may have been suffering from heart disease. Yet, under the urging of the experimenter, they continued to administer the shocks and increase their intensity.

The rationale seems to be that the subjects perceived themselves as carrying out instructions from a respectable scientist in a university, and that no real harm would be permitted. They were protected from any such consequences by the respectability of the researcher. It has been argued that the reports by Rowland and Wells simply verify this phenomena; they need have nothing to do with hypnosis. Their subjects carried out the actions because they were in a respectable university laboratory and reasoned that no real harm would be permitted to result. The "pros" might then counter that a malevolent hypnotist would represent himself as a respectable scientist by distorting his subject's perception of the situation accordingly.

It is doubtful whether the definitive experiments can be

performed which will pin down once and for all whether or not anti-social behavior can be induced through hypnosis. No reputable researcher is going to cause his subjects to engage in criminal behavior simply to prove a point. Accordingly, we are left with indirect substitutes for carefully-controlled laboratory studies.

Reassuring the Patient Who is Fearful of Acting Immorally Under Hypnosis

From the standpoint of a clinician how does one handle the problem if a patient asks, "Doctor, can I be made to do something immoral or criminal under hypnosis?" A good clinician (psychotherapist or hypnotherapist) strives at all times to be honest and authentic with his patients. Accordingly, if the therapist believes that anti-social behavior cannot be induced through hypnosis, then his patients can be so informed.

However, if (like this writer) he believes such behavior is possible, he cannot simply deny the possibility without the risk of cueing to his patient that he is not completely leveling. When the question arises in my own practice I handle it as follows: "You are here because you have been referred by your doctor. He believes I can help you. As a reputable psychologist my job is to do the best possible in solving your problem. Only if you and I trust each other can we be successful in the treatment. In that goal I am bound by the ethical standards of my profession. I want you to know that if at any time you think I am making an unethical or improper suggestion you will immediately alert yourself and emerge from hypnosis." I have never had a patient who, after this, felt the need to pursue the question further.

Handling Therapist's Motivations

In the final analysis, the hypnotherapist must be aware of his own motivations and limitations. For, if the doctor does not trust himself, then how can he expect the patient to? Occasionally during a class or workshop a student will ask, "If you are treating a patient of the opposite sex, should a nurse be in the room?" To which I have always replied, "If you think that in treating such a patient a nurse should be in the room, then *for you* a nurse should be in the room."

Summary

Hypnosis is a fascinating phenomenon concerning which we have many more questions than answers. It permits access to inner mental functioning which may give us greater leverage in dealing with psychological maladjustments. While not harmful in itself, its effective use requires sensitivity, skill and psychological sophistication. Although its power to harm is controversial any modality which can help can also hurt if employed by irresponsible, unskilled or unethical practitioners.

In this volume we have described many therapy techniques involving hypnosis which can aid in treating a wide variety of physiological and psychological conditions. In Volume II of this work (*Hypnoanalytic Technique*) we will consider even more complex procedures for achieving significant personality changes through this modality.

Hypnosis is not charlatanry, nor is it a cure-all. But it does provide a channel through which we are afforded glimpses into man's inner processes and how these affect his health and behavior. It is a tool which can help us to better understand and improve human life.

Outline of Chapter 15.   Precautions, Dangers and Contra-indications

1. Hazards from the use of hypnosis
   a. Inappropriate or improper application of hypnotic techniques
   b. Utilization of hypnosis for the initiation of anti-social behavior
2. Qualifications of hypnotic practitioners
3. Ability of hypnosis to lift repressions and suppressions
4. Possible activation of psychosis
   a. Latent homosexual reactions
   b. Suicide
5. Hazards in stage hypnosis

6. Possibilities for anti-social or unethical use
   a. The factor of dissociation
7. Reassuring the patient who is fearful of acting immorally under hypnosis
8. Handling therapist's motivations

Appendix I.   Societies And Journals

Scientific and Professional Societies in Hypnosis

The Society for Clinical and Experimental Hypnosis
128-A Kings Park Drive
Liverpool, N.Y. 13088
Phone: (315) 652-7299

The American Society of Clinical Hypnosis
2250 East Devon Ave.
Suite 336
Des Plaines, Ill. 60018
Phone: (312) 297-3318

The International Society of Hypnosis
Attn.: Graham D. Burrows, MD, DPM
University of Melbourne
Austin Hospital
Heidelberg, Victoria 3084
Australia

Division 30 (Hypnosis)
The American Psychological Association
1200 Seventeenth St., N.W.
Washington, D.C. 20036

U.S. Scientific Journals in Hypnosis

The International Journal of Clinical and Experimental
    Hypnosis
Editor: Martin T. Orne, M.D., Ph.D.
The Institute of Pennsylvania Hospital
111 North 49th St.
Philadelphia, Pennsylvania 19139

The American Journal of Clinical Hypnosis
Editor: Thurman Mott, Jr., M.D.
Institute of Psychiatry and Human Behavior
Univ. of Maryland School of Medicine
Baltimore, M.D. 21201

Appendix II.   Sources For Advanced Study

A common question asked during courses and workshops is: "If I want to develop my understanding and skill in the field of hypnosis further what additional sources are available?" This writer makes two recommendations: 1. Join one or more of the professional societies in the field. The Society for Clinical and Experimental Hypnosis includes a subscription to *The International Journal of Clinical and International* Hypnosis as part of its membership benefits, and a subscription to *The American Journal of Clinical Hypnosis* accompanies membership in The American Society of Clinical Hypnosis. Through membership in either of these organizations one can also become a member of The International Society of Hypnosis. Both SCEH and ASCH offer beginning and advanced workshops at their annual meetings and at other times.

2. Build up a library of basic works in the field. As noted in the Preface, there are many excellent books in hypnosis. Some emphasize research or theory, others clinical practice. A few texts are devoted to specialized areas such as dental, child, anesthesiology, obstetrics, dermatology, or hypnoanalysis, and some are presented from a certain theoretical viewpoint (behavioral, psychoanalytic, etc.).

The following are suggested for initial acquisition. They have all been written by recognized leaders in the field, include much recent theory, research, and practice.

American Soc. of Clinical Hypnosis. *A syllabus on hypnosis and a handbook of therapeutic suggestions.* Des Plains, Ill.: The Society, 1973.

An inexpensive paperback which presents verbatim excerpts of suggestions used by experienced clinicians in treating a variety of conditions (anxiety, asthma, constipation, enuresis, headache, insomnia, obesity, obstetrics, smoking, study habits, surgery, and many others.)

Bowers, K.S. *Hypnosis for the seriously curious.* Monterey, Calif.: Brooks/Cole, 1976.

A substantial review of research in the field. Paperback edition.

Cheek, D.B. & LeCron, L.M. *Clinical hypnotherapy*. New York: Grune & Stratton, 1968.

Two very experienced clinicians review history, theory, and treatment approaches to a wide variety of disorders.

Crasilneck, H.B. & Hall, J.A. *Clinical hypnosis: Principles and applications*. New York: Grune & Stratton, 2d ed., Rev. 1985.

A solid textbook describing treatment and research in a wide variety of conditions. The strongest current treatise on the use of hypnosis in internal medicine and general practice.

Erickson, M.H., Hershman, S. & Secter, I.I. *The practical application of medical and dental hypnosis*. New York: Julian Press, 1961.

Three former presidents of The American Society of Clinical Hypnosis present (often verbatim) their specific techniques in the treatment of a number of disorders in general medicine, psychiatry, psychology, and dentistry.

Fromm, E. & Shor, R.E. (Eds.), *Hypnosis: Developments in research and new perspectives*. New York: Aldine, 1979.

The most comprehensive and recent work on hypnosis research. Some twenty-five well known researchers review the field. Over 1700 items in the bibliography. A "must" for hypnosis investigators.

Gardner, G.G. & Olness, K. *Hypnosis and hypnotherapy with children*. New York: Grune & Stratton, 1981.

The most complete and up-to-date coverage of hypnosis for children by two authorities in the field. Includes both research and treatment techniques.

Haley, J. (Ed.), *Advanced techniques of hypnosis and therapy: Selected papers of Milton H. Erickson, M.D.* New York: Grune & Stratton, 1967.

A compilation of Erickson's most significant papers and unique treatment approaches.

Hilgard, E.R. Hilgard, J.R. *Hypnosis in the relief of pain*. Los Altos, Calif.: William Kaufman, 1975.

A thorough coverage of research and techniques related to hypnosis in pain. The most comprehensive and solid work available in this area.

Kline, M.B. *Clinical correlations of experimental hypnosis*. Springfield, Ill.: Thomas, 1963.

A collection of significant theoretical and research papers by over 50 prominent contributors.

Kroger, W. *Clinical and experimental hypnosis*. Philadelphia: Lippincott, 1st ed., 1963; 2nd ed., 1977.

An excellent general textbook for the practitioner. Includes detailed therapeutic techniques. The 1st edition (1963) is broader in theoretical orientation. The 2nd edition (1977) reflects a more behavioral approach.

Le Cron, L.M. *Experimental hypnosis*. New York: Macmillan, 1952. (Reprinted in paperback, Citadel Press, 1968).

A collection of significant theoretical, experimental, and clinical papers by a number of the top workers in hypnosis at that time (1952). Republished in 1968 as a relatively inexpensive paperback.

Meares, A. *A system of medical hypnosis*. Philadelphia: Saunders, 1961.

An Australian psychiatrist, a past-president of The International Society of Clinical and Experimental Hypnosis, and a very sensitive clinician, describes in detail many treatment techniques, simple to complex. Comprehensive and readable.

Moss, A.A. *Hypnodontics: Hypnosis in dentistry*. Brooklyn, N.Y.: Dental Items of interest Pub. Co., 1952.

The most complete treatise on dental hypnosis—even though written over 30 years ago.

Schneck, J.M. *Hypnosis in modern medicine*. Springfield, Ill.: Thomas, 1963.

Chapters by 14 authorities. The most comprehensive treatise on hypnosis in general medicine, psychiatry, psychology, and dentistry at that time (1963).

Sheehan, P.W. & Perry, C.W. *Methodologies of hypnosis: A critical appraisal of contemporary paradigms of hypnosis*. Hillsdale, N.J.: Lawrence Erlbaum Associates, 1976.

For the theoretician and researcher. Critically evaluates current concepts concerning the nature of hypnosis. Analyzes strengths and weaknesses in experimental methodologies.

Weitzenhoffer, A.M. *General techniques of hypnotism*. New York: Grune & Stratton, 1957.

A comprehensive, older work whose strength lies in its very detailed description of hypnotic techniques.

Appendix II (Continued)

Much can be learned by reading the contributions of earlier workers, some of them master therapists. All of the following were written more than 30 years ago but were significant contributions of their day. Some of the older treaties exemplify useful treatment approaches which were based on theoretical conceptions of hypnosis no longer current. Others, the more recent ones, still retain much validity and are quoted in present-day literature. Unfortunately (if not recently reprinted), many of these works are no longer in print. However, they can often be found in libraries.

Bernheim, H. *Hypnosis and suggestion in psychotherapy.* New Hyde Park, N.Y.: University Books, 1964. (originally published in 1886 under the title *Suggestive therapeutics.*) Translated by C.A. Herter.
Many case reports. Suggestive techniques described in an informal (1st person) manner. Rich source of the experience of an old master.

Braid, J. *Braid on hypnotism: The beginnings of modern hypnosis.* (Revised Ed. by A.E. Waite), New York: Julian Press, 1960.
Describes hypnotic phenomena, demonstrations of "experiments" and many personal treatment techniques used by this Scottish innovator of the mid-1800's.

Brenman, M. & Gill, M.M. *Hypnotherapy: A survey of the literature.* New York: Int. Univ. Press, 1947.
An early textbook by two analysts from the Menninger Foundation. History, theory, techniques, four case studies, and an experimental study on "Tension Systems."

Esdaile, J. *Hypnosis in medicine and surgery.* New York: Institute for Research in Hypnosis and The Julian Press, 1957 (with an Introduction by William E. Kroger, M.D.). Original copyright 1850, *Mesmerism in India.*
Esdaile, who believed in animal magnetism, describes his induction of hypno-anesthesia in numerous Indian patients. Many good suggestions on technique, plus historical value.

Hull, C. *Hypnosis and suggestibility.* New York: Appleton-Century-Crofts, 1933 (reprinted 1968, New York: Irvington Publishers, Inc).
This treatise by a noted learning theorist (and a past-presi-

dent of The American Psychological Association) surveys most of the experimental studies up to 1933. This book, plus Kline (1963) and Fromm & Shor (1979) will give one a fairly comprehensive picture of hypnosis research over the years.

Janet, P. Psychological healing: *A historical and clinical study.* 2 Vols. New York: Macmillan, 1925.

An old master (and chief competitor of Freud's for the credit in discovering unconscious processes) describes many interesting cases, especially hysterias, treated by hypnosis.

Mesmer, F.A. *Mesmerism: A translation of the original medical and scientific writings of F.A. Mesmer, M.D.* (Translated by G.J. Bloch). Los Altos, Calif.: William Kaufman, 1981.

At last Mesmer's original writings are now available in English.

Watkins, J.G. *Hypnotherapy of war neuroses.* New York: Ronald Press, 1949.

Describes treatment techniques ranging from simple-suggestive to complex-hypnoanalytic. Numerous case chapters (anxiety reactions, phobias, depressions, amnesias, hysterical conversions) presented in almost short-story form. One long hypnoanalytic case with samples of dissociated handwriting.

Wolberg, L.R. *Medical hypnosis: Vol. I. The principles of hypnotherapy. Vol. II. The practice of hypnotherapy.* New York: Grune & Stratton, 1948.

The most complete work of its time. Theory and techniques in Vol. I. Vol. II presents much case material including one long, hypnoanalytic example verbatim.

References

Aaronson, B.S. Hypnosis, time rate perception and personality. *J. of Schizophrenia*, 1968, *2*, 11–41.

Achterberg, J., Simonton, O.C. & Simonton, S. (Eds.), *Stress, psychological factors and cancer*. Fort Worth, Texas: New Medicine Press, 1976.

Alexander, F. Psychological aspects of medicine. *Psychosomatic Med.*, 1939, *1*, 7–18.

Ambrose, G. Hypnotherapy for children. Chap. 7 in J.M. Schneck (Ed.), *Hypnosis in modern medicine*. Springfield, Ill.: Thomas, 1963.

Ambrose, G. & Newbold, G. *A handbook of medical hypnosis: An introduction for practitioners and students*. Baltimore: Williams and Wilkins, 1958.

Ament, P. Time distortion with hypnodontics. *J. Am. Soc. Psychosom. Med. & Dent.*, 1955, *2*, 11–12.

Ament, P. Removal of gagging: A response to variable behavior patterns. *Int. J. Clin. & Exp. Hypn.*, Ja. 1971, *19*, 1–9.

Am. Soc. Clin. Hypn. *A syllabus on hypnosis and a handbook of therapeutic suggestions*. Des Plaines, Ill.: The Society, 1973.

August, R.V. *Hypnosis in Obstetrics*. New York: McGraw-Hill, 1961.

Barber, T.X. Physiological effects of "hypnotic suggestions:" A critical review of recent research (1960–64). *Psychol. Bull.*, 1965, *63*, 201–222.

Barber, T.X. *Hypnosis: A scientific approach*. New York: Van Nostrand Reinhold, 1969.

Barber, T.X. *LSD, marihuana, yoga, and hypnosis*. Chicago: Aldine, 1970.

Barber, T.X. Suggested ("hypnotic") behavior: The trance paradigm versus an alternative paradigm. Chap. 8 in E. Fromm & R.E. Shor (Eds.), *Hypnosis: in research and new perspectives*. New York: Aldine, 1979, pp. 216–271.

Barber, T.X. & Calverly, D.S. Effects of hypnotic induction, suggestions of anesthesia and distraction on subjective and physiological responses to pain. Paper presented at Eastern Psychological Assoc., Philadelphia, April 1969.

Barkley, R.A. et al. The effects of rapid smoking and hypnosis in the treatment of smoking behavior. *Int. J. Clin. & Exp. Hypn.*, 1977, *25*, 7–17.

Bass, M.J. Differentiation of the hypnotic trance from normal sleep. *J. Exper. Psychol.*, 1931, *14*, 382–399.

Bauer, K.E. & McCanne, T.R. An hypnotic technique for treating insomnia. *Int. J. Clin. & Exp. Hypn.*, 1980, *28*, 1–5.

Bauman, F. Hypnosis and the adolescent drug abuser. *Am. J. Clin. Hypn.*, 1970, *13*, 17–21.

Bauman, F. Treatment of incontinent boys with non-obstructive disease. *J. of Urology*, 1974, *3*, 114–116.

Benson, H. et al. The relaxation response and hypnosis. *Int. J. Clin. & Exp. Hypn.*, 1981, *29*, 259–270.

Bernheim, H. *Hypnosis and suggestion in psychotherapy.* New Hyde Park, N.Y.: University Books, 1964. (Originally published in 1886 under the title *Suggestive therapeutics.*)

Bernick, S.M. Relaxation, suggestion and hypnosis in dentistry. *Clin. Pediatr.*, 1972, *11*, 72–75.

Bernstein, D.A. & Glasgow, R.E. Smoking. In Poverleau, O.F. & Grady, J.P. (Eds.), *Behavioral medicine: Theory and practice.* Baltimore: Williams and Wilkins, 1979.

Bernstein, N.R. Observations on the use of hypnosis with burned children on a pediatric ward. *Int. J. Clin. & Exp. Hypn.*, 1965, *13*, 1–10.

Bjorkhem, J. Alcoholism and hypnotic therapy. *Brit. J. Med. Hypnotism*, 1956, 7, No. 4, 23–32.

Blanck, G. & Blanck, R. *Ego psychology: Theory and practice.* New York: Columbia Univ. Press, 1974.

Blum, G.S. & Graef, J.F. The detection over time of subjects simulating hypnosis. *Int. J. Clin. & Exp. Hypn.*, 1971, *19*, 2 11–224.

Bodecker, C.C. Hypnosis in dentistry. *New York State Dent. J.*, 1956, *22*, 226–227.

Bonello, F.J. et al. Hypnosis in surgery. I. The post-gastrectomy dumping syndrome. *Am. J. Clin. Hypn.*, 1960, *2*, 215–219.

Bonica, J.J. Current role of nerve blocks in diagnosis and therapy of pain. In Bonica, J.J. (Ed.), *International symposium on pain. Advances in neurology*, Vol. 4, New York: Raven Press, 1974.

Bowers, K.S. *Hypnosis for the seriously curious*, Monterey, Calif.: Brooks/Cole, 1976.

Bowers, K.S. & van der Meulen, S. A comparison of psychological and chemical techniques in the control of dental pain.

Paper delivered at the Soc. for Clin. & Exp. Hypnosis, Boston, Fall 1972.

Brady, J.P. Metronome-conditioned speech retraining for stuttering. *Behavior Therapy*, 1971, 2, 129–150.

Brady, J.P. et al. Blood pressure reduction in patients with essential hypertension through metronome-conditioned relaxation: A preliminary report. *Behavior Therapy*, 1974, 5, 203–209.

Braid, J. *Neurhypnology, or the rationale of nervous sleep considered in relation with animal magnetism*. London: G. Redway, 1899 (Originally published 1843).

Braid, J. *Braid on hypnotism: The beginnings of modern hypnosis* (Revised ed. by A.E. Waite), New York: Julian Press, 1960.

Bramwell, J.M. *Hypnotism: Its history, practice and theory*. New York: The Institute for Research in Hypnosis and the Julian Press, 1956. (Originally published in 1903 by Grant Richards, England).

Brenman, M. Experiments in the hypnotic production of antisocial and self-injurious behavior. *Psychiatry*, 1942, 5, 49–61.

Breuer, J. & Freud, S. *Studies on hysteria*. New York: Basic Books, 1957.

Brown, E.A. The treatment of bronchial asthma by means of hypnosis as viewed by the allergist. *J. Asthma Res.*, 1965, 3, 101–109.

Burgess, T.O. Hypnosis in dentistry. In L. LeCron (Ed.), *Experimental hypnosis*. New York: Macmillan, 1952, pp. 322–351.

Butler, B. The use of hypnosis in the care of the cancer patient (Part III). *Brit. J. Med. Hypnotism*, 1955, 6, no. 4., 9–17.

Cautela, J.R. Covert sensitization. *Psychol. Rep.*, 1967, 20, 459–568.

Cautela, J.R. Covert extinction. *Behavior Therapy.*, 1971, 2, 192–200.

Cautela, J.R. Covert conditioning in hypnotherapy. *Int. J. Clin. & Exp. Hypn.*, 1975, 23, 15–27.

Cedercreutz, C. & Usitalo, E. Hypnotic treatment of phantom sensations in 37 amputees. In J. Lassner (Ed.), *Hypnosis and Psychosomatic Medicine*. New York: Springer-Verlag, 1967, pp. 65–66.

Charcot, J.M. Sur les divers états nerveux determinés par l'hypnotisation chez les hystériques. *Comptes-Rendus Hebdomadaires des Séances de l'Academie des Sciences, XCIV*

360

(1882) *1*, 403–405.

Charcot, J.M. *Lectures on diseases of the nervous system.* London: New Sydenham Soc., 1889.

Cheek, D.B. Unconscious reactions and surgical risk. *Western J. of Surg., Obst. & Gynecology,* 1961, *69*, 325–328.

Cheek, D.B. Ideomotor questioning for investigation of subconscious "pain" and target organ vulnerability. *Am. J. Clin. Hypn.,* 1962, *5*, 30–41.

Cheek, D.B. Further evidence of persistence of hearing under chemo-anesthesia: Detailed case report. *Am. J. Clin. Hypn.,* 1964, *7*, 55–59.

Cheek, D.B. Personal communication (Dec. 1974) reported in Crasilneck, H.B. & Hall, J.A. Clinical hypnosis: Principles and applications. New York: Grune & Stratton, 1975, p. 275.

Cheek, D.B. & LeCron, L.M. *Clinical hypnotherapy.* New York: Grune & Stratton, 1968.

Coleman, J.C., Butcher, J.N. & Carson, R.C. Abnormal psychology and modern life, (6th ed.). New York: Scott-Foresman, 1980.

Collison, D.R. Which asthmatic patients should be treated by hypnotherapy? *Med. J. of Australia,* 1975, *1*, 776–781.

Collison, D.R. Hypnotherapy in asthmatic patients and the importance of trance depth. In F.H. Frankel & H.S. Zamansky (Eds.), *Hypnosis at its bicentennial.* New York: Plenum Press, 1978.

Conn, J.H. Cultural and clinical aspects of suggestion. *Int. J. Clin & Exp. Hypn.,* 1959, *7*, 175–185.

Conn, J.H. Is hypnosis really dangerous? *Int. J. Clin. & Exp. Hypn.,* 1972, *20,* 61–79.

Conn, J.H. The myth of coercion through hypnosis. *Int. J. Clin. & Exp. Hypn.,* 1981, *19*, 95–99.

Cooke, C.E. & Van Vogt, A.E. *The hypnotism handbook.* Alhambra, Cal.: Borden Publ. Co., 1956, pp. 128–131. (Reprinted in Am. Soc. Clin. Hypn. *A syllabus on hypnosis and a handbook of therapeutic suggestions.* The Society, 1983, pp. 44–45.)

Cooper, L.F. & Erickson, M.H. *Time distortion in hypnosis.* Baltimore: Williams & Wilkins, 1959.

Cooper, L.M. & London, P. The development of hypnotic susceptibility: A longitudinal (convergence) study. *Child Development,* 1971, *42*, 487–503.

Coúe, E. *How to practice suggestion and autosuggestion.* New

York: American Library Service, 1923.

Crasilneck, H.B. & Fogelman, M.J. The effects of hypnosis on blood coagulation. *Int. J. Clin. & Exp. Hypn.*, 1957, *5*, 132–137.

Crasilneck, H.B. & Hall, J.A. *Clinical hypnosis: Principles and applications.* New York: Grune & Stratton, 1975., 2d ed. Rev., 1985.

Crasilneck, H.B. et al. Special indications for hypnosis as a method of anesthesia. *J. Am. Med. Assoc.*, 1956, *162*, 1606–1608.

Crowder, H.M. Hypnosis in the control of tongue thrust swallowing habit patterns. *Am. J. Clin. Hypn.*, 1965, *8*, 10–13.

Davis, L.W. & Husband, R.W. A study of hypnotic susceptibility in relation to personality traits. *J. Abnorm. & Soc. Psychol.*, 1931, *26*, 175–182.

Deabler, H.L. et al. The use of relaxation and hypnosis in lowering high blood pressure. *Am. J. Clin. Hypn.*, 1973, *16*, 75–83.

DeLee, J.B. *Year book of obstetrics and gynecology.* Chicago: Year Book Medical Publishers, 1939.

Dengrove E., A single-treatment method to stop smoking using ancillary self-hypnosis. Discussion. *Int. J. Clin. & Exp. Hypn.*, 1970, *18*, 251–256.

Dengrove, E. (Ed.), *Hypnosis and behavior therapy.* Springfield, Ill.: Thomas, 1976.

Derlega, V.J. & Janda, L.H. *Personal adjustment: The psychology of everyday life.* Morristown, N.J.: General Learning Press, 1978.

Dick-Read, G. *Childbirth without fear.* New York: Heineman, 1968.

Doberneck, R.C. et al. Hypnosis as an adjunct to surgical therapy. *Surgery,* 1959, *46*, 299–304.

Donk, L.J. et al. Toward an increase in reading efficiency utilizing specific suggestions: A preliminary approach. *Am. J. Clin. & Exp. Hypn.*, 1968, *16*, 101–110.

Dorcus, R.M. & Goodwin, P. The treatment of patients with the dumping syndrome by hypnosis. *J. Clin. & Exp. Hypn.*, 1955, *3*, 200–202.

Dorcus, R.M. & Kirkner, F.J. The control of hiccoughs by hypnotic therapy. *J. Clin. & Exp. Hypn.*, 1955, *3*, 104–108.

Duke, R.E., *Hypnotherapy for troubled children.* New York: Irvington, 1984.

du Maurier, George L.P.B. *Trilby.* New York: E.P. Dutton, 1941. (First published in London by J.M. Dent & Sons in 1894).

Dunbar, H.F. *Emotions and bodily changes.* New York: Columbia Univ. Press, 1938.

Edel, J.W. Nosebleed controlled by hypnosis. *Am. J. Clin. Hypn.,* 1959, *2,* 89–91.

Edelstien, M.G. *Trauma, trance, and transformation: A clinical guide to hypnotherapy.* New York: Brunner/Mazel, 1981.

Eichhorn, R. & Tracktir, J. The effect of hypnosis upon gastric secretion. *Gastroenterology,* 1955, *29,* 417–421.

Ellenberger, H.G. *The discovery of the unconscious.* New York: Basic Books, 1970.

Elliotson, J. *Numerous cases of surgical operations without pain in the mesmeric state.* Philadelphia: Lea & Blanchard, 1843.

Erickson, M.H. A study of clinical and experimental findings on hypnotic deafness: I. Clinical experimentation and findings, pp. 127–150; II. Experimental findings with a conditioned response technique, pp. 151–167. *J. Gen. Psychol.,* 1938, *19.*

Erickson, M.H. An experimental investigation of the possible anti-social uses of hypnosis. *Psychiatry,* 1939, *2,* 391–414.

Erickson, M.H. Deep hypnosis and its induction. In L.M. LeCron (Ed.), *Experimental hypnosis.* New York: Macmillan, 1952, pp. 70–112. (Also Citadel Press, 1968)

Erickson, M.H. Special techniques of brief hypnotherapy. *J. Clin. & Exp. Hypn.,* 1954, *2,* 109–129.

Erickson, M.H. Naturalistic techniques of hypnosis. *Am. J. Clin. Hypn.,* 1958, 3–8.

Erickson, M.H. Hypnosis and examination panics. *Am. J. Clin. Hypn.,* 1965, *7,* 356–357. (See also Am. Soc. Clin. Hypn. (1973), p. 106.

Erickson, M.H. An introduction to the study and application of hypnosis for pain control. In J. Lassner (Ed.), *Hypnosis and psychosomatic medicine: Proceedings of the Internat. Congress of Hypnosis and Psychosomatic Med.,* New York: Springer-Verlag, 1967a.

Erickson, M.H. Further experimental investigation of hypnosis: Hypnotic and non-hypnotic realities. *Am. J. Clin. Hypn.,* 1967b, *10,* 87–135.

Erickson, M.H. , Hershman, S. & Secter, I.I. *The practical application of medical and dental hypnosis.* New York: Julian Press, 1961.

Erickson, M.H. & Kubie, L.S. The successful treatment of a

case of acute hysterical depression by return under hypnosis to a critical phase of childhood. *Psychoanalytic Quarterly*, 1941, *10*, 539–609.

Erickson, M.H., Rossi, E.L. & Rossi, S.I. *Hypnotic realities: The induction of clinical hypnosis and forms of indirect suggestion*. New York: Irvington Publishers, 1976.

Esdaile, J. *Hypnosis in medicine and surgery*. New York: Institute for Research in Hypnosis and the Julian Press, 1957. (Original copyright, *Mesmerism in India*, 1850).

Evans, F.J. Hypnosis and sleep: Techniques for exploring cognitive activity during sleep. Chap. 6 in E. Fromm & R.E. Shor (Eds.), *Hypnosis: Developments in research and new perspectives*. New York: Aldine, 1979, pp. 139–183.

Ewen, D.M. Condyloma acuminatum: Successful treatment of four cases by hypnosis. *Am. J. Clin. Hypn.*, 1974, *17*, 73–78.

Federn, P. *Ego psychology and the psychoses*. (E. Weiss, Ed.), New York: Basic Books, 1952.

Ferenczi, S. *Further contributions to the theory and technique of psychoanalysis*. London: Hogarth, 1926.

Field, P. *Hypnotic preparation for surgery*. (audio tape Vol. #53). Orlando, Fla.: Am. Acad. of Psychotherapists, 1974.

Fordyce, W.E. An operant conditioning method for r..anaging chronic pain. *Postgraduate Medicine*, 1973, *53*, 123–128.

Fordyce, W.E. Treating chronic pain by contingency management. In Bonica, J.J. (Ed.), International symposium on pain. *Advances in Neurology*, 1974, Vol. 4, New York: Raven Press, pp. 583–589.

Frankel, F.H. *Hypnosis: Trance as a coping mechanism*. New York: Plenum, 1976.

Frankel, F.H. & Zamansky, H.S. (Eds.). *Hypnosis at its bicentennial: Selected papers*. New York: Plenum Press, 1978.

French, T.M. & Alexander, F. Psychogenic factors in bronchial asthma. *Psychosomatic Med.*, Monograph 4, Washington, D.C.: Nat. Research Council, 1941.

Freud, A. *The ego and the mechanisms of defense*. New York: Int. Univ. Press, 1946.

Freud, S. *Beyond the pleasure principle*. London, Vienna: The Internat. Psychoanalytical Press, 1922.

Freud, S. *A general introduction to psychoanalysis*. New York: Liveright, 1935.

Freud, S. *Collected papers: Vols. I–V*. London: Hogarth Press & The Institute of Psycho-Analysis, 1953.

Fromm, E. & Shor, R.E. (Eds.), *Hypnosis: Developments in research and new perspectives*. New York: Aldine, 1979.

Fromm, E., Brown, D.P., Hurt, S.W., Oberlander, J.Z., Boxer, A.M. & Pfeifer, G. The phenomena and characteristics of self-hypnosis. *Int. J. Clin. & Exp. Hypn.*, 1981, 29, 189–246.

Gardner, G.G. Use of hypnosis for psychogenic epilepsy in a child. *Am. J. Clin. Hypn.*, 1973, 15, 161–169.

Gardner, G.G. Hypnosis with children. *Int. J. Clin. & Exp. Hypn.*, 1974, 22, 20–38.

Gardner, G.G. Childhood, death, and human dignity: Hypnotherapy for David. *Int. J. Clin. & Exp. Hypn.*, 1976, 24, 122–139.

Gardner, G.G. The use of hypnotherapy in a pediatric setting. In E. Gellert (Ed.), *Psychological aspects of pediatric care.* New York: Grune & Stratton, 1978.

Gardner, G.G. Teaching self-hypnosis to children. *Int. J. Clin. & Exp. Hypn.*, 1981, 29, 300–312.

Gardner, G.G. & Olness, K. *Hypnosis and hypnotherapy with children.* New York: Grune & Stratton, 1981.

Garver, R.B. The enhancement of human performance with hypnosis through neuromotor facilitation and control of arousal level. *Am. J. Clin. Hypn.* Jan. 1977, 19, 177–181.

Gibbons, D. *Applied hypnosis and hyperempiria.* New York: Plenum, 1979.

Gill, M. & Brenman, M. *Hypnosis and related states.* New York: Int. Univ. Press, 1959.

Golan, H.P. Control of fear reaction in dental patients by hypnosis: Three case reports. *Am. J. Clin. Hypn.*, 1971, 13, 279–284.

Gordon, J.E. *Handbook of clinical and experimental hypnosis.* New York: Macmillan, 1967.

Gravitz, M.A. & Gravitz, R.F. The collected writings of Milton H. Erickson: A complete bibliography, 1929-1977. *Am. J. Clin. Hypn.*, 1977, 20, 84–94.

Greenson, R.R., & Obermayer, M.D. Treatment by suggestion of verrucae planae of the face. *Psychosomatic Med.*, 1949, 11, 163–164.

Gregory, H.H. *Controversies about stuttering therapy.* Baltimore: University Park Press, 1979.

Grinker, R.R. & Spiegel, J.P. *War neuroses.* Philadelphia: Blakiston, 1945.

Gruenewald, D. Hypnotherapy in a case of nailbiting. *Int. J. Clin. & Exp. Hypn.*, 1965, 13, 209–219.

Hadfield, J.A. Treatment by suggestion and hypnoanalysis. In E. Miller (Ed.), *The neuroses of war.* New York: Macmillan, 1940, pp. 128–149.

Haley, J. (Ed.), *Advanced techniques of hypnosis and therapy: Selected papers of Milton H. Erickson, M.D.* New York: Grune & Stratton, 1967.

Haley, J. *Uncommon therapy: The psychiatric techniques of Milton H. Erickson, M.D.* New York: Norton, 1973.

Hall, J.A. & Crasilneck, H.B. Development of a hypnotic technique for treating chronic cigarette smoking. *Int. J. Clin. & Exp. Hypn.,* 1970, *18,* 283–289.

Hall, W.H. et al. Gastric function during hypnosis and hypnotically-induced gastro-intestinal symptoms. *J. of Psychosomatic Research,* 1967, *11,* 263–266.

Harding, H.C. Hypnosis in the treatment of migraine, In J. Lassner (Ed.), *Hypnosis and psychosomatic medicine.* New York: Springer-Verlag, 1967, pp. 131–134.

Hartland, J. *Medical and dental hypnosis.* Baltimore: Williams & Wilkins, 1966.

Heise, J. *How you can play better golf using self-hypnosis.* Hollywood, Calif., Wilshire Co., 1961.

Heron, W.T. *Clinical applications of suggestion and hypnosis,* 2nd ed. Springfield, Ill.: Thomas, 1953.

Hibbard, W.S. & Worring, R.W. *Forensic hypnosis: The practical application of hypnosis in criminal investigation.* Springfield, Ill.: Thomas, 1981.

Hilgard, E.R. *Hypnotic susceptibility.* New York: Harcourt, Brace & World, 1965.

Hilgard, E.R. Posthypnotic amnesia: Experiments and theory. *Int. J. Clin. & Exp. Hypn.,* 1966, *14,* 104–111.

Hilgard, E.R. *Divided consciousness: Multiple controls in human thought and action.* New York: Wiley, 1977.

Hilgard, E.R. & Hilgard, J.R. *Hypnosis in the relief of pain.* Los Altos, Calif.: William Kaufmann, 1975.

Hilgard, E.R. & Loftus, E.F. Effective interrogation of the eyewitness. *Int. J. Clin. & Exp. Hypn.,* 1979, *27,* 342–357.

Hilgard, J.R. Imaginative and sensory-affective involvements in everyday life and hypnosis. In E. Fromm & R.E. Shor (Eds.), *Hypnosis: Developments in research and new perspectives.* New York: Aldine, 1979, pp. 483–517.

Hilgard, J.R. & Hilgard, E.F. Assessing hypnotic responsiveness in a clinical setting: A multi-item clinical scale and its advantages over single-item scales. *Int. J. Clin. & Exp. Hypn.,* 1979, *27,* 134–150.

Holombo, L.K. *Unilateral hypnotic deafness.* (Unpublished Master's Thesis). Univ. of Montana, 1978.

Hull, C. *Hypnosis and Suggestibility.* New York: Appleton-

Century-Crofts, 1933.

Hunt, W.A. & Bespalec, D.A. An evaluation of current methods of modifying smoking behavior. *J. Clin. Psychol.*, 1974, *30*, 431–438.

Ikemi, Y. et al. Hypnotic experiments on the psychosomatic aspects of gastrointestinal disorders. Chap. 18 in M.V., Kline (Ed.), *Clinical correlations of experimental hypnosis.* Springfield, Ill.: Thomas, 1963, pp. 263–274.

Ikemi, Y. & Nakagawa, S.A. A psychosomatic study of contagious dermatitis. *Kyushu J. of Med. Sc.*, 1962, *13*, 335–352.

Ilovsky, J. & Fredman, N. Group suggestion in learning disabilities of primary grade children: A feasibility study. *Int. J. Clin. & Exp. Hypn.*, 1976, *24*, 87–97.

Jacobs, L. Hypnosis therapy in pediatrics. In Am. Soc. Clin. Hypn., *A syllabus on hypnosis and a handbook of therapeutic suggestions.* Des Plaines, Ill.: The Society, 1973, pp. 71–73.

Jacobson A.M. et al. Raynaud phenomenon: Treatment with hypnotic and operant technique. *J. Am. Med. Assoc.*, 1973, *225*, 739–740.

Jacobson, E. *You must relax.* New York: McGraw-Hill, 1934.

Jacoby, J.D. Practical suggestions for dentists working with the patient in a trance. *Am. J. Clin. Hypn.*, 1967, *10*, 39–43.

Janet, P. *The major symptoms of hysteria.* New York: Macmillan, 1907.

Janet, P. *Psychological healing: A historical and clinical study.* 2 Vol., New York: Macmillan, 1925.

Janis, I.L. *Psychological stress.* New York: Wiley, 1958.

Janis, I.L. et al. *Personality: Dynamics, development, and assessment.* New York: Harcourt, Brace & World, 1969.

Jencks, B. Utilizing the phases of breathing rhythm in hypnosis. In F.H. Frankel & H.S. Zamansky (Eds.) *Hypnosis at its bicentennial.* New York: Plenum, 1978, pp. 169–182.

Johnson, L. Current research in self-hypnotic phenomenology: The Chicago paradigm. *Int. J. Clin. & Exp. Hypn.*, 1981, *29*, 247–258.

Kasanin, J.S. (Ed.) *Language and thought in schizophrenia.* Berkeley and Los Angeles: Univ. of California Press, 1944.

Kelsey, D. & Barrow, J.D. Maintenance of posture by hypnotic suggestion in patient undergoing plastic surgery. *Brit. Med. J.*, 1958, pp. 756–757.

Kihlstrom, J.F. & Evans, F.J. (Eds.), *Functional disorders of memory.* New York: Halsted, 1979.

Kirkner, F.J. & West, P.M. Hypnotic treatment of persistent hiccup: A case report. *Brit. J. Med. Hypnotism*, Spring 1950, *1*, No. 3, pp. 22–24.

Kline, M.V. Situational cardiovascular symptomatology and hypnosis. *Brit J. Med. Hypnotism*, Spring 1950, *1*, No. 3., pp. 33–36.

Kline, M.V. Delimited hypnotherapy: The acceptance of resistance in the treatment of a long standing neurodermatitis with a sensory-imagery technique. *J. Clin. & Exp. Hypn.*, 1953, *1*, No. 4, 18–22.

Kline, M.V. Psoriasis and hypnotherapy: A case report. *J. Clin. & Exp. Hypn.*, 1954, 2, 318–322.

Kline, M.V. (Ed.), *A scientific report on the search for Bridey Murphy*. New York: Institute for Research in Hypnosis and the Julian Press, 1956.

Kline, M.V. *Freud and Hypnosis*. New York: Julian Press and The Institute for Research in Hypnosis, 1958.

Kline, M.V. Hypnotic age regression and psychotherapy: Clinical and theoretical observations. *Int. J. Clin. & Exp. Hypn.*, 1960, 7, 17–35.

Kline, M.V. *Clinical correlations of experimental hypnosis.* Springfield, Ill.: Thomas, 1963.

Kline, M.V. Hypnotic amnesia in psychotherapy. *Int. J. Clin. & Exp. Hypn.*, 1966, *14*, 112–120.

Kline, M.V. et al. *Obesity: Etiology, treatment and management.* Springfield, Ill.: Thomas, 1976.

Kline, M.V. et al. An experimental study of the nature of hypnotic deafness: Effects of delayed speech feed-back. *J. Clin. & Exp. Hypn.*, 1954, 2, 145–156.

Kornfeld, B. Hypnosis as applied in modern dental practice. In *Handbook, of dental practice.* 3rd. ed., Philadelphia: Lippincott, 1958.

Kramer, E. & Tucker, G. Hypnotically suggested deafness and delayed auditory feedback. *Int. J. Clin. & Exp. Hypn.*, 1967, *15*, 37–43.

Krippner, S. & Rubin, D. *Galaxies of life.* New York: Gordon & Breach, 1973.

Kris, E. Ego psychology and interpretation in psychoanalytic therapy. *Psychoanalytic Quarterly*, 1951, *20*, 15–30.

Kroger, W. *Clinical and experimental hypnosis.* Philadelphia: Lippincott, 1963, (1st ed.).

Kroger, W. *Clinical and experimental hypnosis.* Philadelphia: Lippincott, 1977, (2nd ed.).

Kroger, W. *Clinical and experimental hypnosis.* Philadelphia: Lippincott, 1977, (2nd ed.).

Kroger, W.S. & Fezler, W.D. *Hypnosis and behavior modification: Imagery conditioning.* Philadelphia: Lippincott, 1976.

Kroger, W.S. & Freed, S.C. *Psychosomatic gynecology.* Philadelphia: Saunders, 1951.

Kubie, L.S. & Margolin, D. The process of hypnotism and the nature of the hypnotic state. *Am. J. Psychiat.,* 1944, *100,* 611–622.

Kuhner, A. Evaluation of hypnosis in dental therapeutics from the dentist's viewpoint. *J. Am. Soc. Psychosomatic Dent. & Med.,* 1959, *6,* 9–19.

Laguiate, J.K. The use of hypnosis with children with deviant voices. *Int. J. Clin. & Exp. Hypn.,* 1976, *24,* 98–104.

Lait, V.S. A case of recurrent compulsive vomiting. *Am. J. Clin. Hypn.,* 1972, *14,* 196–198.

Lamaze, F. *Painless childbirth.* London: Burke, 1958.

LaScolla, R.L. Chap. 22. Hypnosis with children. In D.B. Cheek & L.M. LeCron, *Clinical hypnotherapy.* New York: Grune & Stratton, 1968, pp. 201–211.

LaScolla, R.L. Treating the teen-age drug abuser with hypnosis. In *A syllabus on hypnosis and a handbook of therapeutic suggestions.* Am. Soc. Clin. Hypn., 1973, pp. 48–49.

Lawlor, E.D. Hypnotic intervention with "school phobic" children. *Int. J. Clin. & Exp. Hypn.,* 1976, *24,* 74–86.

Lea, P. et al. The hypnotic control of intractable pain. *Am. J. Clin. Hypn.,* 1960, *3,* 3–8.

LeCron, L.M. *Experimental hypnosis.* New York: Citadel Press, 1968. (Originally published by Macmillan, 1952).

Levinson, B.W. States of awareness during general anesthesia: Preliminary communication. *Brit. J. Anaesthesiology,* 1965, *37,* 544–546.

Levitt, E.E. & Brady, J.P. Psychophysiology of hypnosis. In J.M. Schneck (Ed.), *Hypnosis in modern medicine.* Springfield, Ill.: Thomas, 1963.

Liebeault, A. *Du summeil et des états analogues considérés surtout au point de vue de l'action moral sur le physique.* Paris: Masson, 1866. (Also Vienna: Deuticke, 1892).

Lim, R.K.S. Pain. *Annual Review of Physiology,* 1970, *32,* 269–288.

London, P. *The children's hypnotic susceptibility scale.* Palo Alto, Calif.: Consulting Psychologists Press, 1963.

Ludwig, A.M. et al. Group hypnotherapy techniques with drug addicts. *Int. J. Clin. & Exp. Hypn.*, 1964, *12*, 53–66.

Malmo, R.B. et al. Electromyographic study of hypnotic deafness. *J. Clin. & Exp. Hypn.*, 1954, *2*, 305–317.

Mann, H. Group hypnosis in the treatment of obesity. *Am. J. Clin. Hypn.*, 1959, *1*, 114–116.

Marchesi, C. The hypnotic treatment of bronchial asthma. *Brit. J. Med. Hypnotism*, 1949, *1*, 14–19.

Marcus, H.W. Chap. 8. Hypnosis in dentistry. In J.M. Schneck, (Ed.), *Hypnosis in modern medicine.* 3rd ed., Springfield, Ill.: Thomas, 1963, pp. 229–279.

Marcuse, F.L. *Hypnosis throughout the world.* Springfield, Ill.: Thomas, 1964.

Margolis, C.G. Hypnotic imagery with cancer patients. *Am. J. Clin. Hypn.*, 1982–83, *25*, 128–134.

Marmer, M.J. *Hypnosis in anesthesiology.* Springfield, Ill.: Thomas, 1959.

Maslach, D. et al. Hypnotic control of peripheral skin temperature: A case report. *Psychophysiology*, 1972, *9*, 600–605.

Mason, A.A. A case of congenital icthyosiform erythroderma of Brocq treated by hypnosis. *Brit. Med. J.*, 1952, *2*, 422–423.

Masters, W.H. & Johnson, V.E. *Human sexual inadequacy.* New York: Little, 1970.

Meares, A. *A system of medical hypnosis.* Philadelphia: Saunders, 1961.

Meares, A. A form of intensive meditation associated with the regression of cancer. *Am. J. Clin. Hypn.*, 1982–83, *25*, 114–121.

Meldman, M.J. Personality decomposition after hypnotic symptom suppression. *J. Am. Med. Assoc.*, 1960, *173*, 359–361.

Mellor, N.H. Hypnosis in juvenile delinquency. *Am. J. Clin. Hypn.*, 1970, *13*, 17–21.

Melzack, R. *The puzzle of pain.* New York: Basic Books, 1973.

Melzack, R. Acupuncture and pain mechanisms. Address, The Soc. for Clin. & Exp. Hypnosis, Montreal, Oct. 13, 1974.

Melzack, R. & Torgerson, W.S. On the language of pain. *Anesthesiology*, 1971, *34*, 50–59.

Melzack, R. & Wall, P.D. Pain mechanism: A new theory. *Science*, 1965, *150*, 971–979.

Mesmer, F.A. *Mesmerism: A translation of the original medical and scientific writings of F.A. Mesmer, M.D.* (Translated by G.J. Bloch). Los Altos, Calif.: William Kaufmann, 1981.

Milgram, S. Behavioral study of obedience. *J. Abn. & Soc. Psychol.*, 1963, 67, 371–378.

Morgan, A.H. & Hilgard, J.F. The Stanford Hypnotic Clinical Scale for Adults. *Am. J. Clin. Hypn.*, 1978/1979, *21*, 134–147.

Morgan, A.H. & Hilgard, J.F. The Stanford Hypnotic Clinical Scale for Children. *Am. J. Clin. Hypn.*, 1978/1979, *21*, 148–169.

Morris, R. Personal communication, 1982.

Moss, A.A. *Hypnodontics: Hypnosis in dentistry.* Brooklyn, N.Y.: Dental Items of Interest Pub. Co., 1952.

Moss, C.S. *The hypnotic investigation of dreams.* New York: Wiley, 1967.

Naruse, G. Hypnosis as a state of meditative concentration and its relationship to the perceptual process. In. M.V. Kline (Ed.), *The nature of hypnosis.* New York: The Institute for Research in Hypnosis & The Postgraduate Center for Psychotherapy, 1962.

Newbold, G. Hypnosis and suggestion in obstetrics. Chap. 7 in R.R. Rhodes (Ed.), *Therapy through hypnosis.* New York: Citadel Press, 1963.

Newman, M. Hypnotic handling of the chronic bleeder in extraction: A case report. *Am. J. Clin. Hypn.*, 1971, *14*, 126–127.

Newman, M. Hypnosis and hemophiliacs. *J. Am. Dent. Assoc.*, 1974, *88*, 273.

Newton, B.W. The use of hypnosis in the treatment of cancer patients. *Am. J. Clin. Hypn.*, 1982-83, *25*, 104–113.

Norris, A., & Huston, P. Raynaud's disease studied by hypnosis. *Dis. Nerv. Sys.*, 1956, *17*, 163–165.

Nuland, W.A. & Field, P.B. Smoking and hypnosis: A systematic clinical approach. *Int. J. Clin. & Exp. Hypn.*, 1970, *18*, 283–289.

O'Connell, D.N., Shor, R.E. & Orne, M.T. Hypnotic age regression: An empirical and methodological analysis. *J. Abn. Psychol. Monographs*, 1970, 76, (3, Pt. 2). 56.

Olness, K. Imagery (self-hypnosis) as adjunct therapy in childhood cancer: Clinical experiment with 25 patients. *Am. J. Pediatric Hematology/Oncology*, 1981, *3*, 313–321.

Orne, M.T. The mechanisms of hypnotic age regression: An experimental study. *J. Abn. Psychol.*, 1951, *46*, 213–225.

Orne, M.T. The nature of hypnosis: Artifact and essence. *J. Abn. Soc. Psychol.*, 1959, *58*, 277–299.

Orne, M.T. Book review of Antisocial or Criminal Acts and Hypnosis: A Case Study by P.J. Reiter. *Int. J. Clin. & Exp. Hypn.*, 1960, *8*, 131–134.

Orne, M.T. On the mechanisms of posthypnotic amnesia. *Int. J. Clin. & Exp. Hypn.*, 1966, *14*, 121–134.

Orne, M.T. Can a hypnotized subject be compelled to carry out otherwise unacceptable behavior: A discussion. *Int. J. Clin. & Exp. Hypn.*, 1972, *20*, 101–117.

Orne, M.T. Pain suppression by hypnosis and related phenomena. In Bonica, J.J. (Ed.), International symposium on pain. *Advances in Neurology*, Vol. 4, New York: 1974, pp. 563–582.

Orne, M.T. On the simulating subject as a quasi-control group in hypnosis research: What, why, and how. Chap. 16 in E. Fromm & R.E. Shor (Eds.), *Hypnosis: Developments in research and new perspectives*. New York: Aldine, 1979a, pp. 518–565.

Orne, M.T. The use and misuse of hypnosis in court. *Int. J. Clin. & Exp. Hypn.*, 1979b, 27, 311–341.

Orne, M.T. & McConkey, K.M. Toward convergent inquiry into self-hypnosis. *Int. J. Clin. & Exp. Hypn.*, 1981, 29, 313–323.

Pavlov, I.P. The identity of inhibition with sleep and hypnosis. *Scientific Monthly*, 1923, *17*, 603–608.

Pavlov, I.P. *Experimental psychology.* New York: Philosophical Library, 1957.

Peale, N.V. *The power of positive thinking.* New York: Prentice-Hall, 1952.

Pearson, R.E. Response to suggestions given under general anesthesia. *Am. J. Clin. Hypn.*, 1961, *4*, 106–114.

Perkins, W. (Ed.), Strategies in stuttering therapy: A symposium. *Seminars in Speech, Language and Hearing.* Issue of Nov. 1980.

Prince, M. *The dissociation of a personality.* New York: Longmans-Green, 1906.

Raginsky, B.B. Chap. 2. Hypnosis in internal medicine and general practice. In Schneck, J.M. (Ed.), *Hypnosis in modern medicine.* Springfield, Ill.: Thomas, 1963a, pp. 29–99.

Raginsky, B.B. Temporary cardiac arrest under hypnosis. Chap. 23 in N.V. Kline (Ed.), *Clinical correlations of experimental hypnosis.* Springfield, Ill.: Thomas, 1963b, pp. 430–455.

Rank, O. *The trauma of birth.* New York: Brunner, 1952.

Reich, W. *Character analysis.* New York: Orgone Inst. Press, 1945.

Reid, A.F. & Curtsinger, G. Physiological changes associated with hypnosis: The effect of hypnosis on temperature. *Int. J. Clin. & Exp. Hypn.*, 1969, *16*, 111–119.

Reiff, R. & Scheerer, M. *Memory and hypnotic age regression.* New York: Int. Univ. Press, 1959.

Reiser, M. *Handbook of investigative hypnosis.* Los Angeles: Lehi, 1980.

Reiter, P.J. The influence of hypnosis in somatic fields of function. Chap. 10 in L.M. LeCron (Ed.), *Experimental hypnosis.* New York: Macmillan, 1952.

Reiter, P.J. Antisocial or criminal acts and hypnosis: A case study. Springfield, Ill.: Thomas, 1958.

Rice, F.G. The hypnotic induction of labor: Six cases. *Am. J. Clin. Hypn.*, 1961, *4*, 119–122.

Rosen, H. *Hypnotherapy in clinical psychiatry.* New York: Julian Press, 1953.

Rosenberg, S.W. Hypnosis in cancer care: Imagery to enhance the control of physiological and psychological "side-effects" of cancer therapy. *Am. J. Clin. Hypn.*, 1982-83, *25*, 122–127.

Rosenthal, R. *Experimenter effects in behavioral research.* New York: Appleton-Century-Crofts, 1966.

Rowland, L.W. Will hypnotized persons try to harm themselves or others? *J. Abn. & Soc. Psychol.*, 1939, *34*, 114–117.

Sacerdote, P. *Induced dreams.* New York: Vantage Press, 1967.

Sacerdote, P. Theory and practice of pain control in malignancy and other protracted or recurring painful illnesses. *Int. J. Clin. & Exp. Hypn.*, 1972, *20*, 1–14.

Sacerdote, P. Teaching self-hypnosis to adults. *Int. J. Clin. & Exp. Hypn.*, 1981, *29*, 282–299.

Samuelly, I. Lamaze method of childbirth, conditioning or hypnosis. *Am. J. Clin. Hypn.*, 1972, *15*, 136–139.

Sanders, S.S. Mutual group hypnosis and smoking. *Am. J. Clin. Hypn.*, 1977, *20*, 131–135.

Sarbin, T.R. & Coe, W.C. *Hypnosis: A social psychological analysis of influence communication.* New York: Holt, Rinehart and Winston, 1972.

Sarbin, T.F. & Slagle, R.W. Hypnosis and psychophysiological outcomes. Chap. 9 in E. Fromm & R.E. Shor, (Eds.), *Hypnosis: Research developments and perspectives.* Chicago: Aldine-Atherton, 1979, pp. 273–303.

Scheibe, K.E. et al. Hypnotically induced deafness and delayed auditory feedback: A comparison of real and simulating subjects. *Int. J. Clin. & Exp. Hypn.*, 1968, *16*, 158–164.

Schneck, J.M. Special aspects of hypnotic regression and revivification. *Int. J. Clin. & Exp. Hypn.*, 1960, *8*, 37–42.

Schneck, J.M. *Hypnosis in modern medicine.*, Springfield, Ill.: Thomas, 1963.

Schneck, J.M. Principles and practice of hypnoanalysis. Springfield, Ill.: Thomas, 1965.

Schreiber, F.R. *Sybil*. New York: Warner Paperback Library, 1974.

Scott, M.J. *Hypnosis in skin and allergic diseases*. Springfield, Ill.: Thomas, 1960.

Secter, I.I. Some notes on controlling the exaggerated gag reflex. *Am. J. Clin. Hypn.*, 1960, 2, 149–153.

Secter, I.I. Tongue thrust and nail biting simultaneously treated during hypnosis. *Am. J. Clin. Hypn.*, 1961, 6, 51–53.

Secter, I.I. Dental surgery in a psychiatric patient. *Am. J. Clin. Hypn.*, 1964, 6, 363–364.

Secter, I.I. Applied psychology in dentistry. *Am. J. Clin. Hypn.*, 1965, 8, 122–127.

Secter, I.I. Swallowing difficulties. In *A syllabus on hypnosis and a handbook of therapeutic suggestions*. Des Plaines, Ill.: Am. Soc. of Clin. Hypnosis, 1973, p. 116.

Selye, H. *The stress of life*. New York: McGraw-Hill, 1956.

Shaw, S.I. *Clinical applications of hypnosis in dentistry*. Philadelphia: Saunders, 1958.

Sheehan, P.W. Incongruity in trance behavior: A defining property of hypnosis? In W.E. Edmonston, Jr. (Ed.), *Conceptual and investigative approaches to hypnosis and hypnotic phenomena*. New York Academy of Sciences, Vol. 296, 1977.

Sheehan, P.W. & Perry, C.W. *Methodologies of hypnosis: A critical appraisal of contemporary paradigms of hypnosis*. Hillsdale, N.J.: Lawrence Erlbaum Associates, 1976.

Sherman, S.E. *Very deep hypnosis: An experiential and electroencephalographic investigation*. Unpublished doctoral dissertation. Stanford Univ., 1971.

Shor, R.E. Three dimensions of hypnotic depth. *Int. J. Clin. & Exp. Hypn.*, 1962, 10, 23–28.

Shor, R.E. *Inventory of self-hypnosis, Form A*. Palo Alto, Calif.: Consulting Psychologists Press, 1978.

Shor, R.E. & Orne, E.C. *Harvard group scale of hypnotic susceptibility*. Palo Alto, Calif.: Consulting Psychologists Press 1962.

Shor, R.E. & Orne, M.T. (Eds.), *The nature of hypnosis: Selected basic readings*. New York: Holt, Rinehart & Winston, 1965.

Simmel, E. War neuroses. In S. Lorand (Ed.), *Psychoanalysis today*. New York: Int. Univ. Press, 1944, pp. 227–248.

Simonton, O.C. & Simonton, S. Belief systems and management of the emotional aspects of malignancy. *J. of Transpersonal Psychol.*, 1975, 7, 29–71.

Sinclair-Geben, A.H. & Chalmers, D. Treatment of warts by hypnosis. *Lancet*, 1959, *2*, 480–482.

Smedley, W.P. & Barnes, W.T. Postoperative use of hypnosis on a cardiovascular service. Termination of persistent hiccups in a patient with an aortorenal graft. *J. Am. Med. Assoc.*, 1966, *197*, 371–372.

Spiegel, H. A single-treatment method to stop smoking using ancillary self-hypnosis. *Int. J. Clin. & Exp. Hypn.*, 1970, *18*, 235–250.

Spiegel, H. An eye-roll test for hypnotizability. *Am. J. Clin. Hypn.*, 1972, *15*, 25–28.

Spiegel, H. & Spiegel, D. *Trance and treatment: Clinical uses of hypnosis* New York: Basic Books, 1978.

Staples, L.M. Relaxation through hypnosis: A valuable adjunct to change anesthesia. *J. Am. Dent. Soc. Anesth.*, Oct. 1958.

Stein, C. Displacement and reconditioning technique for compulsive smokers. *Int. J. Clin. & Exp. Hypn.*, 1964, *12*, 230–238.

Stekel, W. *Frigidity in women* (Vols. 1 & 2). New York: Liverright, 1943.

Stolzenberg, J. Clinical applications of hypnosis in producing hypno-anesthesia control of hemorrhage and salivation during surgery: A case report. *J. Clin. & Exper. Hypn.*, 1955, *3*, 24–27.

Stolzenberg, J. Hypnosis in orthodontics. *Am. J. Orthodontics*, 1959, *45*, 508–511.

Stolzenberg, J. *Dental hypnosis handbook*. Hollywood, Calif.: Wilshire Book Co., 1961.

Strasberg, I.M. Control of gagging by light hypnosis. *Am. J. Clin. Hypn.*, 1960, *2*, 148–149.

Sutcliffe, J.P. "Credulous" and "skeptical" views of hypnotic phenomena: Experiments in esthesia, hallucination, and delusion. *J. Abn. & Soc. Psychol.*, 1961, *62*, 189–200.

Sutcliffe, J.P. "Credulous" and "skeptical" views of hypnotic phenomena: A review of certain evidence and methodology. In R.E. Shor & M.T. Orne (Eds.), *The nature of hypnosis: Selected basic readings*. New York: Holt, Rinehart and Winston, 1965, pp. 124–152.

Tart, C.T. (Ed.), *Altered states of consciousness*. New York: Wiley, 1969.

Tart, C.T. Quick and convenient assessment of hypnotic depth: Self-report scales. *Am. J. Clin. Hypn.*, 1978/79, *21*, 186–207.

Tasini, M.R. & Hackett, T.P. Hypnosis in the treatment of a child with warts. *Am. J. Clin. Hypn.*, 1977, *15*, 12–14.

Theohar, C. & McKegney, F.P. Hiccups of psychogenic origin: A case report and review of the literature. *Comparative Psychiatry*, 1970, *11*, 377–384.

Thigpen, C.H. & Cleckley, H.M. *Three faces of Eve.* New York: McGraw-Hill, 1957.

Thompson, K.F. A rationale for suggestion in dentistry. *Am. J. Clin. Hypn.*, *1963*, *5*, 181–186.

Troffer, S. *Hypnotic age regression and congnitive functioning.* Unpublished doctoral dissertation, Stanford University, 1965.

Trustman, R.B., Dubovsky, S. & Titley, R. Auditory perception during general anesthesia—myth or fact ? *Int. J. Clin. & Expl. Hypn.*, 1977, *25*, 88–105.

Udolf, R. *Forensic hypnosis: Psychological and legal aspects.* Lexington, Mass., D.C. Heath, 1983.

Van Pelt, S.J. Hypnotherapy in medical practice. *Brit. J. Med. Hypnotism*, *1949*, *1*, No. 1, 8–13.

Van Pelt, S.J. The influence of hypnotic suggestion on the heart rate. *Brit. J. Med. Hypnotism.* Spring, 1950, pp. 31–32.

Van Pelt, S.J. Will hypnotism revolutionize medicine? In R.R. Rhodes (Ed.), *Therapy through hypnosis.* New York: Citadel Press, 1963, pp. 232–236.

Vogt. O. Zur Kentnis des Wesens und der psychologischen Bedeutung des Hypnotismus. *Zeitschrift fur Hypnotismus*, 1896, *4*, 32, 122, 229.

Von Dedenroth, T.E.A. The use of hypnosis in 1000 cases of "tobaccomaniacs." *Am. J. Clin. Hypnosis*, 1968, *10*, 194–197.

Wald, A. & Kline, M.V. A university program in dental hypnosis. *J. Clin. & Exp. Hypn.*, 1955, *3*, 183–187.

Watkins, H.H. Hypnosis and smoking: A five-session approach. *Int. J. Clin. & Exp. Hypn.*, 1976a, *24*, 381–390.

Watkins, H.H. Hypnosis in the control of bleeding during facial surgery. Personal communication, 1976b.

Watkins, H.H. Chap. 22, Ego-state therapy. In Watkins, J.G. *The therapeutic self.* New York: Human Sciences Press, 1978, pp. 360-398.

Watkins, H.H. Personal communications, 1979.

Watkins, J.G. Antisocial compulsions induced under hypnotic trance. *J. Soc. & Abn. Psychol.*, 1947, *42*, 256–259.

Watkins, J.G. *Hypnotherapy of war neuroses.* New York: Ronald Press, 1949.

Watkins, J.G. A case of hypnotic trance induced in a resistant subject in spite of active opposition. *Brit. J. Med. Hypnotism*, Summer 1951, *2*, 26–31.

Watkins, J.G. Trance and transference. *J. Clin. & Exp. Hypnosis*, 1954, *2*, 284–290.

Watkins, J.G. *General Psychotherapy*. Springfield, Ill.: Thomas, 1960.

Watkins, J.G. Transference aspects of the hypnotic relationship. Chap. 1 in M.V. Kline (Ed.), *Clinical correlations of experimental hypnosis*. Springfield, Ill.: Thomas, 1963, pp. 5–24.

Watkins, J.G. Symposium on posthypnotic amnesia: Discussion. *Int. J. Clin. & Exp. Hypn.*, 1966, *14*, 139–149.

Watkins, J.G. Hypnosis and consciousness from the viewpoints of existentialism. Chap. III in M.V. Kline (Ed.), *Psychodynamics and hypnosis*. Springfield, Ill.: Thomas, 1967, pp. 15–31.

Watkins, J.G. Antisocial behavior under hypnosis: Possible or impossible? *Internat. J. Clin. & Exper. Hypn.*, 1972, *20*, 95–100.

Watkins, J.G. *The therapeutic self*. New York: Human Sciences Press, 1978.

Watkins, J.G. Further data on the unethical use of hypnosis. (Presented at the Am. Psychol. Assoc. meeting, Los Angeles, Aug. 1985).

Watkins, J.G. & Johnson, R.H. *We, the divided self*. New York: Irvington, 1982.

Watkins, J.G. & Watkins, H.H. The theory and practice of ego-state therapy. Chap. 11 in H. Grayson (Ed.), *Short term approaches to psychotherapy*. New York: Inst. for the Psychotherapies and Human Sciences Press, 1979, pp. 176–220.

Watkins, J.G. & Watkins, H.H. Ego states and hidden observers. *J. Altered States of Consciousness*, 1979-80, *5*, 3–18.

Watkins, J.G. & Watkins, H.H. Ego state therapy. In R. Corsini (Ed.), *Handbook of innovative therapies*. New York: Wiley, 1981.

Watts, A.W. *The way of Zen*. New York: Pantheon, 1957.

Weitzenhoffer, A.M. The production of anti-social acts under hypnosis. *J. Abn. & Soc. Psychol.*, 1949, *44*, 420–422.

Weitzenhoffer, A.M. *Hypnotism: An objective study of suggestibility*. New York: Wiley, 1953.

Weitzenhoffer, A.M. *General techniques of hypnotism*. New York: Grune & Stratton, 1957.

Weitzenhoffer, A.M. & Hilgard, E.R. *Stanford Hypnotic Susceptibility Scale. Forms A & B.* Palo Alto, Calif.: Consulting Psychologists Press, 1959.

Weitzenhoffer, A.M. & Hilgard, E.R. *Stanford Hypnotic Susceptibility Scale, Form C.* Palo Alto, Calif.: Consulting Psychologists Press, 1962.

Weitzenhoffer, A.M. & Hilgard, E.R. *Stanford Profile Scales of Hypnotic Susceptibility.* Forms I & II. Palo Alto, Calif.: Consulting Psychologists Press, 1967.

Wells, W.R. Experiments in the hypnotic production of crime. *J. of Psychology,* 1941, *11,* 63–102.

West, L.J. Psychophysiology of hypnosis. *J. Am. Med.,* 1960, *172,* 672–675.

Wetterstrand, O.G. *Hypnotism, and its application to practical medicine.* (Translated by H.G. Peterson), New York: G.P. Putnam's Sons, 1902.

White, R.W. A preface to the theory of hypnotism. *J. Abn. & Soc. Psychol.* 1941, *36,* 477–505.

Williams, G.W. Hypnosis in perspective. In L.M. LeCron, (Ed.), *Experimental hypnosis.* New York: Citadel Press, 1968, pp. 4–21.

Wolberg, L.R. *Hypnoanalysis.* New York: Grune & Stratton, 1945.

Wolberg, L.R. *Medical hypnosis: Vol. I. Principles of hypnotherapy; Vol. II. Practice of hypnotherapy.* New York: Grune & Stratton, 1948.

Wolberg, L.R. *Hypnosis: Is it for you?* New York: Harcourt-Brace-Janovich, 1972.

Wolfe, L.S. Hypnosis in anesthesiology, Chap. 13 in L.M. LeCron, (Ed.), *Techniques of hypnotherapy.* New York: Julian Press, 1961, pp. 188–212.

Wolfe, L.S. & Millet, J.B. Control of post-operative pain by suggestion under general anesthesia. *Am. J. Clin. Hypn.,* 1960, *3,* 109–112.

Wolpe, J. The systematic desensitization treatment of neuroses. *J. Nerv. & Ment. Dis.,* 1961, *132,* 189–203.

Wookey, E.E. Uses and limitations of hypnosis in dental treatment. *Brit. Dental J.,* Nov. 1, 1938, Vol. 65.

Wright, E. Symposium on posthypnotic amnesia: Discussion. *Int. J. Clin. & Exp. Hypn.,* 1966, *14,* 135–138.

Young, P.C., Antisocial uses of hypnosis. In L.M. LeCron (Ed.), *Experimental hypnosis.* New York: Macmillan, 1952, pp. 376–409. (also Citadel Press, 1968).

Zeig, J.K. *Ericksonian approaches to hypnosis and psycho-therapy.* New York: Brunner/Mazel, 1982.

Zimbardo, P.G. et al. Control of pain motivation by cognitive dissonance. *Science,* 1966, *151,* 217–219.

Zimbardo, P.G., Marshall, G. & Maslach, V. Liberating behavior from time-bound control: Expanding the present through hypnosis. *J. Appl. Soc. Psychol.,* 1971, *1,* 305–323.

SUBJECT INDEX

Abbe Faria, 31, 36
Ablation theory of hypnotic regression, 75
Abortion, 232
  spontaneous, 231
Abreaction, 16, 17, 19, 39, 257, 282
Academy of Psychosomatic Medicine, 24, 251
Age regression, 71, 72, 73, 281
Alcoholism, 284-285, 296
Alpha activity, 32
Altered state of consciousness (awareness), 56, 59, 81
Amenorrhea, 241
American Association for the Advancement of Science, v
American Board of Examiners in Professional Psychology, 23, 28,
American Board of Examiners in Psychological Hypnosis (American Board of Psychological Hypnosis), 23, 28, 228
American Board of Clinical Hypnosis, iv, 28, 228
American Board of Hypnosis in Dentistry, 22, 28, 228
American Board of Medical Hypnosis, 22, 28, 228
American Board of Obstetrics and Gynecology, 22
American Board of Psychiatry and Neurology, 22
American Board of Surgery, 22
American Journal of Clinical Hypnosis, 20, 22, 187, 269, 351
American Medical Association, v, 22
American Psychological Association, v, 20, 22
  Division 30 (hypnosis), 25, 228, 351
American Society of Clinical Hypnosis (ASCH), 20, 22, 25, 28, 228, 267, 351
Amnesia, 38, 40, 49
  faking of, 70
  post-hypnotic, 70, 83
  suggesting, 329
Amputation, 29
Analgesia, 44, 328-331
  suggestins of, 210
Anesthesia, 195, 207-212, 220, 235, 328-331
  glove, 15, 210, 236, 239, 246
  hypnotic, 21, 59, 210
    patient reaction to negative

  suggestions when under, 217
  test for, 236
  transference of, 65, 210, 236
  who administers, 215
Animal magnetism, 3, 5, 8
Anna O., 17
Anorexia nervosa, 15, 211, 265, 272
Anoxia, 238
Anxiety, 255
  in children, 302, 309
  pre-operative, 213
  reaction, 319
  Taylor Scale of Manifest Anxiety, 266
Archaic involvement, 54, 57
Arm drop
  induction, 121-123
  suggestibility test, 94-99, 110
Arm Levitation,
  induction technique, 124-130, 324
  suggestibility test, 104-105, 110
Aristotelian logic, 44
Art therapy, xii
Asthma, 255-257, 302
  in children, 255, 302, 306, 313
Astronomer, Royal, 3
Atavistic regression, 36, 223
Audio tapes (see audio-visual aids).
Audio-visual aids (films, tapes, etc.) vi, xi, 213, 281, 293
Authoritative vs. permissive manner in hypnotherapist, 192, 194
Auto hypnosis (see Hypnosis, self)
Automatic talking, 44
Automatic writing (see also Dissociated writing), 44
Aversion therapy, 275, 284-285, 289
"Awake" trance, 121

Bacquet, 5
Bavarian Academy of Science, 2
Bed wetting, 308-309
Behavior
  behavioral medicine, 171, 271
  behaviorist, 5, 187
  modification, ix, 195
  motor theories, 37-38, 56
  therapy, xii, 162, 248, 327, 335, 336
Berlin Academy of Science, 8
Bible, 195
  Genesis, 222
Bibliotherapy, xii
Biofeedback, 261, 325
Birth,

INDEX OF NAMES